SPINAL CORD INJURY

SPINAL CORD INJURY

Edited by
N. Eric Naftchi, Ph.D.
New York University Medical Center
Institute of Rehabilitation Medicine, N.Y.

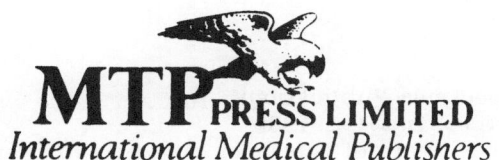

MTP PRESS LIMITED
International Medical Publishers

Published in the UK and Europe by
MTP Press Ltd.
Falcon House
Lancaster, England

Published in the US by
SPECTRUM PUBLICATIONS, INC.
175-20 Wexford Terrace
Jamaica, N.Y. 11432

ISBN-13: 978-94-011-6307-1   e-ISBN-13: 978-94-011-6305-7
DOI: 10.1007/978-94-011-6305-7

CONTRIBUTORS

SUSAN J. ABRAHAMS
New York University Medical Center
Institute of Rehabilitation Medicine
New York, New York

JULIUS AXELROD
Laboratory of Clinical Science
National Institute of Mental Health
Bethesda, Maryland

JOAN L. BARDACH
New York University Medical Center
Institute of Rehabilitation Medicine
New York, New York

G. BAUTZ
Department of Pharmacology
Hoffman-LaRoche, Inc.
Nutley, New Jersey

M.V. BENJAMIN
Department of Neurosurgery
New York University Medical Center
New York, New York

M. BERARD
New York University Medical Center
Laboratory of Biochemical Pharmacology
New York, New York

R.T. BERGERON
University Hospital
New York, New York

A. BIGNAMI
Department of Neuropathology
Veterans Administration Hospital
West Roxbury, Massachusetts

DONG SUN CHU
New York University Medical Center
Institute of Rehabilitation Medicine
New York, New York

D. DAHL
Spinal Cord Injury Service
West Roxbury Veterans Administration Hospital
Boston, Massachusetts

MARGARET DEMENY
New York University Medical Center
New York, New York

HARRY B. DEMOPOULOS
Department of Pathology
New York University Medical Center
Bellevue Hospital
New York, New York

N. DIFERRANTE
The Institute of Rehabilitation & Research
Houston, Texas

EUGENE S. FLAMM
Department of Neurosurgery
New York University Medical Center
Bellevue Hospital
New York, New York

S. FRANCO
Department of Pharmacology
Hoffman-LaRoche, Inc.
Nutley, New Jersey

AJAX GEORGE
Bellevue Hospital
New York, New York

D.W. HORST
Department of Pharmacology
Hoffman-LaRoche, Inc.
Nutley, New Jersey

P.E. KAPLAN
Rehabilitation Institute of Chicago
Chicago, Illinois

AGNES KIRSCHNER
New York University Medical Center
Laboratory of Biochemical Pharmacology
New York, New York

MICHAEL KREBS
Department of Physical Medicine
Baylor College of Medicine
Houston, Texas

I. KRICHEFF
New York University Medical Center
University Hospital
New York, New York

J.P. LIN
New York University Medical Center
University Hospital
New York, New York

E.W. LOWMAN
New York University Medical Center
Institute of Rehabilitation Medicine
New York, New York

DONNA MANNING
New York Hospital
Payne-Whitney
New York, New York

J.M. MILLER, III
Spain Rehabilitation Hospital
Birmingham, Alabama

N. ERIC NAFTCHI
New York University Medical Center
Laboratory of Biochemical Pharmacology
New York, New York

K.M.W. NIEMANN
Spain Rehabilitation Hospital
Birmingham, Alabama

FRANK PADRONE
New York University Medical Center
Institute of Rehabilitation Medicine
New York, New York

NORMAN PAY
St. Francis Hospital
Radiology Department
Wichita, Kansas

CLAUDIO PETRILLO
New York University Medical Center
Institute of Rehabilitation Medicine
New York, New York

K.T. RAGNARSSON
New York University Medical Center
Institute of Rehabilitation Medicine
New York, New York

J. RANSOHOFF
Department of Neurosurgery
New York University Medical Center
Bellevue Hospital
New York, New York

M. RODRIQUEZ
Rehabilitation Institute of Chicago
Chicago, Illinois

V. SAHGAL
Rehabilitation Institute of Chicago
Chicago, Illinois

W. SCHLOSSER
Department of Pharmacology
Hoffman-LaRoche, Inc.
Nutley, New Jersey

M.L. SELIGMAN
Department of Pathology
Bellevue Hospital
New York, New York

G.H. SELL
New York University Medical Center
Institute of Rehabilitation Medicine
New York, New York

J. SINGH
The Institute for Rehabilitation & Research
Houston, Texas

S.R. SNIDER
Neurological Institute
College of Physicians and Surgeons of
    Columbia University
New York, New York

SAMUEL L. STOVER
Spain Rehabilitation Hospital
Birmingham, Alabama

V. SUBARAMI
Rehabilitation Institute of Chicago
Chicago, Illinois

J. TUCKMAN
New York University Medical Center
Laboratory of Biochemical Pharmacology
New York, New York

LINDA L. VACCA
Department of Pathology
Medical College of Georgia
Augusta, Georgia

ANNA VIAU
New York University Medical Center
Institute of Rehabilitation Medicine
New York, New York

JACQUELINE L. CLAUS-WALKER
The Institute for Rehabilitation & Research
Houston, Texas

G. FREDRICK WOOTEN
Laboratory of Clinical Science
National Institute of Mental Health
Bethesda, Maryland

C. WURSTER
Rehabilitation Institute of Chicago
Chicago, Illinois

CONTENTS

FOREWORD

We shall not, and those who come after us must not, accept
the goals that were not reached yesterday as unsurmountable
today or tomorrow. We will strive to render the world of the
paralyzed-on-wheels but a transitory stop, and settle for
nothing short of optimal recovery.

N. Eric Naftchi

In man, the process of "encephalization" culminates in almost complete
control of the brain over the lower centers. Transection of the spinal cord
severs the extensions of its nerve fiber tracts running to and from various
brain centers. Although there is some confusion on the meaning of spinal
shock, it is supposed to last from two to three weeks or longer in man,
compared with less than a few minutes in the frog. This is a testimony to
the complexity of the suprasegmental control in higher animals. Since the
brain exerts its control over the internal environment through several
monoamine, amino acids, and peptide neurotransmitters, it should not be
surprising if the metabolism of these transmitters is found to be drastically
altered along with other physical and metabolic dysfunctions which ensue
following the spinal cord section.

In spite of the major strides in rehabilitation of traumatic spinal cord
injury, our knowledge of the etiology underlying the diverse neurophysiologic
derangements remains limited. For instance, we are just becoming aware
of some of the changes in the "milieu interieur." The constancy of this
internal enviroment is ordinarily integrated between normal functioning
of the central and autonomic nervous systems on the one hand, and the
endocrine glands on the other. We still have much to learn about the fate
of the biogenic amine, amino acid, and peptide neurotransmitters in the
CNS after a spinal cord transection. Do their biosynthesis, metabolism,
storage, release, and re-uptake mechanisms change? If so, how do these
changes affect the hypothalamic-hypophyseal relationship, vasomotor, and
temperature regulating centers. In turn, how do the foregoing alterations
affect the functions of the endocrine glands, the target organs, and the
circulatory system? What are the causes of stress intolerance, spasticity,
calciuria, osteoporosis, trohpic skin ulcers, and so on?

This foreword, therefore, will serve as a cursory review of three
major areas of dysfunction encountered in spinal-cord-injured humans. It
will also suggest some future areas of research directed towards elucidation
of the pathophysiology of spinal cord injury. Finally, this investigator
suggests boldly that re-education and restoration of sensory-motor function
should be our ultimate aim. It is in the realm of possibility and must be
vigorously pursued.

A frequent and serious complication of spinal cord injury, occurring
immediately after the onset of the lesion, is the loss of bone minerals and

bone matrix. This loss of bone (resorption) results from a concomitant loss of calcium and hydroxyproline. The latter is a major amino acid found in collagen which is the main component of the bone matrix. The progressive loss of bone leads to osteoporosis and a negative calcium balance.

In spinal cord injury, extremely rapid and progressive loss of bone is often associated with kidney stone formation, pathologic fractures, and the development of ectopic bone. The purposes of the studies on bone demineralization were to: determine when the process of loss begins, find the extent and duration of the loss, find the reason for the loss, and retard and/or prevent the loss.

The results of our work and those of other investigators have shown that hypercalciuria occurs in spinal cord injury during the first six months postinjury and that the calcium excretion becomes less severe thereafter presumably due to increased patient activity. A longitudinal investigation of the degree of calcium and hydroxyproline loss, measured at weekly intervals, in paraplegic and quadriplegic subjects was conducted. The data from our longitudinal study show that the increase in urinary calcium starts almost immediately after the onset of injury. The elevated urinary calcium cannot simply be attributed to prolonged inactivity since the degree of calciuria is greater in spinal-cord-injured persons than in normal control subjects following prolonged bed rest.

Total urinary hydroxyproline is used as a sensitive index and quantifier of bone collagen metabolism. An increase in urinary hydroxyproline following spinal cord injury indicated collagen breakdown and bone resorption. In our longitudinal studies, we found that the excretion of hydroxyproline was greater and of longer duration in quadriplegics than in paraplegics. The correlation between hydroxyproline and calcium excretion in spinal-cord-injured subjects, without concomitant marked increases in serum alkaline phosphatase, indicates that the loss of calcium and hydroxyproline is consistent with bone resorption.

Thyrocalcitonin usually counteracts parathormone to keep plasma and bone exchange of calcium at a constant level. This hormone's effect is produced by the inhibition of bone resorption, especially when bone resorption is stimulated by the parathyroid hormone. Parathyroid hormone is also known to increase urinary excretion of hydroxyproline. Possibly, the main effect of thyrocalcitonin in humans is to protect against excessive bone loss due to parathyroid hormone.

In our studies on animal models with spinal cord injury, administration of thyrocalcitonin to paraplegic rats resulted in a marked improvement of calcium, phosphorus, and magnesium balances that were depressed following spinal cord injury. Another significant finding was that after transection of the spinal cord at the T_5 level, the survival rate in thirty untreated male Wistar rats was 25 percent. Death usually occurred within eight to fourteen days after transection although the urinary bladder was expressed three times daily. Autopsy revealed hydronephrosis of the kidneys which occurred either bilaterally, or, more often, unilaterally on the right side. Thyrocalcitonin administered subcutaneously increased the survival rate to 80 percent and markedly reduced the indicence of hydronephrosis.

Another complication of spinal cord injury is heterotopic ossification (myositis ossificans, extraskeletal, ectopic, or periarticular bone) which occurs in 16 to 53 percent of spinal-cord-injured victims. This condition starts as an inflammatory reaction causing edema, chrondrogenesis, and osteogenesis. Its etiology may possibly be related to autonomic dysfunctions commencing with the appearance of venous thrombosis and arteriovenous shunts in the affected area. The intimate association of osteoporosis with periarticular ossification indicates that excessive calcium loss from bones is one of the predisposing factors in the formation of ectopic bone. In a preliminary study, the effect of thyrocalcitonin on ectopic bone was studied in three subjects. One paraplegic subject with long duration periarticular ossification of both hips was treated for a month with thyrocalcitonin. The serum ionized calcium, which is the exchangeable calcium between bone and plasma, decreased significantly after thyrocalcitonin therapy while the total calcium did not change appreciably. The results of ^{18}F scintimetry revealed that, after one month of thyrocalcitonin treatment, the enormous uptake observed before treatment had diminished to insignificant amounts in the affected areas. Clinically the range of motion in the above paraplegic subject increased by 25 degrees (from -35 to -10) and localized pain was significantly decreased. These results were not duplicated in the two other paraplegic subjects with short duration heteroptopic ossification. The response to thyrocalcitonin therapy may be different in an immature periarticular bone compared with that of one almost grown to maturity. The maturity of the heterotopic ossification is also of great importance in surgical intervention as well; surgery performed too early results in the regrowth of the extraskeletal bone. Immature periarticular bone may require a larger dose of thyrocalcitonin.

Another pharmacologic agent, diphosphonate, administered in large doses, was found to block or retard the progressive soft tissue ossification in adults and children with myositis ossificans progressiva and prevented the recurrence of calcification after surgical removal of ectopic bone. Thyrocalcitonin and diphosphonate ameliorating effects on heterotopic ossification must be compared for efficacy as well as minimum side effects.

A further complication following spinal cord injury is the formation of renal calculi (kidney stones). Formation of kidney stones appears to be favored when the concentrations of sodium and potassium in the urine is decreased and that of calcium is increased.

Based on speculation that a low calcium diet may reduce hypercalciuria and prevent renal calculi and periarticular bone formation, the calcium intake of paraplegic and quadriplegic patients is often restricted. Findings of rapid bone mineral loss following spinal cord injury lead to the conclusion, however, that a low calcium diet may exacerbate bone resorption leading to the early development of osteoporosis.

In our recent study of the effect of a calcium diet, rats fed on high calcium diets had normal calcium balance following spinal cord transection as compared with a significantly depressed calcium balance in rats on normal calcium diets. Rats fed high calcium diets also retained more calcium than animals receiving the normal calcium ration. The testes and prostates in paraplegic rats fed a normal calcium diet were atrophied compared with the controls. No atrophy was observed in rats fed a high calcium diet. The data indicate that the occurrence of urinary tract infections was more prevalent and of longer duration in paraplegic rats fed a normal calcium diet than in those fed a high calcium diet. Furthermore, hydronephrosis occurred in several paraplegic rats fed the regular calcium diet but not in animals fed the high calcium diet. Examination of the kidneys and bladders in the transected rats fed a high calcium diet revealed no evidence of renal or bladder calculi.

Spinal cord injuries in the human male result in various degress of testicular atrophy and sterility in the majority of subjects and, in some cases, gynecomastia. The occurrence of mammary hypertrophy which is found occasionally in men with spinal cord injury may appear as early as three months or as late as five years after the onset of injury. Testicular atrophy is reported to occur in over 50 percent of human males. Metabolic and hormonal disturbances causing the impairment of fertility in spinal man are not yet fully understood.

It is well known that in patients with spinal cord lesions above the sympathetic outflow, body heat regulation becomes extremely irregular due to the loss of sympathetic hypothalamic control of sweating and the skin blood flow regulation. There is no explanation as to why some patients with spinal cord injury develop stress intolerance, gynecomastia, testicular, atrophy, amenorrhea, etc., all manifestations of disturbed functioning of the endocrine system.

In our recent studies, concentrations of testosterone, luteinizing hormone (LH), and follicle stimulating hormone (FSH) in the serum of ten paraplegic and ten quadriplegic subjects were measured once a week for a period of four months from the onset of injury. In paraplegic subjects, serum FSH and testosterone levels were significantly lower than those of the age-matched normal controls for a period of two and six weeks after spinal cord injury, respectively. Following the above periods of time, serum concentrations of both hormones were not significantly different from those of the controls. In paraplegic subjects, serum LH concentrations were also within control levels. By contrast, in quadriplegic subjects, serum FSH was depressed for three weeks while testosterone and LH concentration remained significantly lower than those of the controls during the entire four month test period. Furthermore, in another group of ten chronic (one to six years after the onset of injury) paraplegic and ten chronic quadriplegic subjects, serum FSH concentrations were comparable to those of the normal controls. Although serum LH concentrations were at control levels in chronic paraplegic they were significantly depressed in chronic quadriplegic subjects.

Whether the depressed serum testosterone was due to a primary testicular deficiency or to a decreased secretion of LH from the pituitary gland causing less stimulation of testicular Leydig cells remains to be investigated. In addition, it is not known whether low serum LH levels are due to pituitary deficiency or to a low level of pituitary stimulation by the hypothalamic LH releasing hormone. The low concentrations of the latter hormone could result from altered feedback involved in the function of the hypothalamic-pituitary-gonadal axis which is permanently disturbed in the acute and chronic quadriplegic subjects.

The purpose of biochemically stressing subjects is to determine the extent of remaining function, (i.e., the ability to respond to different degrees of stress). In this study, we wished to compare the response of spinal-cord-injured subjects to insulin induced hypoglycemia with that of controls.

The response to insulin induced hypoglycemia in spinal cord injury showed that 30 minutes after insulin administration glucose decreased by 70 percent in the controls and paraplegics but only 40 percent in quadriplegic subjects. Correlating with glucose findings, plasma epinephrine levels increased fifteen fold in the controls, five fold in paraplegics, and were unchanged in quadriplegic subjects. The peak epinephrine release came after that of hypoglycemia at 45 minutes postinsulin administration.

The results indicate a dampening of physiological and reduced hypoglycemic response in quadriplegic subjects possibly due to lower demand for glucose utilization and/or insulin receptor subsensitivity as a result of the loss of supraspinal control and curtailment of sympathetic outflow.

Autonomic hyperreflexia, characterized by paraxysmal hypertension, has been well documented ever since Head and Riddoch and Guttmann and Whitteridge first described the symptoms in quadriplegia. Patients with high level spinal cord injury, above the sympathetic outflow, at the level of thoracic six vertebra (T_6), very often develop spontaneous hypertensive crisis due to any one of several noxious stimuli. These stimuli usually arise from the urinary bladder because of cystitis or kidney stone formation or from the rectum because of constipation or rectal impaction. Since quadriplegic patients are generally hypotensive, the high pressures that develop represent pressure changes of a magnitude that can cause cerebrovascular accident and death of the subject.

Occurrence of paroxysmal hypertension and its associated and documented mortality in quadriplegic subjects during episodic autonomic dysreflexia is well known. We have shown that the severity of the attacks are comparable to the activity of serum dopamine-β-hydroxylase (DBH) and plasma norepinephrine concentration.

Dopamine-β-hydroxylase is the enzyme that synthesizes neurotransmitter norepinephrine from its precursor, dopamine. Evidence has been accumulated to show that both DBH and norepinephrine are released simultaneously from sympathetic nerve endings. The activity of both DBH in serum and norepinephrine in plasma are used as indicators of sympathetic activity.

The excretion of catecholamine (norepinephrine, dopamine, and epinephrine) metabolites in 52 randomly chosen subjects suffering from chronic spinal cord injury was significantly higher than that of 36 normal control subjects. Eighteen subjects with spinal cord injury were followed longitudinally for six months from the date of onset of injury. A long-term decrease in serum DBH activity occurred in quadriplegic subjects when compared with their initial level (just after the onset of injury). Another group of ten chronic quadriplegic subjects were kept as free as possible from conditions that would cause autonomic overactivity. Endogenous plasma norepinephrine levels in this group were also significantly lower than those of ten normal control subjects. The high excretion of catecholamine metabolites found in the first group of randomly selected spinal-cord-injured subjects, therefore, must be due to many subclinical, undetected episodes of autonomic dysreflexia.

Systemic arteriolar vasoconstriction during hypertensive crises in spinal man are due to "reflex" sympathetic activity in the distal cord stump, and the action of the postganglionic neurotransmitter, norepinephrine. We also established that the severe elevations of arterial pressure during this syndrome are associated with an unchanged cardiac output and a great increase in total peripheral resistance. Thus, the primary cardiovascular mechanism of the hypertensive episodes is systemic arteriolar vasoconstriction.

These findings provide the basis for the pharmacological treatment of the acute hypertensive crises and for maintaining normal blood pressures in those subjects who are chronically prone to repetitive, overt and/or subclinical hypertensive episodes. Aside from pheochromocytoma, this is the first time that a causative neurotransmitter has been unequivocally indentified in hypertension. Therefore, nitropruside or a short-acting ganglion blocker, trimethaphan camphorsulfonate, are most satisfactory for reducing arterial blood pressure during acute hypertensive episodes of autonomic dysreflexia. The use of antihypertensive medication such as long-acting ganglionic blocking agents, alpha adrenergic receptor blocking drugs and guanethidine, are potentially dangerous in quadriplegic patients because they can produce exaggerated postural hypotension and, therefore, may bring about catastrophic episodes of myocardial and cerebral ischemia.

In order to determine whether impaired sympathetic nerve response and/or impaired renin release are responsible for orthostatic hypotension in patients with cervical spinal cord lesions, serum dopamine-β-hydroxylase (DBH) activity and plasma renin activity (PRA) were examined during passive tilting in six quadriplegic patients and in six normal control types and degrees of stresses.

The investigation will involve longitudinal, repetitive measurements of the effects of different levels of spinal cord lesion on (1) the concentrations of the catecholamines, serotonin, dopamine-β-hydroxylase activity, other peptide neurotransmitters, and Na^+, K^+, and Ca^{++} in the blood and cerebrospinal fluids, and the catecholamine and serotonin metabolites in the urine; (2) the reactivity of peripheral blood vessels to intravenously infused 1-norepinephrine; (3) the uptake, release, and excretion of intravenously infused labelled-norepinephrine in spinal-cord-injured subjects and controls; (4) the cardiovascular, endocrinological, and biochemical responses to the stresses of head-up tilt, hypovolemia and insulin-induced hypoglycemia in spinal-cord-injured subjects and controls for each respective stress test.

The results from the above investigation and those in animal models will provide information about the disturbances in basic biological mechanisms caused by spinal cord injury and how they change after the onset of injury. This knowledge will permit more definitive estimation of the beneficial effects of currently used methods of rehabilitation, and the logical introduction of new pharmacological agents in this process. Thus, the conclusions from such investigations may hasten the rehabilitation of spinal-cord-injured subjects, make it more complete and, thus, prevent relapses and re-hospitalization.

The neuroendocrinological functional changes in paraplegic and quadriplegic subjects must be studied in depth. The major hormones such as ACTH, LH, FSH, TSH, vasopressin, cortisol, testosterone, thyroxine, etc. must be analyzed in the serum of spinal-cord-injured subjects by the most sensitive and specific methods available. These techniques include radioimmunoassay and high pressure liquid chromatography. Immunocytochemistry must be used for localization of hormones in tissues. Thus, changes in negative feedback due to the degree of loss of supraspinal control will be measured and correlated with the time after the onset of spinal cord injury. Furthermore, the adaptive mechanisms to physical (head-up tilting, hypovolemia) and biochemical (insulin-induced hypoglycemia) stresses, and the degree of their deficiencies in spinal-cord-injured subjects require elucidation.

Our preliminary results on hypothalamic corticotrophic releasing hormone (CRF) and vasopressin seem to suggest that they act synergistically in the release of ACTH and that, in subjects with high-level spinal cord injury, the diurnal rhythm may be curtailed. The data indicate that the interruption of the afferent stimuli to the brain after spinal cord injury affects the CNS control of ACTH secretion and thus the release of cortisol.

Even in persons with intact spinal cords, receiving drugs which reduce normal compensatory reflex sympathetic nervous system activity, a small degree of blood loss can cause severe hypotension and syncope when supine. Although this question has not been adequately studied in spinal-cord-injured subjects, it must be presumed that those with high lesions are inordinately sensitive to blood loss.

The investigations of the physical and biochemical stresses in spinal-cord-injured humans are essential in order to identify the basic deficiencies, excesses and conditions of supersensitivity and/or subsensitivity which would result from the loss of supraspinal control and disturbance in negative feedback systems after spinal cord injury.

The results from previous studies have delineated some of the derangements in the metabolism of biogenic amines, disruption of other neurotransmitters, and autonomic impairment of cardiovascular regulation subjects. Serum DBH was measured by an isotopic enzymatic method and PRA by radioimmunoassay. Following head-up tilting, quadriplegic subjects demonstrated a prompt significant decrease in mean arterial pressure (MAP) and an increase in heart rate. Dopamine-β-hydroxylase activity and PRA increased significantly in 15 minutes following tilt. In normal subjects, although heart rate increased, mean arterial pressure was unchanged and DBH and PRA did not increase significantly during head-up tilt. The findings of increased DBH during tilt hypotension in quadriplegic subjects provide evidence that reflex sympathetic nerve stimulation persists despite cervical cord transection. Increased PRA may be attributed to decreased renal perfusion pressure and increased sympathetic stimulation during tilt hypotension. In another study, we found that responses of eight paraplegic subjects to head-up tilt were not significantly different from those of eight normal controls but glomerular filtration rate (GFR) and renal plasma flow (RPF) were significantly lower in nine quadriplegics in the supine position. During tilt, RPF decreased significantly, but the fall in GFR was not significant. In all three groups, the GFR during head-up tilt was similar, indicating that in spite of the great loss of supraspinal sympathetic control, quadriplegic subjects apparently equally constrict their afferent and efferent renal arterioles during orthostatic stress and thus prevent excessive fall of GFR. These data further suggest that orthostatic hypotension in quadriplegic patients cannot be attributed solely to the failure of the sympathetic nervous system or the renin-angiotensin system to respond to the stimulus of orthostasis (erect posture).

Investigations of dysfunction of the endocrine and autonomic nervous system, and mineral metabolism must be continued in order to explain and treat the causes of the various disorders discussed. The long-term goals of our investigation of dysfunction in mineral metabolism are (1) to develop and standardize a method which measures the extent of osteoporosis in spinal-cord-injured subjects by computerized tomography; (2) to determine longitudinally the degree of bone demineralization in patients with paralysis due to spinal cord lesion by use of computerized tomography as early as possible after the onset of spinal cord injury and once a month for three months thereafter; (3) to initiate the treatment of paraplegic and quadriplegic subjects with thyrocalcitonin and diphosphonates immediately after the onset of injury in order to determine which drug is more efficacious in preventing osteoporosis and other complications such as renal and bladder stone formation and development of periarticular bone with the least amount of side effects; (4) to investigate the effect of thyrocalcitonin and diphosphonate therapy on periarticular bone formation and to prevent its restrictive, debilitating effects, either by inhibiting the formation of extraskeletal bone, or once formed, causing its resorption or maturation by pharmacologic means; (5) to measure the effect of dietary calcium on the amelioration or exacerbation of complications associated with dysfunction of mineral metabolism in animal models of spinal cord injury. If these results demonstrate conclusively that a high calcium diet has ameliorating effects, the experiment must be extended to humans under strict dietary control.

The long-term aim of our research in autonomic nervous dysfunction has been to measure the effects of different levels of spinal cord injury on the metabolism of catecholamines in man and to correlate these changes with the associated degrees of impairment of neural, endocrinal and cardiovascular functions. That is, to delineate the autonomic function of the spinal cord and sympathetic nervous system below the transection. These studies should be of particular importance with reference to the ability of the spinal-cord-injured subjects to tolerate and adapt to different in paraplegic and quadriplegic subjects. Similar investigations regarding the interrelationships between neural, neuroendocrinal, and cardiovascular mechanisms are necessary to provide the basic knowledge required for more adequate means of rehabiliating and re-educating spinal-cord-injured patients based on sound medical principles.

N. Eric Naftchi

SECTION ONE

Molecular Mechanisms of
Acute Traumatic Spinal
Cord Injury

1

Glial Fibrillary Acidic Protein (GFA) and Neuroglial Scarring, A Review

A. BIGNAMI and D. DAHL

A major goal of spinal cord injury research is to promote a vigorous growth of axons in mammalian spinal cord following transection, which is comparable to the regeneration that occur in fish and amphibia. The studies of Windle suggest that axons in the mammalian spinal cord are capable of regenerating and that the growth is aborted because of a dense neuroglial and connective tissue scar that develops at the site of transection. Yet, by the use of pharmacological agents (steroid hormones, pyrogenic drugs), it is possible to "loosen" the scar and thus allow regeneration to proceed for a longer period (Windle, 1956; Windle et al., 1956). More recently, similar conclusions have been reached by Matinian and Andreasian (1976).

During the past seven years at the Palo Alto Veterans Administration Hospital and in the newly constituted Spinal Cord Injury Research Laboratories at the West Roxbury Veterans Administration Hospital in Boston, we have been investigating one basic aspect of neuroglial scarring, which is the accumulation of cytoplasmic filaments within astrocytes, based on the assumption that fibrous gliosis not only provides a mechanical barrier but also interferes with other glial functions that may be relevant to axonal regeneration, such as the supply of trophic factors (Varon, 1975). *In vivo* and *in vitro* studies have recently provided an experimental basis for this assumption. When a piece of peripheral nerve is surgically removed and a graft from another nerve is inserted between the stumps, regenerating axons from the proximal stump will grow into the graft and reach the distal stump. As shown by Aguayo and Spencer at the Winter Conference in Brain Research in January 1978, the situation is reversed when optic nerve, a CNS tract of myelinated fibers, is used as the graft. Regenerating peripheral axons will not enter the optic nerve but rather grow at the periphery of the graft. This "barrier" effect is still observed when all myelin has been removed from the optic nerve and, thus, appears to be due to the dense fibrous gliosis, resulting from Wallerian degeneration, rather than to the persistance of degenerated myelin. With regard to *in vitro* studies, several lines of evidence indicate that neuroglia can stimulate neurite outgrowth, while there appears to be a reverse relation between neuronal viability and fibrous transformation of glia in monolayer and aggregating cultures of mammalian CNS (Kozak et al., 1977, 1978a).

With the exception of the pioneer investigations of Bairati (1957), very little work had been done in the past on the biochemistry of glial filaments. In these studies, two main methodological approaches are possible. One approach is based on the isolation of filaments from brain, the main difficulty residing in the separation of different types of brain filaments (glial and neuronal) (Benitz et al., 1976) and also in the stability of brain filaments after isolation, so that protein can be solubilized only with detergent, urea or guanidine hydrochloride at high concentrations. (Huneeus and Davison, 1970; Shelanski et al., 1971; Davison and Winslow, 1974; Yen et al., 1976).

In the approach that has been followed in most of our studies, the protein subunit of glial filaments is isolated from extracts of brain tissue. Due to the lack of any known enzymatic activity or binding properties (such as colchicine for tubulin), the recognition of this protein that is called glial fibrillary acidic protein (GFA) was originally based on immunological techniques. Antibodies were first prepared against protein that was isolated from multiple sclerosis plaques, (Uyeda et al., 1972; Bignami and Dahl, 1974a) a tissue markedly enriched in glial filaments, and, after the development of adequate purification procedures, they were prepared against protein that was isolated from normal material (Dahl and Bignami, 1976b, 1977a).

Although work that is aimed at reconstituting glial filaments from GFA in solutions is still in progress, direct and indirect evidence indicates that GFA is indeed the major, if not the only, constituent of glial filaments. This evidence can be summarized as follows: (1) GFA is the main fraction of the water-soluble and insoluble proteins in neuroglial scar tissue, constituting up to 35% of the total water-soluble protein in old multiple sclerosis plaques (Dahl and Bignami, 1974); (2) Using GFA antiserum, glial filaments are stained by the immuno-peroxidase technique at the electron microscopic level (Schachner et al., 1977); (3) In bovine brain, GFA protein and the major polypeptide of isolated filaments have similar electrophoretic mobility, tryptic peptide maps, and immunological properties (Yen et al., 1976; Benitz et al., 1976).

Isolation

The use of gliosed human brain originally allowed the isolation of GFA protein (Eng et al., 1971). Essentially, no experimental procedure will result in the tremendous enrichment in fibrous astrocytes that has been observed in old multiple sclerosis plaques. However, the limitations associated with the use of autopsy material soon became apparent (Dahl and Bignami, 1974). It was first observed that GFA protein, which is isolated from the human brain, was heterogenous and that different preparations varied in polypeptide composition. Since heterogeneity was not related to the isolation procedure but rather to the material used, the possibility was considered that GFA could vary in polypeptide composition, depending on the stage of gliosis. Although this possibility has not been completely ruled out, it has now become apparent that the heterogeneity of human GFA is to a large extent the result of post-mortem autolysis. Degradation of the higher molecular weight components into the lower molecular weight species could be obtained by *in situ* proteolysis in tissues and homogenates (Dahl and Bignami, 1975a), and the major factor, which appeared to be related to the band pattern in a series of 30 human brains, was the time interval between death and autopsy. The initial work on GFA protein from gliosed human brain required relatively simple procedures, such as buffer extraction and ammonium sulfate precipitation, in order to obtain purified preparations (Eng et al., 1971; Uyeda et al., 1972).

Using normal material as the source, these procedures did not allow satisfactory purification, therefore, new methods were developed.

GFA protein from human brain and from urea extracts of bovine brain is isolated by hydroxyapatite chromatography as the main step in purification (Dahl and Bignami, 1975a, 1976b; Chan et al., 1976). Preparations of comparable purity can also be obtained by DEAE - Sephadex column chromatograhy (Dahl and Bignami, 1973a). Traditional isolation procedures cannot be used to isolate nondegraded protein from buffer extracts of rapidly frozen material because of the risk of tubulin contamination (Bignami et al., 1978).

Homogeneous preparations that are not contaminated with tubulin have been recently obtained by immunoaffinity chromatography from buffer extracts of bovine brain rapidly frozen after slaugter (Rueger et al., 1978a).

The molecular weight of nondegraded bovine GFA ranges from a high of 53,000 to a low of 50,000, depending on the gel system (Rueger et al., 1978b). This has been substantiated by guanidine-agarose chromatography and sedimentation equilibrium in 6 M GuHC1, giving a molecular weight of 49,000 (± 3,500) and 53,750 (± 2,500), respectively (Huston and Bignami, 1977). The essential agreement of these measurements proves that the reduced protein in SDS and the reduced and carboxymethylated species in 6 M GuHC1 are, respectively, binding the standard amount of SDS and are denatured to a random coil by concentrated guanidine, GFA from autopsy specimen comprises material that may exhibit as many as eight distinctive bands on 12.5% SDS gels. The highest observed molecular weight for GFA among these specimen co-migrates with bovine GFA, with the other species ranging down to 40,500 (± 1,000). The lower bands can be enriched at the expense of the upper bands by prior incubation of tissues and homogenates, and thus the high mol. wt. species yield those of lower weight by specific proteolytic breakdown. Polypeptides in the 45,000 - 40,500 range are more resistant to further degradation and, thus, are selectively enriched in autopsy specimen.

Degradation

Our data indicated the existence of two distinct degradative pathways for GFA protein (Dahl and Bignami, 1975a; Dahl, 1976a). In one type best demonstrated in homogenates incubated at pH 6.0 and 6.5 or at pH 8.0 with the addition of certain inhibitors, GFA protein is rapidly destroyed with loss of immunological activity. The other type of degradation is observed in tissues that are incubated at room temperature, as a result of *post-mortem* autolysis, and in homogenates that are incubated in phosphate buffer pH 8.0 at 24°C and 37°C. It presents a characteristic disc-electrophroetic pattern of multiple closely spaced bands, suggesting that small fragments are cleaved from the original polypeptide chain, in successive steps of degradation. All preparations, degraded or nondegraded, are immunologically indistinguishable, as indicated by disc immunodiffusion and by microcomplement fixation. The final products of this type of degradation, a polypeptide 40,500 (± 1,000) mol. wt. is remarkably resistant to tissue autolysis and is still present after many days of incubation of spinal cord *in vitro* (Dahl and Bignami, 1976b). The degraded protein has a unique aminoterminal sequence Ala-Gly-Phe, (Dahl and Bignami, 1975a) which has been confirmed and extended to include five additional residues (Lys-Glu-Thr-Gly-Ala) by automated Edman degradation procedures (Dahl and Moo Penn, unpublished results).

Astroglial Differentiation

The onset of differentiation has been related to the production of proteins that are unique to a single-cell type in many developmental studies. As indicated by immunofluorescence studies (Bignami et al., 1972; Bignami and Dahl, 1974a) and, more recently, with peroxidase labeled antiserum at the light microscopic (Ludwin et al., 1976) and electron microscopic levels (Schachner et al., 1977), GFA protein is selectively located in astroglia. Therefore, we have conducted a series of investigations to study the differentiation of this type of neuroglia in various regions of the central nervous system, both in normal animals and neurological mutants. (The differential staining of neuroglial with the traditional methods of neurohistology is often difficult to achieve in the immature brain.)

In the cerebral and spinal cord white matter, our findings indicate a close correlation between the appearance of GFA protein and myelination in a period of intense cell multiplication (Bignami and Dahl, 1973; 1975), thus suggesting the existence of a matrix cell (glioblast) from which both the oligodendrocyte (myelin-forming cell) and the astrocyte (GFA-producing cell) originate (Privat, 1975). GFA expression is not retarded in mutant mice with deficient myelination, quaking and jimpy (Bignami and Dahl, 1974c; Jacque et al., 1974; 1976), indicating that astroglial differentiation is not dependent on myelination and that in these mutants the defect in myelination is strictly associated with abnormalities of the oligodendroglial cell line.

As assessed by immunofluorescence with GFA antiserum, Bergmann glia differentiation precedes neuronal migration from the external granular layer but is not delayed in the weaver mouse (Bignami and Dahl, 1974d), thus indicating that the reduced rate of granule cell migration in this neurological mutant is not due to the absence of Bergmann fibers (Rakic and Sidman, 1973).

A distinctive change in the morphology of astrocytes could be demonstrated in the granular layer of the hippocampus, during development, i.e., a radial system of fibers later transforming into astrocytes of mature appearance (Bignami and Dahl, 1974a). Radially disposed glial fibers extending from the ventricle to the external surface of the brain are a well-known feature of the fetal brain (Rakic, 1972). These fibers could not be demonstrated in the rat telencephalon during normal development but only as a response to injury (Bignami and Dahl, 1974b, 1976). As in the granular layer of the hippocampus, reactive radial glia later transformed into astrocytes of typical stellate shape. Radially disposed fibers spanning the entire width of cerebrum from the ventricular zone to the external surface have been demonstrated by immunofluorescence with GFA antisera in human fetuses as early as the 10th and 11th week (Antanitus et al., 1976). This important finding convincingly demonstrates that neuroglia are present at an early stage of development, which is contrary to the widely held belief that neurogenesis precedes gliogenesis.

Immunogenicity

Antisera to GFA protein were originally obtained against antigen isolated from multiple sclerosis plaques (Uyeda et al., 1972; Bignami and Dahl, 1974a). Due to the difficulty in obtaining such pathological material and in following the development of better purification procedures that allow the isolation of highly purified protein from normal brain, an immunization program was initiated in rabbits to study the immunogenic properties of different GFA preparations (Dahl and Bignami, 1976b). Antisera that are comparable in strength to those previously obtained against multiple sclerosis plaques could only be prepared using highly degraded protein in the 40,000 mol. wt. range. No immunological response at all was seen with nondegraded GFA protein. Antisera that is comparable in specificity to those obtained with degraded protein could be also prepared with nondegraded protein that has been heated in sodium dodecyl sulfate and with the cyanogen bromide digest of nonimmunogenic preparations (Dahl and Bignami, 1977a). In this respect it is interesting to note that all GFA preparations from mammalian brain, degraded and nondegraded, share a cyanogen bromide peptide in the myoglobin range (17,200), retaining full immunological activity (Dahl and Bignami, 1975a, 1976b).

Phylogeny

The earliest phylogenetic studies of GFA protein were mainly immuno-chemical, due to the difficulty in obtaining purified preparations from normal material with the methods that were then available. It was shown that antiserum to human GFA protein cross-reacted with brain extracts from all classes of vertebrates with the exception of the lamprey, a jawless cartilagineous fish believed to be a direct descendent of the earlier vertebrates (Dahl and Bignami, 1973b). However, even at this time, differences between GFA in mammalian and submammalian vertebrates were already apparent as indicated by the reaction of incomplete identity with antihuman GFA serum, indicating that submammalian GFA proteins were deficient in some antigenic determinants that are present in the human protein. Improvement in the purification procedures has allowed the isolation of proteins from the chicken, turtle, frog, and fish, which share common properties with mammalian GFA protein and are extremely susceptible to limited *in situ* proteolysis but also have distinctive features (Dahl, 1976b). The major differences that have been detected so far are in the immunological properties. Antisera directed against purified chicken protein react with turtle although with spur formation but not with mammalian protein. Since the glial filaments have essentially the same electron microscopic appearance in mammalian and submammalian vertebrates, it is possible that such comparative studies of GFA protein may reveal the conservative parts of the molecule by stabilizing the conformation of the monomeric species and by favoring its aggregation to form filaments.

On more biological grounds, the cross-reactivity between mammalian and submammalian GFA has allowed comparative studies on the expression of this protein as a response to injury. Since GFA is the major protein of scarred (gliosed) nerve tissue and considering that glial scarring (Windle, 1956; Clemente, 1964 and 1970) is probably a major factor preventing regeneration in the mammalian CNS, these studies may in the future lead to a point where practical issues could be possible.

In the rat, injury to the brain that is produced by stabbing is followed by the most remarkable transformation of the neuroglial cells, located in the cerebral isocortex and corpus striatum (Bignami and Dahl, 1974b, 1976). These cells, which contain small amounts of GFA protein under normal conditions, become intensely immunofluorescent with GFA antisera within 36-48 hours after injury. Whether this is due to an increased rate of synthesis or to decreased degradation is still not known. The transformation of cortical neuroglia into immuno-fluorescent cells is still presistent many months after injury, indicating that the change is irreversible. In submammalian vertebrates the neuroglial response to injury as assessed by immunofluorescence by GFA antiserum is extremely limited (Bignami and Dahl, 1976) and is altogether absent in fish spinal cord that is undergoing regeneration after transection (Bignami et al., 1974).

In Vitro Studies

Antisera to GFA protein have been extensively used to investigate the *in vitro* differentiation of astroglia (Antanitus et al., 1975; Sipe et al., 1975; Bissell et al., 1974 and 1975; Bock et al., 1975, 1977; VandenBerg et al., 1975 and 1976; Vraa-Jensen et al., 1976; Manoury et al., 1976; Gilden et al., 1976).

The C6 glioma contains minimal amounts of GFA protein when grown in suspension or monolayer culture, while the concentration dramatically increases when the cells are reaggregated on sponge foam (Bissell et al., 1974, 1975). It is interesting to note that these high levels of GFA could not be correlated with filament formation by electron microcopy, a situation comparable to round cell neuroblastoma in culture where tubulin is a major fraction and microtubules are scarce (Morgan and Seeds, 1975).

In collaboration with Kozak, M.D., and Eppig, M.D., at the Jackson Laboratory, we have explored the possibility of utilizing tissue culture procedures to study the relations between GFA production and neuronal viability. Dissociated cells from fetal mouse brain and neonatal cerebellum differentiate *in vitro* when grown in reaggreating cultures, as originally shown by Moscona (1961) for a variety of tissues. While aggregates of mouse fetal cerebrum maintain their viability for long periods in culture (Kozak et al., 1978a), in aggregates of neonatal cerebellum one finds the progressive degeneration of neurons and their gradual replacement with fibrous neuroglia after 10 days *in vitro*. (Kozak et al., 1977). If poly-L-lysine is added to the culture medium, either for the entire culture period or during the period of accelerated gliosis, the neuronal character is stabilized (Kozak et al., 1978b).

Comparison with Neurofilament Protein

Most biochemical studies of neurofilament proteins were, until recently, based on the isolation of these structures, either by dissecting the axoplasm from the giant axons of invertebrates or by fractionation of bovine white matter, using the myelin sheath to float the axons and, subsequently, stripping the myelin from the axons by osmotic shock (Shelanski et al., 1971). These studies have demonstrated that the mammalian filament is clearly distinguishable in its properties from the filament protein of invertebrates, although the neurofilaments from all these species have similar ultrastructural appearance. In the squid, the subunit is an acidic protein of approximately 80,000 (Huneeus and Davison, 1970). In the *Myxicola infundibulum*, a marine worm, neurofilaments are composed of high molecular weight chains above 100,000 (Gilbert et al., 1975; Lasek and Krishnan, 1975) while the electrophoretic mobility on sodium dodecyl sulfate gels of the major neurofilament protein from bovine brain indicates a molecular weight in the 50,000 range (Shelanski et al., 1971; Davison and Winslow, 1974; Yen et al., 1976; DeVries et al., 1976; Benitz et al., 1976). Recent evidence suggests that the differences in molecular weight between mammalian and invertebrate neurofilament proteins are more apparent than real and that the high molecular weight proteins are oligomers of the 50,000

mol. wt. species (Shook and Norton, 1975; Lasek and Wu, 1976).
According to Gilbert et al. (1975), the slow components are rapidly
degraded to the 50,000 mol. wt. species by a calcium-activated protease.
The conversion of a major 100,000 dalton species into products in the
50,000 dalton range has been similarly observed in myelin free axons
isolated from rabbit peripheral nerve following *in vitro* incubation in
elevated calcium (Frankel and Koenig, 1977).

Neuronal and glial filaments belong to a class of cytoplasmic filaments
that are intermediate in size between actin microfilaments and microtubules,
the 100 Å filament. Experimental data, which have become available in
the last few years, suggest that there might be a relationship between
the protein subunits of different types of intermediate filaments.

The first indication that neuronal and glial filaments are made of
similar proteins came from comparative studies of the overall polypeptide
composition of the optic nerves in normal and blind rats five months
after removal of the eyes (Dahl and Bignami, 1975b), at a time when
myelinated nerve fibers have disappeared and are replaced by glial
fibers (Vaughn et al., 1970; Vaughn and Pease, 1970). Apart from the
disappearance of myelin proteins after longstanding Wallerian degeneration
(Bignami and Eng, 1973), the disc-gel patterns by SDS-acrylamide gel
electrophoresis of normal and gliosed nerves were remarkably similar,
suggesting that the major proteins of glial and neuronal filaments have
the same molecular weight.

More direct evidence of the similarity between the building blocks of
glial and nerve filaments has been provided by the direct comparison
of the major protein fraction constituting neurofilaments, isolated from
bovine brain, with GFA protein, isolated from extracts of the same
tissue, (Yen et al., 1976) and with CNS fractions, enriched in glial
fibers (Benitz et al., 1976). Neurofilament and GFA proteins not only
have the same molecular weight and similar peptide maps that, contrary
to a previous report (Johnson and Sinex, 1974), are different from
tubulin but also cross-react with a line of complete identity by double
immunodiffusion when tested against antisera to GFA and neurofilament
proteins. The immunological cross-reactivity is difficult to explain,
considering that extensive experience in different laboratories has
shown that using both fluorescein and peroxidase-labeled antisera, the
immunohistochemical staining with GFA antibodies, is restricted to
astroglia while nerve fibers are not stained (Bignami et al., 1972;
Bignami and Dahl, 1974a; Antanitus et al., 1975 and 1976; Ludwin et
al., 1976; Schachner et al., 1977). A possible explanation of the
phenomenon may reside in the facts that neurofilament preparations
also contain glial filaments and that antisera against these preparations
are directed against the more antigenic glial component (Benitz et al.,
1976; DeVries et al., 1976).

Comparison of the disc-gel electrophoretic pattern of the axonal
fraction and of glial preparations selectively enriched in GFA protein
have confirmed the observation that both neurofilaments and glial filaments
share a major protein in the 50,000 mol. wt. range (Benitz et al.,
1976). High molecular weight bands are more prominent in the axonal
than in the glial fraction.

Using a different approach to the problem, procedures used to
isolate GFA protein were applied to extracts of sciatic nerves under
the assumption that closely related proteins will follow similar purification
procedures. Peripheral nerves do not contain astroglia, while the
large myelinated axons are very rich in neurofilaments both in the
central and peripheral nervous system.

The isolated protein did not react with GFA antisera but appeared to be related to GFA protein as indicated by comigration experiments on SDS-acrylamide gel electrophoresis, the type of degeneration resulting from *in situ* proteolysis, amino acid composition, and cyanogen bromide peptide mapping (Dahl and Bignami, 1976a).

The antigen that was isolated by hydroxyapatite chromatography from human sciatic nerve was selectively localized by immunofluorescence to neurofibrils in rat and chicken CNS, and the same was true for an antigen that was isolated from 8 M urea extracts of chicken brain by the same procedure (Dahl and Bignami, 1977b). In addition, the reaction of complete identity by immunodiffusion between human and chicken suggested that the neurofilament protein is highly conservative in phylogeny. The localization of the human and chicken antigens to neurofilaments was recently confirmed by the intense immunofluorescent staining of aluminum-induced neurofibrillary tangles (Dahl and Bignami, 1978). These are structures that are formed almost exclusively of neurofilaments (Terry and Peña, 1965). A similar immunofluorescent pattern, which is selective neurofibrillary staining, has been also demonstrated with antisera that are raised against neurofilaments, isolated from peripheral nerve (Schlaepfer and Lynch, 1977). The major protein in these preparations is 68,000 mol. wt. (Schlaepfer, 1977).

REFERENCES

Antanitus, D.S., Choi, B.H. and Lapham, L.W. Immunofluorescence staining of astrocytes *in vitro* using antiserum to glial fibrillary acidic protein. *Brain Research 89:*363-367 (1975).

Antanitus, D.S., Choi, B.H., and Lapham, L.W. The demonstration of glial fibrillary acidic protein in the cerebrum of the human fetus by indirect immunofluorescence. *Brain Research 103:*613-616 (1976).

Bairati, A. Propriétés biophysiques des fibres névrogliques. *C.R. Ass. Anat. 44:*113-119 (1957).

Benitz, W.E., Dahl, D., Williams, K.W. and Bignami, A. The protein composition of glial and nerve fibers. *FEBS Letters 66:*285-289 (1976).

Bignami, A., and Dahl, D. Differentiation of astrocytes in the cerebellar cortex and the pyramidal tracts of the newborn rat. An immunofluorescence study with antibodies to a protein specific to astrocytes. *Brain Research 49:*393-402 (1973).

Bignami, A., and Dahl, D. Astrocyte-specific protein and neuroglial differentiation. An immunofluorescence study with antibodies to the glial fibrillary acidic protein. *J. Comp. Neur. 153:*27-38 (1974a).

Bignami, A., and Dahl, D. Astrocyte-specific protein and radial glia in the cerebral cortex of newborn rat. *Nature 252:*55-56 (1974b).

Bignami, A., and Dahl, D. Glial fibrillary acidic protein in mutant mice with deficiency of myelination: Quaking and jimpy. *Acta Neuropath. (Berl.) 28:*269-272 (1974c).

Bignami, A., and Dahl, D. The development of Bergmann glia in mutant mice with cerebellar malformations: Reeler, staggerer and weaver. Immunofluorescence study with antibodies to the glial fibrillary acidic protein. *J. Comp. Neur. 155:*219-230 (1974d).

Bignami, A., and Dahl, D. Astroglial protein in the developing spinal cord of the chick embryo. *Develop. Biol. 44:*204-209 (1975).

Bignami, A., and Dahl, D. The astroglial response to stabbing. Immunofluorescence studies with antibodies to astrocyte-specific protein (GFA) in mammalian and submammalian vertebrates. *Neuropathology and Applied Neurobiology 2:*99-111 (1976).

Bignami, A., Dahl, D. and Rueger, D.C. Isolation of neurofilament and glial filament proteins from water and urea extracts of nerve tissue.   In *Mechanisms, Regulation and Special Functions of Protein Synthesis in the Brain*, S. Roberts, A. Lajtha and W.H. Gispen, editors.   Elsevier, Amsterdam, 1978 (in press).

Bignami, A., and Eng, L.F.   Biochemical studies of myelin in Wallerian degeneration of rat optic nerve.   *J. Neurochem. 20:*165-173 (1973).

Bignami, A., Eng, L.F., Dahl, D., and Uyeda, C.T.   Localization of the glial fibrillary acidic protein in astrocytes by immunofluorescence. *Brain Reserach 43:*429-435 (1972).

Bignami, A., Forno, L., and Dahl, D.   The neuroglial response to injury following spinal cord transection in the goldfish.   *Exp. Neurol. 44:*60-70 (1974).

Bissell, M.G., Rubinstein, L.J., Bignami, A., and Herman, M.M. Characteristics of the rat C-6 glioma maintained in organ culture systems.   Production of glial fibrillary acidic protein in the absence of gliofibrillogenesis.   *Brain Research 82:*77-89 (1974).

Bissell, M.G., Eng, L.F., Herman, M.M., Bensch, K.G., and Miles, L.E.M.   Quantitative increase of neuroglia-specific GFA protein in rat C-6 glioma cells *in vitro*.   *Nature 255:*633-634 (1975).

Bock, E., Jørgensen, O.S., Dittmann, L. and Eng, L.F.   Determination of brain-specific antigens in short term cultivated rat astroglial cells and in rat synaptosomes.   *J. Neurochem. 25:*867-870 (1975).

Bock, E., Møller, M., Nissen, C., and Sensenbrenner, M.   Glial fibrillary acidic protein in primary astroglial cell cultures derived from newborn rat brain.   *FEBS Lett. 83:*207-211 (1977).

Chan, P.H., Huston, J.S., Moo-Penn, W., Dahl, D. and Bignami, A. Biochemical studies related to CNS regeneration: Isolation and characterization of urea-soluble gliofibrillary protein.   In *Proceedings of the Second Annual Maine Biomedical Science Symposium*.   (July 8-10, 1976) University of Maine Press, Vol. 2, pp. 496-524.

Clemente, C.D.   Regeneration in the vertebrate central nervous system. *Int. Rev. Neurobiol. 6:*257-301 (1964).

Clemente, C.D.   Structural regeneration in the mammalian central nervous system and the role of neuroglia and connective tissue.   In *Regeneration in the central nervous system*, W.F. Windle, ed. Thomas, Springfield, p. 147, 1970.

Dahl, D.   Glial fibrillary acidic protein from bovine and rat brain. Degradation in tissues and homogenates.   *Biochim. Biophys. Acta 420:*142-154 (1976a).

Dahl, D.   Isolation and initial characterization of glial fibrillary acidic protein from chicken, turtle, frog, and fish central nervous system. *Biochem. Biophys. Acta 446:*41-50 (1976b).

Dahl, D., and Bignami, A.   Glial fibrillary acidic protein from normal human brain.   Purification and properties.*Brain Research 57:*343-360 (1973a).

Dahl, D., and Bignami, A.   Immunochemical and immunofluorescence studies of the glial fibrillary acidic protein in vertebrates.   *Brain Research 61:*279-293 (1973b).

Dahl, D., and Bignami, A.   Heterogeneity of the glial fibrillary acidic protein in gliosed human brains.   *J. Neurol. Sci. 23:*551-563 (1974).

Dahl, D., and Bignami, A.   Glial fibrillary acidic protein from normal and gliosed human brain.   Demonstration of multiple related polypeptides.   *Biochim. Biophys. Acta 386:*41-51 (1975a).

Dahl, D., and Bignami, A.   Protein differences associated with the loss of myelinated axons and fibrillary gliosis in rat optic nerves following Wallerian degeneration.   *FEBS Letters 51:*313-316 (1975b).

Dahl, D., and Bignami, A.   Isolation from peripheral nerve of a protein similar to the glial fibrillary acidic protein.   *FEBS Letters 66:*281-

284 (1976a).

Dahl, D., and Bignami, A. Immunogenic properties of the glial fibrillary acidic protein. *Brain Research* 116:150-157 (1976b).

Dahl, D., and Bignami, A. Effect of sodium dodecyl sulfate on the immunogenic properties of the glial fibrillary acidic protein. *J. Immunol. Methods* 17:201-209 (1977a).

Dahl, D., and Bignami, A. Preparation of antisera to neurofilament protein from children brain and human sciatic nerve. *J. Comp. Neur.* 176:645-658 (1977b).

Dahl, D., and Bignami, A. Immunochemical cross-reactivity of normal neurofibrils and aluminum-induced neurofibrillary tangles. Immuno-fluorescence study with antineurofilament serum. *Exp. Neurol.* 58: 74-80 (1978).

Davison, P.F., and Winslow, B. The protein subunit of calf brain neurofilament. *J. Neurobiol.* 5:119-133 (1974).

DeVries, G.H., Eng, L.F., Lewis, D.H., and Hadfield, M.G. The protein composition of bovine myeline-free axons. *Biochim. Biophys. Acta* 439:133-145 (1976).

Eng, L.F., Vanderhaeghen, J.J., Bignami, A., and Gerstl, B. An acidic protein isolated from fibrous astrocytes. *Brain Research* 28: 351-354 (1971).

Frankel, R.D., and Koenig, E. Identification of major indigenous protein components in mammalian axons and locally synthesized axonal protein in hypoglossal nerve. *Exp. Neurol.* 57:282-295 (1977).

Gilbert, D.S., Newby, B.J., and Anderton, B.H. Neurofilament disguise, destruction and discipline. *Nature* 256:586-589 (1975).

Gilden, D.H., Wroblewska, Z., Eng, L.F., and Rorke, L.B. Human brain in tissue culture. Part 5. Identification of glial cells by immunofluorescence. *J. Neurol. Sci.* 29:177-184 (1976).

Huneeus, F.C., and Davison, P.F. Fibrillary proteins from squid axons. I. Neurofilament protein. *J. Mol. Biol.* 52:415-428 (1970).

Huston, J.S., and Bignami, A. Structural properties of the glial fibrillary acidic protein. Evidence for intermolecular disulfide bonds. *Biochim. Biophys. Acta* 493:97-103 (1977).

Jacque, C.M., Jorgensen, O.S., and Bock, E. Quantitative studies of the brain specific antigens S-100, GFA, 14-3-2, D1, D2, D3 and C1 in quaking mouse. *FEBS Letters* 49:264-266 (1974).

Jacque, C.M., Baumann, N.A., and Bock, E. Quantitative studies of the brain specific antigens FFA, 14-3-2, synaptin C1, D1, D2, D3 and D5 in jimpy mouse. *Neurosci. Letters* 3:41-44 (1976).

Johnson, L., and Sinex, F.M. On the relationship of brain filaments to microtubules. *J. Neurochem.* 22:321-326 (1974).

Kozak, L.P., Eppig, J.J., Dahl, D., and Bignami, A. Ultrastructural and immunohistological characterization of a cell culture model for the study of neuronal-glial interactions. *Devel. Biol.* 59:206-227 (1977).

Kozak, L.O., Dahl, D., and Bignami, A. Glial fibrillary acidic protein in reaggregating and monolayer cultures of fetal mouse cerebral hemispheres. *Brain Res.* (1978a, in press).

Kozak, L.P., Eppig, J.J., Dahl, D., and Bignami, A. Enhanced neuronal expression in reaggregating cells of mouse cerebellum cultured in the presence of poly-L-lysine. *Devel. Biol.* (1978b) (in press).

Lasek, R.J., and Krishnan, N. Identification of the proteins constituting 10 nm neurofilaments from the giant axon of Mixicola. Transactions of the American Society for *Neurochemistry* 6:106 (1975).

Lasek, R.J., and Wu, J.-Y. Immunochemical analysis of the proteins comprising myxicola (10 nm) neurofilaments. *Neuroscience Abstracts Vol. II*, Pt. 1, p. 40 (1976).

Ludwin, S.K., Kosek, J.C., and Eng, L.F. The topographical distribution of S-100 and GFA proteins in the adult rat brain: An immunohistochemical study using horseradish peroxidase-labeled antibodies. *J. Comp. Neur. 165:*197-208 (1976).

Manoury, R., Delpech, A., Delpech, B., Vidard, M.N., and Vedrenne, C. Presence of neurospecific antigen NSA 1 in fetal human astrocytes in long-term cultures. *Brain Res. 112:*383-387 (1976).

Matinian, L.A., and Andreasian, A.S. Enzyme therapy in organic lesions of the spinal cord. *Brain Information Service*, UCLA, Los Angeles, 1976.

Morgan, J.L., and Seeds, N.W. Tubulin constancy during morphological differentiation of mouse neuroblastoma cells. *J. Cell Biol. 67:*136-145 (1975).

Moscona, A. Rotation-mediated histogenetic aggregation of dissociated cells. *Exp. Cell Res. 22:*455-475 (1961).

Privat, A. Postnatal gliogenesis in the mammalian brain. *Int. Rev. Cytol. 40:*281-323 (1975).

Rakic, P. Mode of cell migration to the superficial layers of fetal monkey neocortex. *J. Comp. Neurol. 145:*61-84 (1972).

Rakic, P., and Sidman, R.L. Weaver mutant mouse cerebellum: Defective neuronal migration secondary to abnormality of Bergmann glia. *Proc. Nat. Acad. Sci. U.S.A. 70:*240-244 (1973).

Rueger, D.C., Dahl, D., and Bignami, A. *Purification of a brain specific astroglial protein by immunoaffinity chromatography.* 1978a (submitted for publication).

Rueger, D.C., Dahl, D., and Bignami, A. *Comparison of bovine glial fibrillary acidic protein with tubulin,* 1978b (submitted for publication).

Schachner, M., Hedley-Whyte, E.T., Hsu, D.W., Schoonmaker, G., and Bignami, A. Ultrastructural localization of glial fibrillary acidic protein in mouse cerebellum by immunoperoxidase labeling. *J. Cell Biol. 75:*67-73 (1977).

Schlaepfer, W.W. Immunological and ultrastructural studies of neurofilaments isolated from rat peripheral nerve. *J. Cell Biol. 74:* 226-240 (1977).

Schlaepfer, W.W. and Lynch, R.G. Immunofluorescence studies of neurofilaments in the rat and human peripheral and central nervous system. *J. Cell Biol. 74:*241-250 (1977).

Shook, W.J., and Norton, W.T. On the composition of axonal neurofilaments, Transactions of the American Society for *Neurochemistry 6:* 274 (1975).

Shelanski, M.L., Albert, S., DeVries, G.H., and Norton, W.T. Isolation of filaments from brain. *Science 174:*1242-1244 (1971).

Sipe, J.C., Rubinstein, L.J., Herman, M.M., and Bignami, A. Ethylnitrosourea-induced astrocytomas. Morphological observations on rat tumors maintained in tissue and organ culture system. *Lab. Inv. 31:*571-579 (1975).

Terry, R.D., and Pena, C. Experimental production of neurofibrillary degeneration. 2. Electron microscopy, phosphatase histochemistry and electron probe analysis. *J. Neuropath. Exp. Neurol. 24:*200-210 (1965).

Uyeda, C.T., Eng, L.F., and Bignami, A. Immunological study of the glial fibrillary acidic protein. *Brain Research 37:*81-89 (1972).

VandenBerg, S.R., Herman, M.M., Ludwin, S.K., and Bignami, A. An experimental mouse testicular teratoma as a model for neuroepithelial neoplasia and differentiation. *Am. J. Path. 79:*147-168 (1975).

VandenBerg, S.R., Ludwin, S.K., Herman, M.M., and Bignami, A. *In vitro* astrocytic differentiation from embryoid bodies of an experimental mouse testicular teratoma. *Am. J. Path. 83:* 197-206 (1976).

Varon, S. Nerve growth factor and its mode of action. *Exp. Neurol. 48:* 75-92 (1975).

Vaughn, J.E., Hinds, P.L., and Skoff, R.P. Electron microscopic studies of Wallerian degeneration in rat optic nerves. I. The multipotential glial. *J. Comp. Neur. 140:* 175-206 (1970).

Vaughn, J.E., and Pease, D.C. Electron microscopic studies of Wallerian degeneration in rat optic nerve. II. Astrocytes, oligodendrocytes and adventitial cells. *J. Comp. Neuro. 140:* 207-226 (1970).

Vraa-Jensen, J., Herman, M.M., Rubinstein, L.J., and Bignami, A. *In vitro* characteristics of a fourth ventricle ependyoma maintained in organ culture systems: Light and electron microscopy observations. *Neuropath. and Applied Neurobiol. 2:* 349-364 (1976).

Windle, W.F. Regeneration of axons in the vertebrate central nervous system. *Physiol. Rev. 36:* 427-440 (1956).

Windle, W.F., Littrell, J.L., Smart, J.O., and Toralemon, J. Regeneration in the cord of spinal monkeys. *Neurology 6:* 420-428 (1956).

Yen, S.-H., Dahl, D., Schachner, M., and Shelanski, M.L. Biochemistry of the filaments of brain. *Proc. Nat. Acad. Sci. U.S.A. 73:* 529-533 (1976).

2

Positive and Negative Contrast Myelograph in Spinal Trauma

N.T. PAY, A.E. GEORGE, M.V. BENJAMIN,
R.T. BERGERON, J.P. LIN and I. KRICHEFF

Spinal cord trauma has been successfully treated by cooling of the spinal cord (Albin et al., 1968; Negrin, 1965; Tomasula et al., 1069) and the administration of steroids (Hedeman and Sil, 1974; Tomasula et al., 1969) and low molecular weight dextran and catecholamine blockers (Hedeman and Sil, 1974) as well as by aggressive surgical procedures such as early decompression and dorsal midline myelotomy (Tomasula et al., 1969) in laboratory animals. In view of these

Table I: Protocol

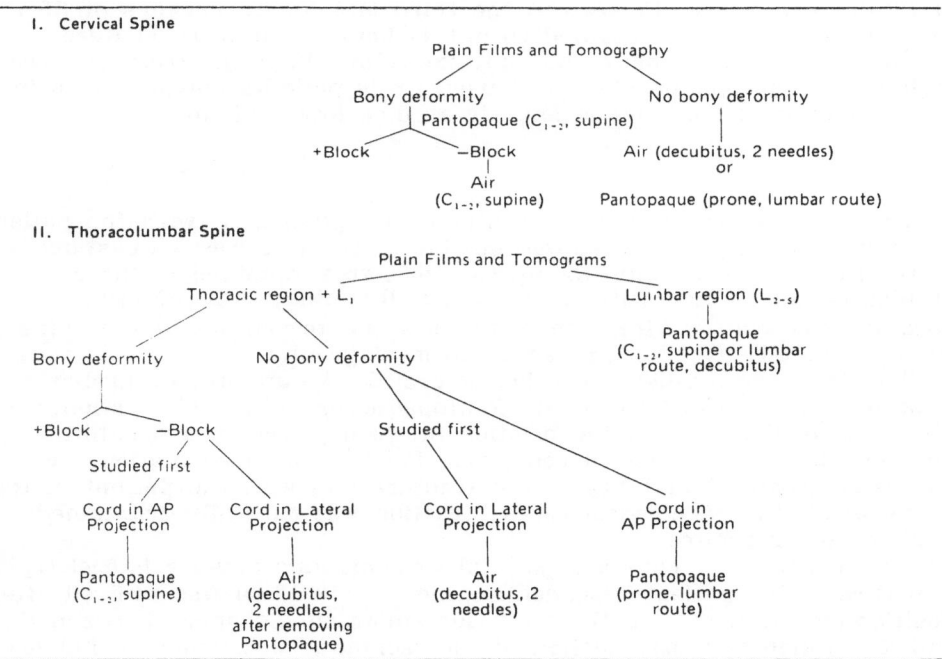

[1] From the Departments of Radiology (Section of Neuroradiology) and Neurosurgery, New York University Medical Center, New York, N. Y. Revised manuscript accepted for publication in December 1976.

Presented at the Fourteenth Annual Meeting of the American Society of Neuroradiology, Atlanta, Ga., May 18–22, 1976.

Supported in part by the Spinal Cord Clinical Research Center, NINDS NS 10164–03.

This paper is reprinted from RADIOLOGY 123: 103-111, April 1977.

encouraging results, it has become important to radiographically define the spinal cord and the integrity of the spinal canal in traumatic conditions although the role of myelography has been generally limited and poorly defined and has even been described as harmful and nondiagnostic (Braakman and Penning, 1971). We have reviewed our clinical material to determine the need for and the role of positive as well as negative contrast myelography in spinal trauma, and we have formulated a tentative protocol for the evaluation of spinal cord injuries based on clinical and radiographic findings.

MATERIAL

Following commencement of the NYU-Bellevue Spinal Cord Trauma Study (SCTS) in December 1973, we began an ongoing review of the radiologic management and diagnostic results obtained in patients admitted to the study. Thus, our approach to these cases evolved and changed as we gained experience. This report encompasses a review of 60 patients admitted to the SCTS.

Of the 36 patients with cervical spine injuries, 32 were males in the first four decades of life. There were 13 in the first two decades of life and 15 in the third and fourth decades. Most (22 patients) had been studied within 24 hours, some as long as 11 weeks from the time of injury. Positive contrast material (Pantopaque[2]) alone was used in 20 patients, and negative contrast material (air) alone in 3. Combined Pantopaque and air studies were obtained in 13 patients.

Twenty-four patients with thoracolumbar trauma were studied, 18 of whom were males; 15 were in the third and fourth decades of life. Thirteen patients were studied within 24 hours of injury; 11 were studied more than 24 hours but not exceeding 12 weeks from the time of injury. Pantopaque alone was used in 20 patients and air alone in 4. No combined Pantopaque and air studies were obtained.

METHOD

Trauma patients were initially studied by plain films with the patient maintained strictly in the supine position. If there was a question of fracture or dislocation, tomograms were then obtained. These studies were also done with the patient still supine, with the least possible movement. After the plain films and tomograms of the spine were evaluated, we then proceeded to myelography.

Patients were studied by either lateral C_{1-2} puncture or lumbar puncture with instillation of air, Pantopaque or both. The patients were examined in the supine position or were placed in a decubitus position, but were never placed prone for the initial evaluation. We observed greater instability at the fracture site with the patient in the prone position. In cervical cases, traction was carefully maintained during the procedure.

Cervical positive contrast material was introduced via a lateral C_{1-2} puncture. The patient remained supine and 10-12 ml was utilized after positioning the needle in the posterior subarachnoid space between C_1 and C_2, which is a modification of the technique described by Kelley (1968). We preferred the lateral C_{1-2} approach because the patient could remain supine during the whole study, obviating undue movement

---

[2]Iodophendylate (Lafayette Pharmaceutical, Inc., Lafayette, Ind.).

to another position, which could enhance and aggravate cord compression at an unstable site.   Cervical traction could also be maintained constantly, which would have been awkward and difficult if the head were tilted down to allow Pantopaque to gravitate up to the cervical level from a usual lumbar approach.   In the majority of cases, a tilt of 10-20° of the patient's feet downwards (Fowler position) enhanced the flow of contrast material down to the fracture site, and might retard intracranial spillage, yet without interfering with the application of cervical traction.

Thoracic and thoracolumbar positive contrast studies were performed from below in the conventional manner, keeping the patient in a decubitus position for preliminary evaluation.   Only when the information needed by the neurosurgeon could not be obtained in any other manner and there was no evidence of cord compression was the patient placed prone.

Cervical air myelography was performed in the supine or in the decubitus position either by C_{1-2} puncture or by the two-needle technique of Lodin (1966), with air instillation from below and CSF removal from above,   This same technique was utilized for thoracic air myelography.   Tomographic imaging by linear or hypocycloid motion was necessary for cord visualization in air myelography.

RESULTS

We have divided our cases into two groups, according to the presence or absence of bony deformity.   Bony deformity is defined as radiological evidence of any fracture extensive enough to disrupt the bony "ring" (composed of the vertebral body, pedicles, lamina and facets) of the vertebral segment and of any dislocation affecting the canal's integrity which ultimately determines spinal stability.   Bony deformity is initially determined by plain films and tomograms of the injured site.

Although bony deformity may be present in gunshot wound cases, ligamentous integrity is usually not totally disrupted (Norrell, 1975) and relative stability is maintained.   Thus, unless the injury was massive and extensively disruptive, we have included our gunshot injuries under the group with no bony deformity.

I.   Patients with Bony Deformity

A.   Cervical Spine Injury (24 patients):   Sixteen patients were studied by Pantopaque alone, one patient by air alone and 7 by a combination of air and Pantopaque.   All of these patients had complete neurologic deficits.

Extradural compression by bony fragments at the fracture site or by dislocation was readily evaluated by plain films and tomography. The presence or absence of spinal cord swelling was of significance but was quite hard to determine in the setting of bony deformity.

In addressing ourselves to this problem, we analyzed the 6 surgically verified cases of cord swelling involving the lower cervical spinal cord; 3 cases were studied by Pantopaque alone, and two of these examinations were diagnostic.   Three cases were studied by a combination of air and Pantopaque.   Only one of these was diagnostic of cord swelling, and this diagnosis was made by air myelography after the Pantopaque study failed to delineate the cord.

The following phenomena contribute to the difficulty of making a diagnosis of cord swelling.

Pantopaque Myelography: In the presence of a block from extradural compression by bony fracture fragments, dislocation, ridges or hematoma, the anteroposterior view of the compressed spinal cord simulates intrinsic cord swelling or hematoma when such lesions are not present (Fig. 1). The corresponding lateral view in the supine position

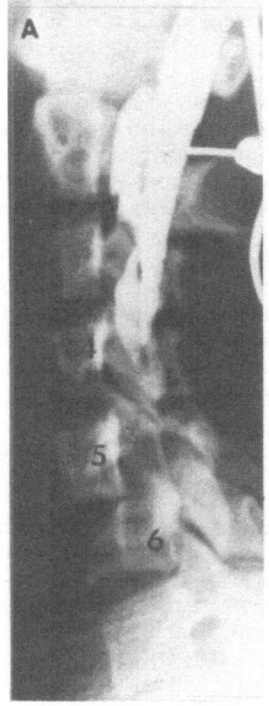 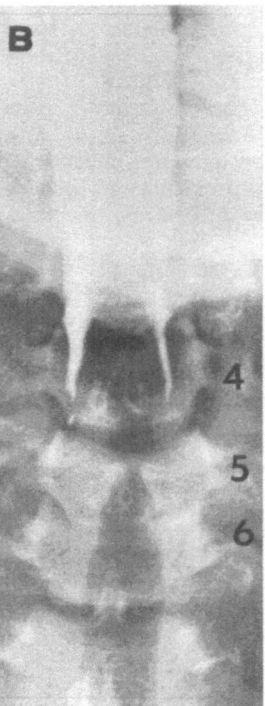

Fig. 1. A.   Laterial Pantopaque myelogram through the lateral C_{1-2} route reveals a block at the level of the midvertebral body of C_4.   A subluxation at C_{5-6} with bilateral locked facets is seen.   Surgically verified cord swelling was present.
B.   Corresponding AP Pantopaque myelogram shows two tapering contrast columns at the site of the block which is consistent with but not specific for spinal cord swelling.   Cord flattening from extradural compression, without cord swelling, may have the same appearance.

is usually inadequate for it does not demonstrate the anterior and the posterior subarachnoid spaces or the spinal cord well.   It is often observed that only a small amount of Pantopaque can be used since a large amount (sufficient to outline the entire cord shadow) will likely "spill" into the head.   This is a limitation of Pantopaque in the study of cervical spinal cord injury.   Four out of 6 surgically verified cases of cervical cord swelling with blocks and bony deformities were in this category.

In only one case were we able to unequivocally diagnose cord swelling with Pantopaque.   Two features were present in this case:

(a) Spinal cord widening was seen in two views—a cardinal diagnostic sign of cord swelling (Fig. 2).

(b) A block was present at more than one vertebral body level above the site of dislocation with no evidence of extradural compression (Fig. 2).   This implies spinal cord swelling which is extensive enough

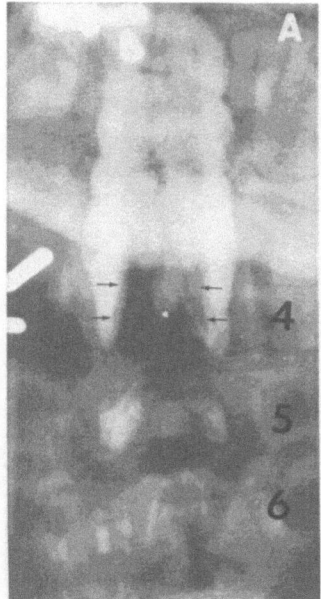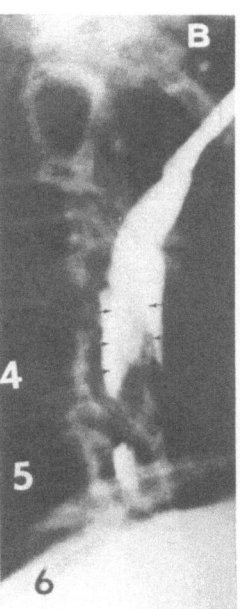

Fig. 2,A and B. Widening of the spinal cord (↑) at the site of a block at C$_{4-5}$ seen in *two views* (AP and lateral), instead of only one, is more strongly confirmatory of spinal cord swelling, as was proved in this case. A subluxation at the level of C$_{5-6}$ has been reduced.

to cause a block at a level some distance from the known site of dislocation. Bony deformity does not necessarily imply a block to Pantopaque or air. In 11 cases with bony deformities, no block was defined with either of these materials.

In the absence of a block, Pantopaque slips by the injured site and no adequate evaluation of the spinal cord and canal can be made. In this group, only one case of verified cord swelling could be diagnosed preoperatively; Pantopaque delineated the C$_{5-6}$ swollen cord segment with uneven and irregular margins (Fig. 3). Three out of 4 cases of cord swelling were missed in these patients without block because Pantopaque, in an amount sufficient to outline the entire cord margin, was not present. If a sufficiently adequate amount is used, it would likely "spill" intracranially. This limitation in the use of Pantopaque in cervical cord injuries should be reemphasized.

Air Myelography: In the presence of a complete block, an evaluation of the injured site usually cannot be made with air if the patient is kept supine for the air collects anteriorly and, despite continued injection, will not outline the posterior subarachnoid space. The antero-posterior (AP) view is of little value even with tomography. The air column in the anterior subarachnoid space tapers at the site of injury which may be due to either spinal cord swelling or to posterior extradural compression (Fig. 4). Thus, we prefer the decubitus position for our air studies since the posterior subarachnoid space may also be filled.

In the absence of a block, the cord outline is best studied by air, with the patient in a decubitus position. However, in a patient with bony deformity, we are loath to turn the patient from the supine to the decubitus position due to the instability at the injured site, and we attempt the examination first with the patient supine. In one patient

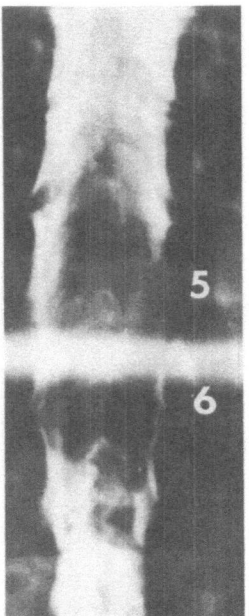

Fig. 3. Pantopaque flows past the C_5 and C_6 compression fracture sites, outlining a swollen cord, with irregular, uneven margins. After a C_{5-6} laminectomy and dural decompression, a "pulped" cord at the C_{5-6} level was seen with hemorrhage in the cord substance.

with a gunshot injury who was examined in the decubitus position, we noticed persistence of air within the cord shadow representing "air trapping" in the injured and torn portions of the cord (Fig. 5). This case was included in the unstable bony deformity group because of a previous laminectomy at C_6 and C_7.

    B. *Thoracolumbar Spine Injury* (12 patients): There were 12 patients in this group with bony deformity. Nine were studied with Pantopaque alone, 2 with air alone and one patient with both air and Pantopaque. Surgically verified cord swelling was diagnosed preoperatively in only one patient who had been studied by Pantopaque alone in the supine position and intrinsic cord widening was demonstrated a full vertebral level above the site of anterior extradural compression. Spinal cord swelling was observed in both the AP and lateral projections.

    Two patients with T_{12}–L_1 surgically verified cord swelling were studied by air. The true size of the conus medullaris could not be accurately estimated. Severe extradural compression and associated dislocation were present; these factors may have accounted for the poor visualization of the conus.

    One half of the total number of patients, i.e., 6 of 12 patients, did not demonstrate a block. The single case of surgically verified cord swelling studied by Pantopaque alone demonstrated a block, while the other 2 cases studied with air alone demonstrated no block. The majority of patients had complete neurologic deficits.

II. Patients Without Bony Deformity

    A. *Cervical Spine Injury* (12 patients): There were 12 patients in

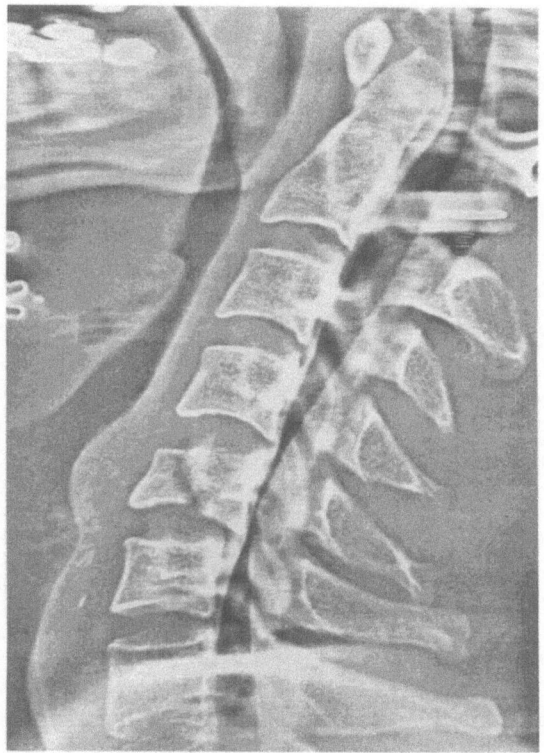

Fig. 4.   A xeromyelogram utilizing air through the lateral C_{1-2} route
in the supine position shows the anterior subarachnoid space and the
anterior cord margin well, but not the posterior subarachnoid space.
A C_5 vertebral body fracture is seen.

this category; 6 had both air and Pantopaque studies, 4 had Pantopaque
studies alone and 2 had air studies alone.   There were 2 cases of
surgically verified cord swelling; both were diagnosed preoperatively
by air in the decubitus position.   Air usually bathed the cord, showing
all its margins while Pantopaque failed because it slipped by the
affected cord segment in the absence of a block.   Pantopaque could
not be used in sufficient amounts because of the likelihood of intracranial
spillage as was previously emphasized.   Unlike the group with bony
deformities, in whom extradural compression may be suspected from the
routine plain films and tomograms, myelography in the group without
bony deformities in indispensable in establishing the presence or absence
of extradural non-bony compression.
     Extradural compression was diagnosed in 3 cases.   Bony ridges alone
were present in 2 cases and were easily shown by both air and Pantopaque.
In 1 case, a ridge and a herniated disk were demonstrated only by
Pantopaque in the prone position after a supine air study had failed to
yield diagnostic results (Fig. 6).   Most patients had no block, the only
cases showing a block being these 3 with ridges.   Six of these 12
patients had incomplete motor neurologic deficits with favorable prognoses
in most cases.
     B.   *Thoracolumbar Spine Injury* (12 patients):   There were 12
patients in this category without bony deformity.   Eleven patients were
studied by Pantopaque alone and one patient by air alone.   No combined

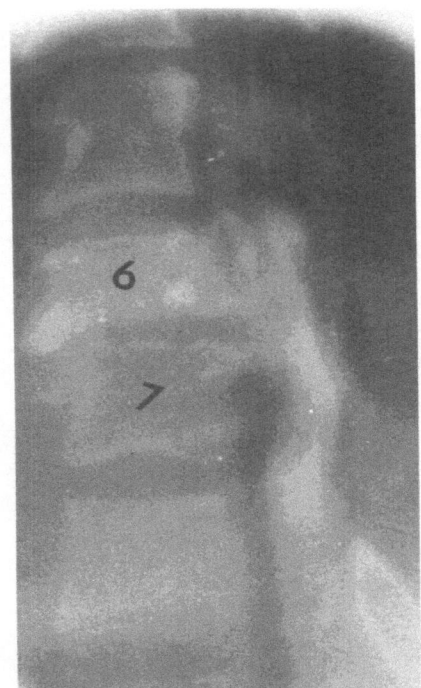

Fig. 5. Air myelogram done two weeks after a laminectomy at C_6 and C_7 for a gunshot would reveals "air streaking" within the cord. Spondylotic changes are also seen. At autopsy, swelling and necrosis of the spinal cord from C_5 to T_1 were seen.

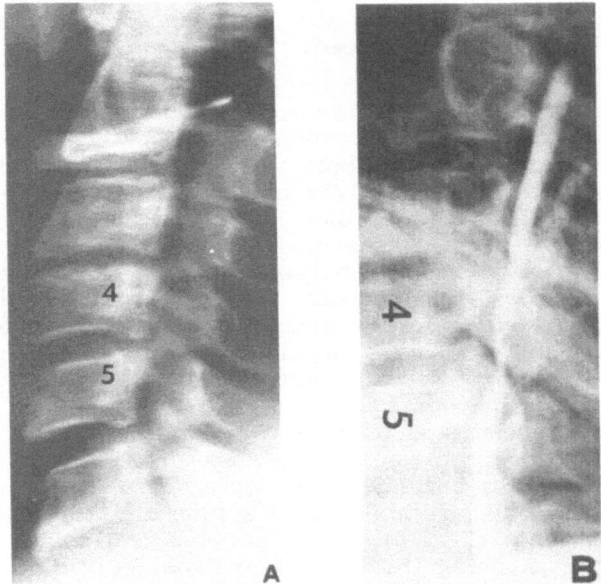

Fig. 6. A. Air myelography does not clearly delineate the anterior subarachnoid space at the C_{4-5} level.
B. Prone Pantopaque myelography shows an extruded disk and bony ridge at C_{4-5} displacing the Pantopaque column posteriorly.

studies were done.   All patients were paraplegic except one.

There were 4 cases of surgically verified cord swelling.   All were studied by Pantopaque alone, but a correct preoperative diagnosis was made in only one case.   Misdiagnosis in the other 3 patients was due to: (a) insufficient Pantopaque; (b) an upper lumbar block which prevented the Pantopaque from reaching the lower thoracic cord, and (c) a clot on the left side of the spinal cord at T_{3-4} which prevented filling of the gutter on that side.

Posterior extradural compression by hematoma (Fig. 7) and tear of the ligamentum flavum were demonstrated by Pantopaque in 2 patients. Complete blocks were present in both cases of extradural compression and in one case of cord swelling.

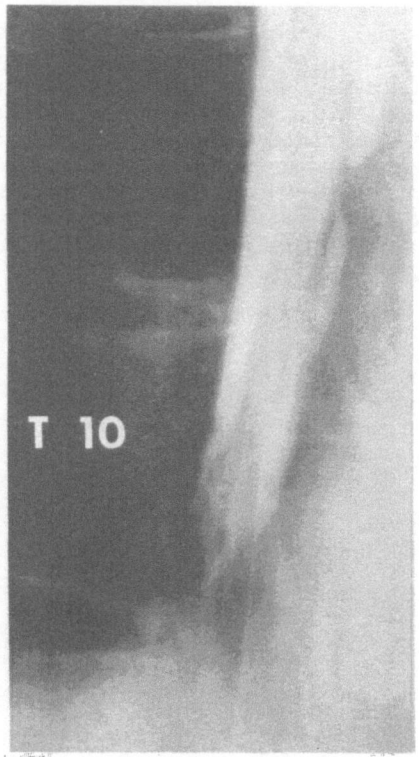

Fig. 7. The lateral view shows absence of filling of the posterior subarachnoid space by Pantopaque at the T_{10} level. The cord is displaced anteriorly. On the AP view (which is not shown), two thin contrast columns in the lateral gutters mimicked the appearance of spinal cord widening. At surgery, posterior epidural hematoma was found, without any spinal cord swelling.

DISCUSSION

Protocol

On the basis of our experience, we have devised a protocol for the diagnostic work-up of spinal trauma patients. Each case is individualized according to several factors:

1.   The presence or absence of radiologically demonstrable deformity of the bony spinal canal.

2. The relative diagnostic merits of air and Pantopaque.

3. Evidence that placing a patient in the prone position may compromise the spinal cord by producing or worsening bony displacements.

In the presence of bony deformity, instability of the spinal column should be highly suspected. The determination of instability preoperatively (Norrell, 1975) unfortunately is speculative in most cases. The *in vitro* criteria developed in the laboratory (White et al., 1976) may not apply *in vivo*. But this critical and often very difficult determination must be made as quickly as possible before any further steps are taken. Thus, if the patient demonstrates bony deformity at the trauma site, he or she is maintained strictly in the supine position and myelography is accomplished by C_{1-2} puncture. Traction should be maintained throughout the examination.

Injuries at T_{1-9} and L_{2-5} are relatively more stable than cervical injuries due to the stabilizing effect of the bony thorax and lower torso muscles, respectively (Norrell, 1975). If bony deformities are present at these levels, these patients may be moved from the supine to the decubitus position, but they should not be placed prone even if their fracture sites are relatively more stable. In our experience, bony displacements in the supine position have been accentuated in the prone position (Fig. 8). The increased displacement predisposes to increased cord compression in T_{1-9} injuries and impingement on the nerve roots of the cauda equina in L_{2-5} injuries.

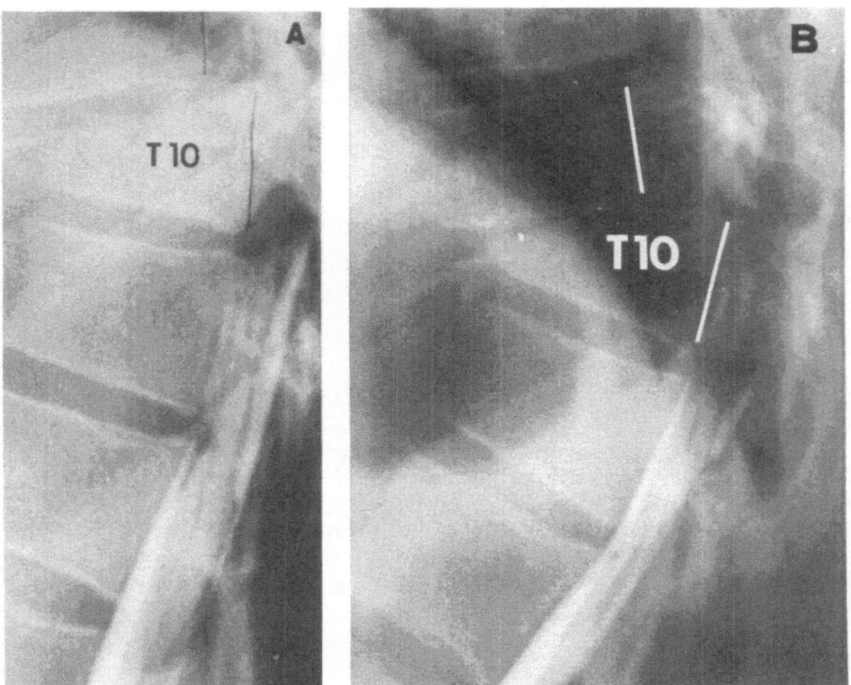

Fig. 8. A. Pantopaque myelography in the supine position shows a complete block at the T_{10-11} level. The T_{10} vertebral body is compressed and posteriorly displaced.
B. With the patient prone, T_{10} is seen to be more posteriorly displaced than in the supine position.

If no bony deformity is demonstrated, the patient may be moved into the decubitus or even into the prone position. Thus, in the cervical area, the patient may be positioned in the decubitus position and studied by air with the neck maintained in a cervical collar. Prone Pantopaque studies may be used to rule out the presence of anterior extradural compression by bony ridges or extruded disks.

The presence of bony deformity mandates a determination of the presence or absence of a block. This is quickly demonstrated by Pantopaque *via* a C_{1-2} puncture with the patient in the supine position. In patients with bony deformities, the block is usually due to extradural compression and reduction of the deformity is the first objective of treatment (Norrell, 1975). Our most recent cases of subluxation have been reduced immediately by spinal traction under fluoroscopic control.

The information gained from supine Pantopaque C_{1-2} myelography is limited generally to determining the presence or absence of a block. With the small volumes of Pantopaque which have been used, the lateral view does not outline the anterior or posterior subarachnoid spaces consistently (Fig. 9), and the AP view is not helpful either because two thin columns of Pantopaque in the posterior gutters are usually demonstrated, mimicking spinal cord swelling which may or may not be present.

Although a complete block is studied most easily and quickly with Pantopaque, cord swelling is hard to assess. Severe compression of the cord hinders the diagnostic value of both Pantopaque and air.

In the cervical area, in the absence of a block, air may be introduced *via* the C_{1-2} route (supine) to delineate the anterior subarachnoid space and cord. Unfortunately, the posterior subarachnoid space is not consistently demonstrated, and the patient may have to be placed in the decubitus position. The merits of air cervical myelography in spinal trauma have been noted by Heinz and Goldman (1972) and Rossier et al. (1975).

In the thoracic area including the L_1 vertebral segment, in the absence of a block or bony deformity, the spinal cord up to the conus medullaris may be visualized by Pantopaque in the frontal projection and air in the lateral projection. These complementary qualities of air and Pantopaque have been described by Di Chiro (1964); thus, combined air and Pantopaque myelography may be necessary. Amipaque[3] (Fig. 10), a new water soluble myelographic contrast medium presently under controlled clinical investigation, may show the spinal cord to good advantage in both the frontal and lateral projections and may be more extensively used in the evaluation of spinal trauma in the future.

Pantopaque alone has been preferred by our group in the lumbar area (L_{2-5}) since it can readily delineate a block by extradural compression.

In a separate category, we have found air to be extremely useful in the evaluation of chronic cord trauma including long-standing spondylosis in which atrophy of the spinal cord is suspected (Fig. 11). Even in the presence of severe bony deformity, surgical decompression is contraindicated if spinal cord atrophy is demonstrated. Therefore, we feel that air myelography is the procedure of choice in the evaluation of chronic spinal cord trauma.

CONCLUSIONS

Pantopaque is the preferred contrast medium in our experience for establishing the presence of a block in patients with cervical and thoracic

---

[3]Metrizamide (Sterling-Winthrop Research Institute, Rensselaer, New York).

26 PAY et al.

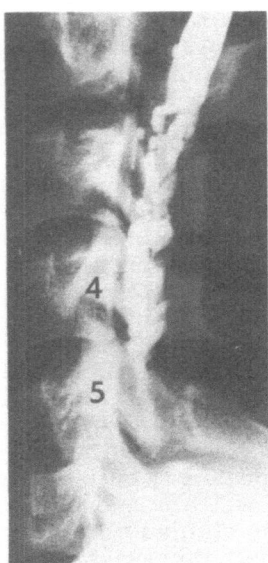

Fig. 9. A supine C_{1-2} Pantopaque myelogram shows no clear delineation of the subarachnoid spaces. The column is blocked at the C_{4-5} level. A compressed C_5 vertebral body is present.

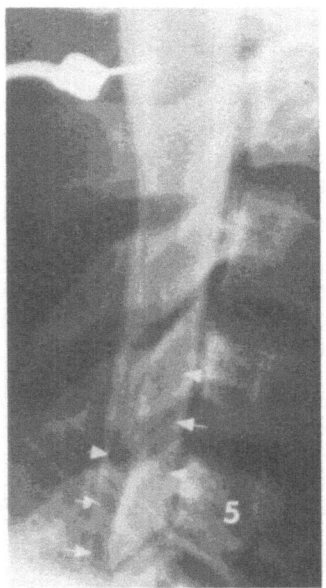

Fig. 10. Lateral view of an Amipaque myelogram shows localized spinal cord widening (↑) from the C_{4-5} to C_{5-6} levels. The cord swelling is maximal opposite the C_5 vertebral body fracture. Fifteen milliliters of 200 mg/100 ml Amipaque was instilled through a lateral C_{1-2} needle. The patient was in a 60° Fowler position, supine, and on 18 pounds traction applied through head tongs.
The anteroposterior view showed insufficient contrast density. We have subsequently increased the Amipaque concentration to 270 mg/100 ml, which has resulted in very satisfactory visualization of the spinal cord.

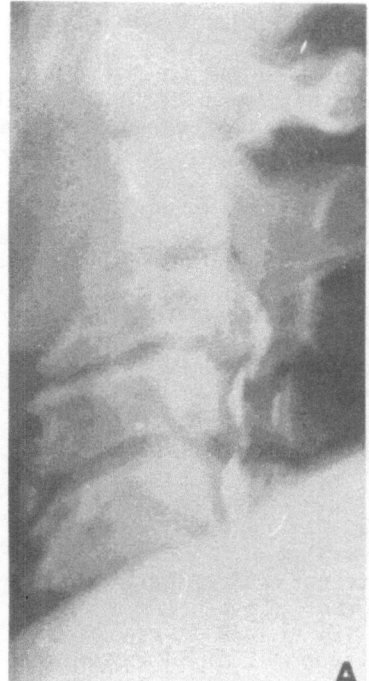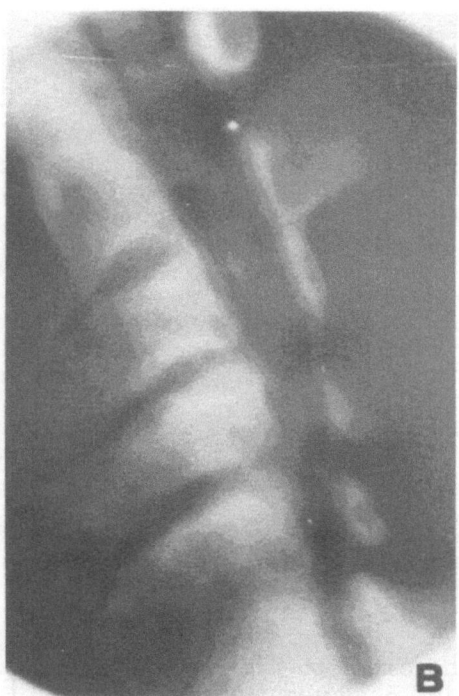

Fig. 11. A. Prone Pantopaque myelography shows multiple extradural defects from bony ridges due to cervical spondylosis. The cord margins are not demonstrated.
B. Decubitus air myelography shows a markedly atrophied spinal cord. The lower cervical canal is markedly compromised by the hypertrophic spondylotic changes.

trauma who manifest bony deformity, in cervical trauma without bony deformity (in the prone position), in delineating the thoracic spinal cord in the frontal projection and in lumbar spine injuries.

Air is preferred in cervical trauma without bony deformity, and to delineate the thoracic spinal cord in the lateral projection. If there is no block to the flow of Pantopaque in a patient with cervical spine injury with bony deformity, air may be used to delineate the anterior subarachnoid space and the anterior cord margin. In chronic trauma, air may be used to demonstrate cord atrophy.

Lateral C_{1-2} puncture for the introduction of positive contrast material is the technique of choice in patients with cervical injury. This approach permits the patient to remain supine throughout the initial myelographic evaluation and avoids tilting the patient's head down, a position which makes the maintenance of cervical traction most difficult.

REFERENCES

Albin, M.S., White, R.J., Acosta-Rua, G., et al. Study of functional recovery produced by delayed localized cooling after spinal cord injury in primates. *J. Neurosurg.* 29: 113-120 (1968).
Braakman, R., Penning, L. Injuries of the Cervical Spine. Amsterdam, Excerpta Medica Foundation, p. 118 (1971).

Di Chiro, G., Fisher, R.L. Contrast radiography of the spinal cord. *Arch. Neurol. (Chicago) 11:*125-143 (1964).

Hedeman, L.S., Sil, R. Studies in experimental spinal cord Trauma. Part 2: Comparison of treatment with steroids, low molecular weight dextran and catecholamine blockade. *J. Neurosurg. 40:*44-51 (1974).

Heinz, E.R., Goldman, R.L. Role of gas myelography in neurologic diagnosis. *Radiology 102:*629-634 (1972).

Kelley, D., Alexander, E. Lateral cervical puncture for myelography. *J. Neurosurg. 29:*101-110 (1968).

Lodin, H. Two-needle oxygen myelography. *Acta Radiol. (Diag)4:* 62-64 (1966).

Negrin, J., Jr. Local hypothermia in spinal cord traumatic lesions. [In] Proceedings Third International Congress of Neurological Surgeons. Copenhagen, Excerpta Medica, International Series, pp. 377-381 (1965).

Norrell, H.A. Fractures and dislocations of the spine. [In] Rothman, R.H., Simeone, F. The Spine, Philadelphia, W.B. Saunders Co., pp. 529-566 (1975).

Raynor, R.B. Discography and myelography in acute injuries of the cervical spine. *J. Neurosurg. 35:*529-535 (1971).

Rossier, A.B., Berney, J., Rosenbaum, A.E., et al. Value of gas myelography in early management of acute cervical spinal cord injuries. *J. Neurosurg. 42:*330-337 (1975).

Tomasula, J.J., Crescito, V., Goodkin, R., et al. A survey of the management of experimental spinal cord trauma. [In] Proceedings of the Seventeenth Veterans Administration Spinal Cord Injury Conference, pp. 12-15 (1969).

White A.A., Southwick, W.O., Punjabi, M. Clinical instability in the lower cervical spine. *Spine 1:*15-27 (1976).

3

Effect of Pharmacological Agents on Normalization of Molecular and Histologic Dysfunction Following Traumatic Injury to the Spinal Cord

N.E. NAFTCHI, M. DEMENY, H. DEMOPOULOS, and E. FLAMM

INTRODUCTION

Despite impressive achievements in the rehabilitation of spinal cord injured subjects, the following important areas of research have not been adequately investigated: (1) the general underlying pathophysiologic problems that occur in traumatically paralyzed subjects who undergo osteoporosis, periarticular bone formation, episodic hypertensive crises, and so forth; (2) mitigation of serious dysfunction by vigorous pharmacologic or surgical intervention to preserve as much sensory and motor function as possible, or both; and (3) the possibility of the elimination of paralysis *per se.*

Traumatic injury to the spinal cord leads to the immediate cessation of propagation of action potential. The ability to walk requires the maintenance of a small number of the long tracts of the spinal cord. Furthermore, pathophysiologic alterations do not occur immediately after impact. If we were cognizant of the exact pathophysiologic events, it would seem possible to decrease the rate of permanent paralysis after acute spinal cord injuries and to preserve some degree of motor function by appropriate intervention.

The sequence of morphologic changes that result from impact injuries to the spinal cord in experimental animal models are similar to those that take place in most human spinal cord injuries. The cell membranes of neurons, glia, and blood vessels undergo irreversible pathologic changes that lead to degeneration of the spinal cord and include mechanical, vascular, and free radical chemical processes.

In spinal cord trauma models, blood flow to the impacted segment is markedly decreased, suggesting that ischemia may be an important pathogenic mechanism (Griffiths, 1976). The diminished blood flow may be due to vasospasm or microvascular occlusions, or both.

The spinal cord and the rest of the central nervous system (CNS) more than other vital organs, have strict requirements for membrane integrity. The blood-CNS barriers maintain a unique environment for the CNS by excluding certain substances and enhancing the transport of others such as ascorbic acid. Therefore, membrane lipids and proteins must be physicochemically intact in order to maintain the structural integrity of the excitable membranes involved in conduction and transmission.

Minor perturbations in the configuration of strategic membrane molecules, the lipids that help maintain the active shape of key enzymes

29

such as Na^+, K^+-ATPase, adenylate cyclase, and prostaglandin synthetase, can have detrimental consequences. Altering the fluidity of the lipids will affect synaptosome formation and the coupling of transmitter-receptors (Strittmatter et al., 1979).

Biogenic amines released within the spinal cord after trauma were implicated to contribute to the formation of the lesion. The mechanism proposed for this enhancement of deterioration was based, in part, on the general knowledge of the necrotizing effect of norepinephrine (NE) when infiltrated in tissues (Osterholm and Mathews, 1972a; Osterholm and Mathews, 1972b). Catecholamine metabolism was previously reported to be altered in humans after spinal cord injury (Naftchi et al., 1972; Naftchi et al., 1974; Naftchi et al., 1978). Therefore, we decided to undertake a quantitative measurement of the turnover rate of biogenic amines in the traumatized spinal cord (Naftchi et al., 1974). We, also, studied the effect of the membrane stabilizing and anti-inflammatory drugs epsilon aminocaproic acid (EACA) and the methyl prednisolone sodium succinate (MP) on biogenic amines and their possible ameliorating effect, both histologically and functionally, on animal models after traumatic spinal cord injury (Naftchi et al., 1974). Some of the enzymes involved in catecholamine synthesis and metabolism were studied in the spinal cord. The activity of L-aromatic-amino acid decarboxylase, a ubiquitous nonphospholipid-dependent-enzyme, and monamine oxidase (MAO) and dopamine-β-hydroxylase (DBH), two membrane-bound phospholipid-dependent enzymes, was determined. Finally, pathologic changes in the spinal cord were visualized by light microscopy.

MATERIALS AND METHODS

Eighty-six immunized mongrel cats of either sex, ranging in weight from 2.5 to 2.8 kg, were used in eight experimental groups.

Preparation of Animals

Intravenous pentobarbital (30 mg/kg) was used for anesthesia. Animals underwent laminectomy from T-7 to T-11. A 400 gm-cm force was delivered to the exposed dura at the ninth thoracic segment in the experimental groups.

Arterial blood pressure was continuously monitored in all animals. The blood pressure was permitted to stabilize for one hour before laminectomy and trauma. Averaged evoked cortical sensory action potentials were recorded from the region of the sigmoid gyrus during stimulation of the contralateral peroneal nerve before and after impact to ascertain the adequacy of the trauma. (see Figure 1.)

One hour after impact, a 3 cm portion of the cord, centered at the level of the impact, was removed in a temperature-controlled room (40°C). The specimens were divided into three equal portions: labelled rostral, middle, and caudal.

Concentrations of norepinephrine (NE), dopamine (DA), serotonin (5-hydroxytryptamine, 5-HT), and histamine in the spinal cords were determined for the five groups of cats. One group underwent laminectomy only. A second untreated group received a 400 gm-cm impact at the T-9 level. These animals were compared with three groups treated with EACA, MP, and a combination of EACA and MP after similar trauma. One hour after trauma, the biogenic amines were measured in each of the three 1 cm cord segments.

In animals treated with drugs, each received an intravenous priming dose of EACA (1 gm) or MP (3 mg) one hour before contusion or both. Animals were then maintained on a continuous infusion of EACA (350 mg/hour) and MP (1.5 mg/hour), separately, or in combination until the time of sacrifice

L-tyrosine (2,6-^{3}H, 45 Ci/mM, New England Nuclear) was administered intravenously to three groups of cats (10 cats/group). One hour after injection of tyrosine (1 mCi/kg) each experimental animal received a 400 gm-cm impact to the exposed dura at the ninth thoracic segment (T9). The animals were sacrificed one hour (Group 6), two hours (Group 7), and three hours (Group 8) after contusion of the spinal cord.

A 3 cm portion of the spinal cord centered at the level of impact (T9) was removed in a temperature-controlled room (4°C) at the appropriate times (vida infra) after the injection of tritiated precursors. The specimens were divided into three (1 cm) equal parts. These spinal cord segments, labelled rostral, middle, and caudal, were immediately frozen on dry ice or in liquid nitrogen and were stored at -25°C until analyzed. The total disappearance rate of ^{3}H-radioactive compounds from the blood and the specific activities of DA and NE on each one cm segment of the spinal cord were determined.

Determination of Endogenous Biogenic Amines

The tissues were homogenized in acidified butanol. After centrifuging the homogenate, catecholamines from the supernatant were extracted into water and adsorbed on alumina. Norepinephrine and dopamine were eluted from alumina and were assayed fluorometrically as described previously (Naftchi et al., 1974).

Analysis of Labelled Dopamine and Norepinephrine

The metabolites of ^{3}H-L-tyrosine, ^{3}H-dopamine, and ^{3}H-norepinephrine were analyzed as follows: each 1 cm segment of spinal cord was homogenized in acidified butanol, centrifuged, and the catecholamines contained in the supernatant were extracted into water and adsorbed on alumina as above. The eluate was adjusted to pH 2 and applied to a column of Dowex W-X4 (200-400 mesh, 5mm x 2 cm). Norepinephrine and dopamine were eluted with 1 N HCl and 2 N HCl, respectively. Eluates containing NE or DA were quantitatively transferred to a counting solution (Aquasol, New England Nuclear) and the radioactivity was determined in a liquid scintillation spectrometer (Searle). The entire procedure was carried out in a temperature-controlled room (4°C).

L-Aromatic-Amino Acid Decarboxylase Activity

A spinal cord segment was homogenized in 5 volume (w/v) ice cold 0.05 Tris HCl buffer pH 6.0 containing 0.1% (v/v) Triton X-100 in a glass teflon homogenizer. The homogenate was centrifuged in a refrigerated centrifuge at 10,000 g for 10 minutes, and the supernatant was decanted for the enzyme assay (Lamprecht and Coyle, 1972). An aliquot of the supernatant was incubated in a closed system with the carboxyl-labelled substrate, L-3,4-dihydroxyphenylalanine (L-^{14}C dopa). The activity of L-aromatic-amino acid decarboxylase (L-AAD) was determined by measuring the $^{14}CO_2$ product liberated by TCA and was captured in plastic wells that contained filter paper soaked in Hyamine;

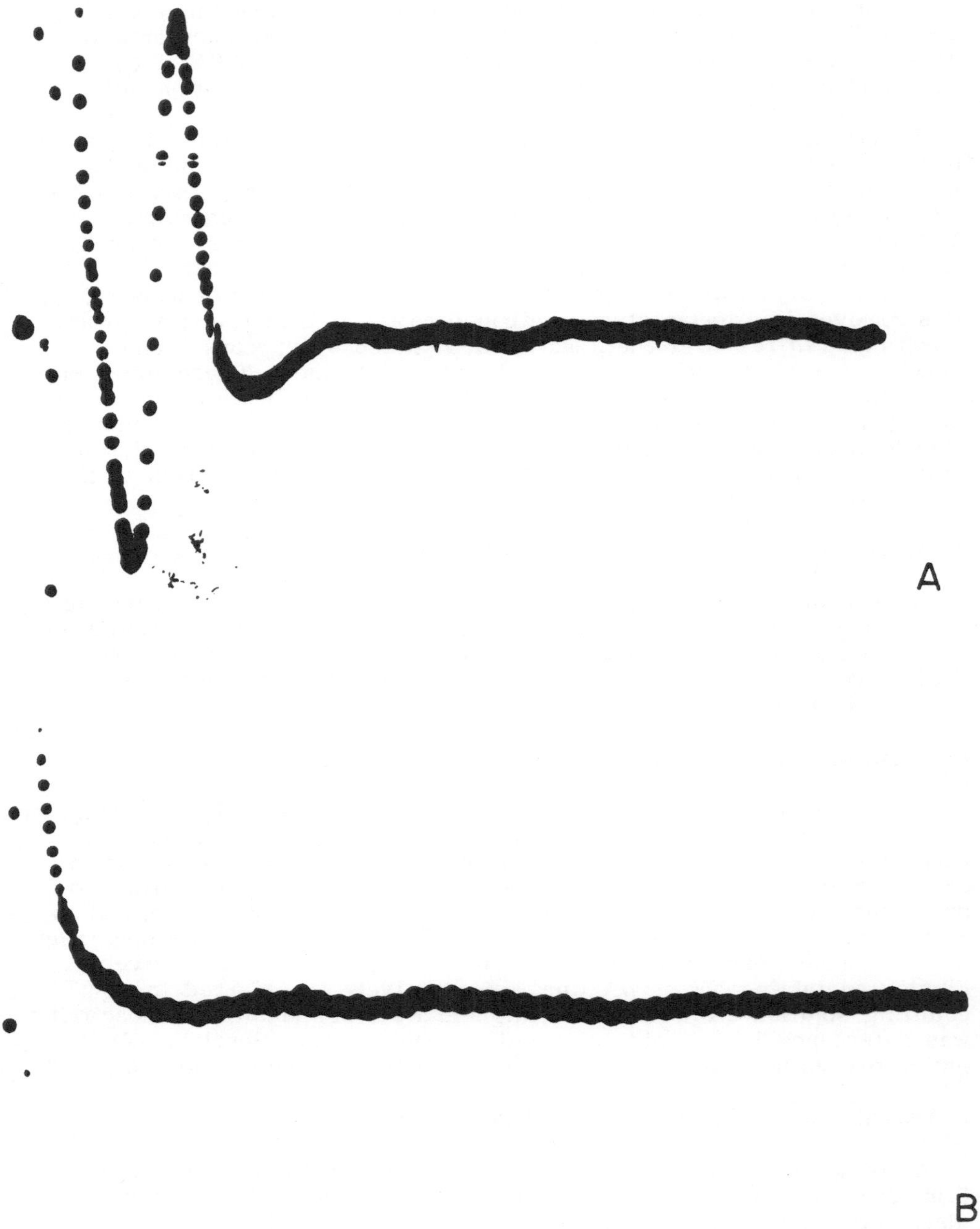

Fig. 1. Somatosensory evoked potentials (SEPs) are obtained by electrical stimulation of the sciatic nerve, with electrodes over the corresponding cerebral cortex. The top curve represents a pre-impact SEP. Immediately post-impact, the SEPs flatten as shown in the bottom curve. Permanent paraplegia is indicated if within 3 to 24 hours post-impact, SEPs do not return.

the entire well was then dropped into a scintillation vial containing Aquasol and was counted in a liquid scintillation spectrometer. The units of L-AAD are given in nmoles CO_2/g tissue/hour.

Dopamine-β-Hydroxylase Activity

The spinal cord segments were homogenized and centrifuged as described for L-AAD, except that the Tris buffer was 0.005 M. The assay is based on β-hydroxylation of the substrate phenylethylamine by dopamine-β-hydroxylase (DBH) to phenylethanolamine (Molinoff et al., 1971). The latter is converted to ^{14}C-labelled N-methylphenyl-ethanolamine by purified bovine adrenal phenylethanolamine-N-methyl-transferase in the presence of the active methyl donor s-adenosyl-methionine methyl-^{14}C. Dopamine-β-hydroxylase units are given in nmoles N-methylphenylethanolamine/g tissue/hour.

Monoamine Oxidase Activity

The spinal cord segments were homogenized in 10 volume 0.005 M phosphate buffer pH 7.0, and the enzyme activity was assayed on an aliquot of the homogenate. The method is based on the oxidative deamination of tritiated substrate ^{3}H-tyramine to tritiated product ^{3}H-p-hydroxyphenylacetic acid (Jarrot, 1971). After separation of the product by extraction with ethyl acetate, the radioactivity was measured in a liquid scintillation spectrometer. Units of enzyme activity are given in nmoles of p-hydroxyphenylacetic acid/g tissue/hour.

RESULTS

There were 10 animals in each group listed below. The concentrations of biogenic amines measured in the treated groups were compared with those of the impacted, but untreated, animals. Results were only considered significant if, by comparison with the untreated animals, the probability was below 5% ($p < 0.05$). The results are expressed as mean ± standard deviation for each group of 10 animals.

Arterial Blood Pressure

Feline arterial carotid pressure increased during laminectomy and impact (Figure 2). The results after pretreatment with MP for one hour were similar to those of the untreated group. Pretreatment with EACA, however, depressed the arterial blood pressure. During laminectomy the blood pressure was depressed further for a short time, and the impaction of the cord raised the blood pressure only to the low levels, that were acheived after infusion of EACA (Figure 2). The results after pretreatment with combined EACA and MP were similar to that with trimethephan camphorsulfonate, a ganglion-blocking drug; after stabilizing at a lower level, the arterial blood pressure did not change appreciably during laminectomy or impact except that it was depressed during impact in animals that were receiving the combined MP-EACA therapy.

Effect of Trauma on Biogenic Amine Concentrations

Group 1: laminectomy

A concentration gradient, proceeding along the rostral caudal axis, was observed for NE, DA, and histamine (Figure 3).

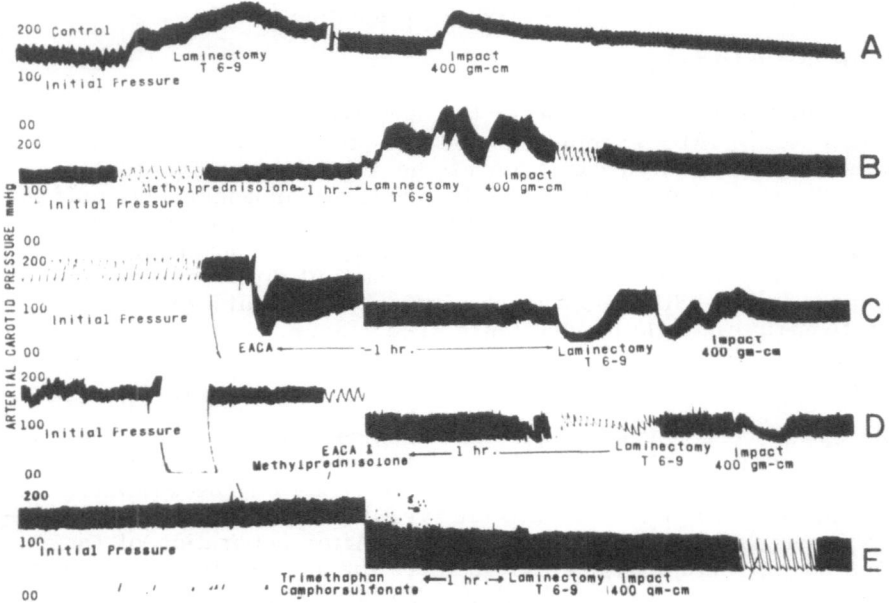

Fig. 2. Segments of an actual record of arterial carotid pressure in five cats. *A)* During laminectomy at T6-T9, arterial blood pressure (BP) rises sharply. After restoration of the BP to the initial level, a 400 gm-cm impact at T7 again causes a rise in BP. *B)* One hour after pretreatment with methylprednisolone (MP), both laminectomy and impact result in a significant rise in BP. *C)* One hour of pretreatment with epsilon aminocaproic acid (EACA) causes a decrease in BP during both laminectomy and impact followed by an increase over the stabilized prelaminectomy BP. *D)* Combined treatment with EACA and MP reduces the BP significantly. Laminectomy does not affect the BP, but after spinal cord contusion, BP is depressed. *E)* After pretreatment with the ganglion blocking drug trimethaphan comphorsulfonate, neither laminectomy nor impact causes a change in BP.

Group 2: impact

The gradient for biogenic amines was not present after impact. The NE concentration was the same in all three segments (Figure 3*A*). The concentration of DA (Figure 3*B*) was significantly increased after impact in all three segments of the cords, compared with specimens obtained after laminectomy alone (Group 1). Similarly, a significant rise in histamine concentrations was observed (Figure 3*C*). The levels of serotonin, however, remained unchanged in all segments of the cord.

Group 3: epsilon aminocaproic acid (EACA)

Treatment with EACA produced a significant decrease in the concentration of norepinephrine in the impacted (middle) segment and significantly decreased both DA and histamine concentrations below that of untreated animals. Again, the concentrations of serotonin

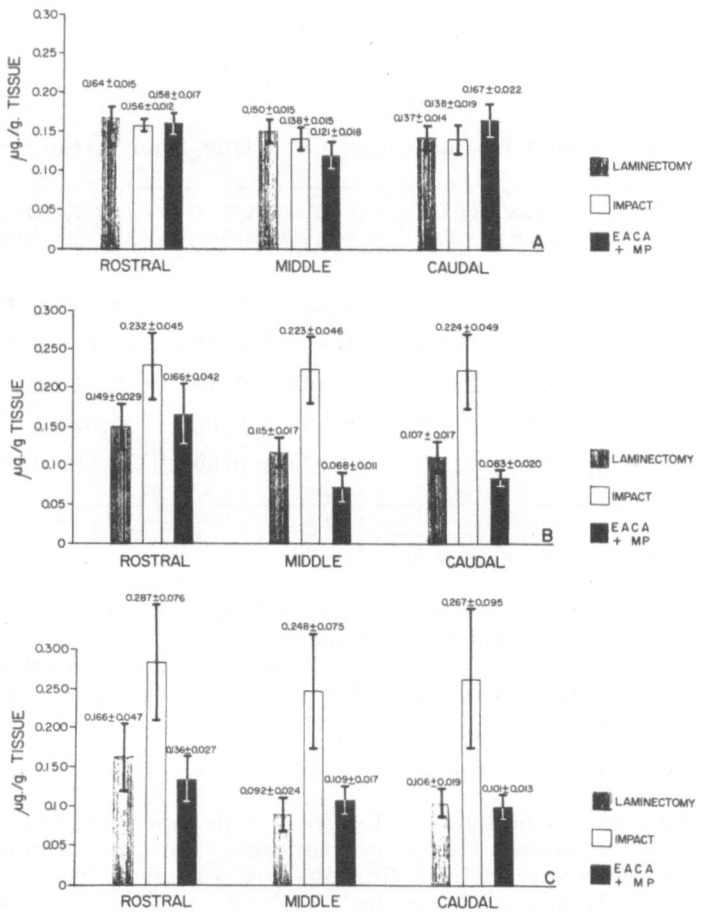

Fig. 3. Concentration gradients for norepinephrine (A), dopamine
(B), and histamine (C) content of the cat spinal cord. Each bar
represents mean ± SD, μg/g, tissue in 10 cats. After laminectomy
from T-7 to T-11, the animal's spinal cord was contused by dropping
a 20 gm weight from a height of 20 cm at T-9, the middle segment.
Each segment represents 1 cm of the spinal cord. A. A concentration
gradient for norepinephrine exists along the rostral caudal axis. This
gradient is disrupted after contusion of the spinal cord but is rees-
tablished during therapy with EACA and MP, only in the middle contused
1 cm segment. B. After contusion the dopamine gradient is abolished,
and the dopamine content of all segments rises significantly to approximately the same level. Administration of EACA and MP reestablishes
the gradient; the dopamine concentration in all segments is significantly
reduced. C. The histamine content shows similar patterns of changes
to those described for dopamine.

Reprinted with permission of the Journal of Neurosurgery 40: 55, Jan 1974.

remained unchanged in all segments (Table I).

Group 4: methyl prednisolone sodium succinate (MP)

The results with MP treatment were similar to those obtained with
EACA alone (Group 3) with the exception of histamine, the concentration
of which was significantly reduced only at the impacted site in the cord.

TABLE I

Serotonin Concentrations in the Spinal Cord One Hour After Trauma

GROUP	ROSTRAL (μg/gm)	MIDDLE (μg/gm)	CAUDAL (μg/gm)
1. laminectomy	0.693 ± 0.044	0.684 ± 0.045	0.672 ± 0.074
2. impact	0.625 ± 0.106	0.692 ± 0.159	0.614 ± 0.074
3. EACA	0.765 ± 0.104	0.668 ± 0.107	0.530 ± 0.067
4. MP	0.746 ± 0.043	0.732 ± 0.062	0.639 ± 0.055
5. EACA and MP	0.715 ± 0.127	0.623 ± 0.062	0.629 ± 0.051

Group 5: combined EACA and MP

There was no significant change in concentration of NE and 5-HT (Figure 3 and Table I). This form of therapy produced a significant reduction of the concentration of DA in all segments, compared with Group 2. The concentration of histamine was significantly lower in all three segments of the cord.

Group 6-8: infusion of tritiated tyrosine

The circulating levels of labelled L-tyrosine dropped by 80% from the zero time concentrations within five minutes after the administration of the labelled precursors. These findings are similar to those of Wurtman et al. (1970) using (Coyle and Axelrod, 1972) C-L-dopa in the whole mouse.

The circulating levels of total radioactivity reached a plateau 10 minutes after injection and remained fairly constant for four hours. There was no appreciable difference between the experimental and laminectomy control groups.

Effect of Trauma on the Biosynthesis of Dopamine and Norepinephrine from ^{3}H-L-tyrosine Precursor (Groups 6-8)

There was no appreciable difference in concentrations of ^{3}H-NE among the three 1 cm segments of the spinal cord of the control groups. Nor was there an appreciable variation among those of the experimental groups. The disappearance rate of ^{3}H-NE and ^{3}H-DA from the spinal cord was linear in the control groups. The decay curve of ^{3}H-NE was slower than that of ^{3}H-DA; the half lives of ^{3}H-DA and ^{3}H-NE were about 3.5 and 4 hours, respectively. Between one and two hours after injection of ^{3}H-tyrosine the molar ratio of the tritiated DA to tritiated NE in the spinal cord of the control was approximately 1.3; from each fmole (mole x 10^{-15}) of DA about 0.8 fmole NE was synthesized (Figure 4). In control Group 8 (four hours after injection) the concentrations of ^{3}H-DA and ^{3}H-NE decreased to levels approximately 60% of those in control Group 6 (two hours after injection, Figure 4).

One hour after spinal cord trauma the ^{3}H-DA concentration was 15% below that of laminectomy control (Group 6), but it had reached a plateau two hours after (Group 7) and was 17% above that of the control three hours after contusion of the spinal cord (Group 8). By comparison,

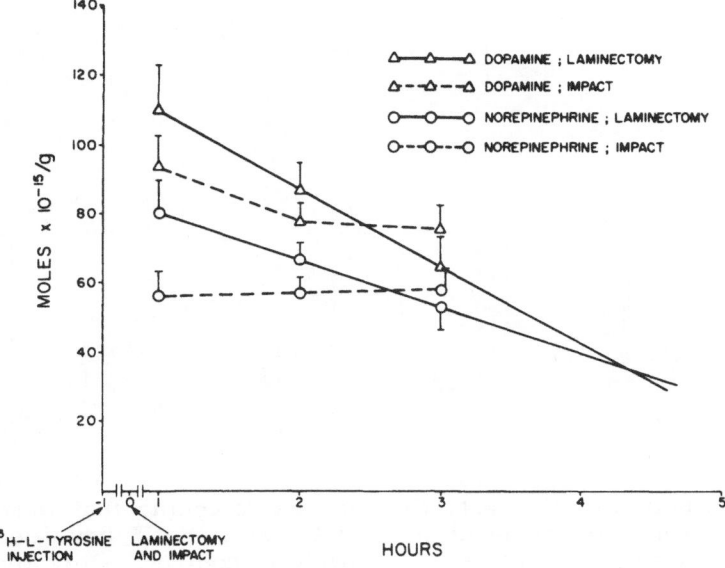

Fig. 4. After injection of 3H-2',6'-tyrosine, the half-lives of 3H-DA
and 3H-NE in the spinal cord are 3.5 and 4 hours, respectively (solid
lines). Two hours and one hour after impact, their respective
biosynthesis and degradation stopped (dotted line).

the 3H-NE levels were 30% lower than those of the corresponding
laminectomy control (Group 6, one hour after trauma) and remained
relatively unchanged thereafter in all experimental groups (Figure 3).
One hour after impact the radioactive counts incorporated from 3H-L-
tyrosine into 3H-DA were reduced from 5.4 nCi/g in the control Group
6 to 4.4 nCi/g in the experimental Group 6. Since after impact the
endogenous DA concentrations were twice those of the control, the
specific activity was sharply reduced after impact (Figure 5). Radioactivity incorporated into 3H-NE decreased from about 4.0 nCi/g to 3.1
nCi/g. The endogenous concentrations, however, did not change
appreciably. Therefore, the specific activity of NE was not significantly
altered (Figure 5).

Metabolic Enzymes

The activity of the enzymes in laminectomy control Group 6 and its
corresponding experimental group (two hours after impaction of the
spinal cord) is shown in Table II. There was no appreciable change
in the activities of L-AAD and DBH. In the impacted group, the
monoamine oxidase (MAO) activity was significantly lower than that of
the control.

Light Microscopy

The post-impact alterations that lead to permanent paraplegia occur
over a period of hours. The most marked tissue change is the gradual
development of hemorrhage in the central gray matter. In the first
15-30 minutes, there are only scattered petechial hemorrhages in the
gray, and, by 60 minutes, some of these have enlarged and coalesced.

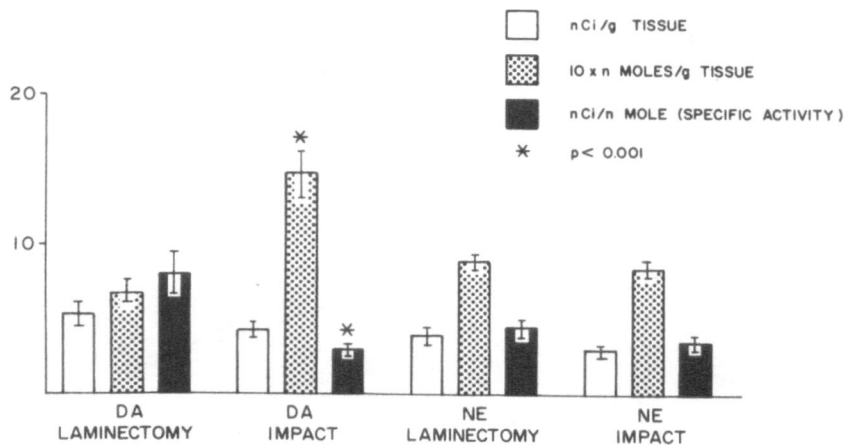

Fig. 5. One hour after impact, the radioactive counts that were incorporated from 3H-L-tyrosine into 3H-DA and 3H-NE have decreased somewhat, compared with those of laminectomy control. Only the specific activity of dopamine is significantly reduced; endogenous DA increased sharply after impact.

TABLE II

Effect of Spinal Cord Trauma on Activity of the
Enzymes of Catecholamine Pathways

	L-AAD	DBH	MAO
Control	143 ± 12.6	26.5 ± 1.3	2048 ± 66
Two hours post impact	127 ± 8.7	23.7 ± 2.1	1672[*]± 58

units of enzyme activity - nmoles/g wet tissue/hour
*$p < 0.01$

The long tracts show no evidence of morphologic change at this time except for enlargement of the periaxonal space in a small percentage of the myelinated fibers, as seen ultrastructurally. The amount of blood extravasated in the gray appears to reach maximum at about three to four hours, and, by this time, there may be petechial hemorrhages in the white matter, in the long tracts. Approximately 25% of the myelinated fibers show enlargement of the periaxonal space and fraying of the myelin by six hours. At 24-36 hours, the gray matter has undergone hemorrhagic necrosis and the long tracts show extensive structural degeneration (Figures 6A and 6B).

DISCUSSION

A traumatic injury to the spinal cord causes a marked reduction in the blood flow of the impacted segment. The diminished blood flow may be due to vasospasm or microvascular occlusion, or both. Progressive vascular changes, which include ischemic focal hemorrhages

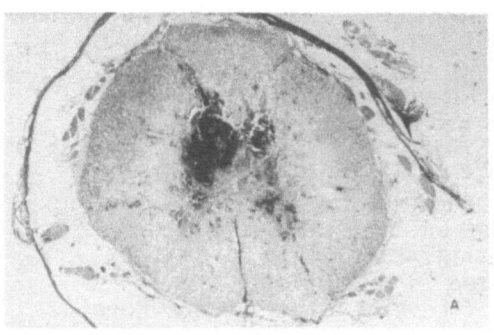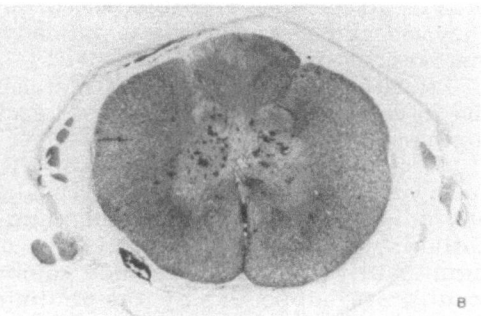

Fig. 6. A. Light microscopy of a cross section of the spinal cord at
the impact site six hours post impact in a control cat. Extensive
central gray hemorrhage and white matter edema has occurred at the
site of impact. B. A cross-section of the spinal cord six hours post
impact in a cat treated with epsilon aminocaproic acid and methyl
prednisolne. Compared with the impacted control (Figure 2A), there
is diminished central gray hemorrhaging and edema. Hematoxyline and
Eosin stained. Magnification 20X.*

and collapsed vessels, lead to pathological alterations in the membrane
lipids that are termed free radical reactions. The latter reactions
adversely affect the lipid-dependent enzymes and disturb the endothelium,
causing hemorrhagic necrosis of the central gray matter. Microvascular
endothelial pathology, which is studied by scanning electron microscopy,
correlates with the reduction in blood flow, progressive tissue degeneration, and free radical damage. (See Chapter Four).

A significant rise in the concentrations of DA within the spinal cord
was noted (Figure 3). These findings may be explained by the fact
that the enzyme that was responsible for the conversion of DA to NE
exerts its biosynthetic effect in the central nervous system only when
membrane-bound (Coyle and Axelrod, 1972). Trauma to the cord may
alter this state and thereby reduce DBH activity. Dopamine and
norepinephrine, released from the storage vesicles after trauma, are
subject to degradation by MAO and catechol-O-methyl transferase.
Dopamine levels remain higher than those of NE because its turnover
to NE is curtailed owing to a reduction in DBH activity within the
traumatized spinal cord. The biosynthesis of DA, however, continues
since dopa decarboxylase is not membrane-bound. In addition, tyrosine
hydroxylase activity is decreased, possibly due to an increase in
availability of the free intraneuronal norepinephrine, which would
reduce its activity through end-product feedback inhibition (Levitt
et al., 1965).

These results may partially explain the elevated urinary levels of
homovanillic acid, the major metabolite of DA, that has been found in
man as early as two days after spinal cord injury. The urinary levels
may reflect changes in peripheral metabolism of biogenic amines after
trauma (Naftchi and Tuckman, 1979; Naftchi et al., 1976).

Treatment with MP preserves membrane integrity (Rothman and
Engelman, 1972; Weissman, 1965). This may explain the reduction in
DA concentration after treatment with MP. Under these conditions,

*Reprinted from Advances in Experimental Medicine: A Centenary Tribute to Claude
Bernard, H. Parvez and S. Parvez, eds. Copyright 1980 Elsevier/North Holland
Biomedical Press.

DBH may remain in a relatively bound form and the turnover of DA to NE is not appreciably altered. EACA, by virtue of its antiproteolytic activity, may also preserve membrane integrity by neutralizing lysosomal enzymes and thus act synergistically with MP. This is supported by histological findings (Figure 6).

Elevated levels of DA and histamine after trauma and their role in the development of a spinal cord lesion are not known and deserve further elucidation.

A rise in the concentration of NE one hour after impact was not observed, nor was there a concomitant decrease in the levels of DA as was noted by others (Osterholm and Mathews, 1972a; Osterholm and Mathews, 1972b). By contrast, the concentration of DA increased significantly, and NE remained unchanged in this period. These results are supported by the findings of several other investigators (de la Torre et al., 1974; Hedeman et al., 1974; Vise et al., 1974).

After trauma the amount of radioactivity incorporated from ^{3}H-DA and ^{3}H-NE was sharply reduced when compared with that of laminectomy controls (Figures 4 and 5). The rise in the levels of endogenous DA in all segments of the spinal cord in Group 7 cats may reflect a reduction in the activity of DBH, which in the central nervous system synthesizes NE effectively only when membrane-bound (Coyle and Axelrod, 1972). Trauma to the cord may alter this state and thereby reduce DBH activity. DA and NE, released from the storage vesicles after trauma, are subject to degradation by MAO and catechol-0-methyl transferase. The specific activity of DA in Group 7 (one hour after impact) was sharply lower than that of corresponding laminectomy control groups, owing to a dilution of the labelled DA in a larger pool of endogenous DA that is accumulated after trauma because of impaired DBH activity. Monoamine oxidase, a membrane-bound mitochondrial enzyme that catabolizes intraneuronal DA and NE to their corresponding dihydroxy acid metabolites, cannot be implicated in reducing the amount of ^{3}H-DA, since it would also catabolize the endogenous DA comparably, and the specific activity of DA would, therefore, remain relatively unchanged.

Analysis of MAO activity *in vitro* demonstrates that two hours after impact, activity of the enzyme is significantly reduced (Table II). The reduction in specific activity of DA after contusion of the spinal cord also indicates that the activity of tyrosine hydroxylase is decreased Tyrosine hydroxylase is the rate-limiting enzyme that converts tyrosine to dopa in the biosynthetic pathway of NE (Levitt et al., 1965). After trauma, the incorporation of radioactivity from ^{3}H-L-tyrosine into ^{3}H-DA is reduced. Table II shows that the activities of L-AAD and DBH after impact, although lower, are not significantly different from those of the control. The reason for this apparent paradox is that *in vivo* the concentration of molecular oxygen, a primary substrate for tyrosine hydroxylase, DBH, and MAO, is sharply reduced, due to local circulatory stasis and hypoxia or anoxia. *In vitro* provided with all cofactors, including oxygen, DBH activity in the spinal cord two hours after impact remains relatively unchanged; within this time interval little denaturation has taken place in DBH protein.

The finding of large amounts of endogenous DA in the nontraumatized spinal cord indicates that DA in the spinal cord does not serve only as a substrate for DBH but may be stored in specific dopaminergic storage pool(s) and possibly serve as an inhibitory neurotransmitter of internuncial neurons. If all DA in the spinal cord served only as a substrate for DBH rather than being stored in specific dopaminergic storage reserves, endogenous DA would be expected to be rapidly transformed to NE and stored in noradrenergic vesicles.

The results demonstrate that (1) not only tyrosine hydroxylase is present but also the whole complement of the NE synthesizing enzymes exists in the spinal cord. As early as five minutes after administration of L-2',6'-ditritio-tyrosine, both DA and NE are detected, and 15 minutes after injection they are found in measurable amounts in the spinal cord at the level of thoracic seventh to eleventh (T7-T11) dermatomes. The rate of axoplasmic flow is too low to account for the formation of ^{3}H-DA and ^{3}H-NE in the brain stem neurons and subsequent transport to the T7-T11 level. (2) There is a reduction in the activity of L-AAD as evidenced by lower amounts of ^{3}H-DA formed from the ^{3}H-L-tyrosine precursor. (3) The activity of the membrane-bound enzymes DBH and mitochondrial MAO is curtailed, probably due to circulatory stasis, hypoxia, and disruption of the membrane integrity. This condition results in the accumulation of DA and no change in NE concentration within the limits of the experimental time (one to three hours after spinal cord trauma). (4) Slopes of the disappearance rate of ^{3}H-DA and ^{3}H-NE, which plateau but do not become positive (Figure 3), indicate that little ingress of circulating ^{3}H-DA and ^{3}H-NE occurs after traumatic spinal cord injury. This statement is supported by our preliminary experiments infusing ^{3}H-DA in cats; this biogenic amine does not cross the blood-spinal cord barrier. An intravenous dose of ^{3}H-DA, which was calculated to be five times higher than the amount that was expected to be synthesized from a similar dose of ^{3}H-2',6'-tyrosine that was used in the experiments, was administered to six cats. The concentration (fmole) of ^{3}H-DA recovered from the spinal cord of traumatized cats was corrected for the residual ^{3}H-DA background (blank) found in the spinal cord of the laminectomized control groups. The latter experiments demonstrated that the amount of circulating ^{3}H-DA, which could have entered the traumatized spinal cord after the injection of ^{3}H-2',6'-tyrosine, was only 1-3% of the total ^{3}H-DA synthesized in the spinal cord from the precursor. (5) The restoration of impaired NE synthesizing enzymes by membrane stabilizing drugs, such as epsilon aminocaproic acid and methyl prednisolone sodium succinate, further suggests that the changes seen after trauma may be secondary to a more diffuse process of membrane dysfunction. From these results it is difficult to support a direct etiologic role for catecholamines in the production of the pathophysiologic events that are seen after spinal cord injury.

Membrane dysfunction and pathology after trauma is evidenced by a reduction in the activity of the phospholipid dependent, membrane-bound mitochondrial enzyme monoamine oxidase (Table II) and the formation of microglobules and noncellular material on the endothelial lining. Impact injury results in physiologic and structural alterations, which in turn lead to pathologic free radical reactions within the membrane (Figure 7).

SUMMARY AND CONCLUSION

Concentration of norepinephrine, dopamine, serotonin, and histamine were determined in the spinal cords of five groups of cats. One group underwent laminectomy only; a second untreated group received a 400 gm-cm impact at the T-9 level. These were compared with three groups that were treated with epsilon aminocaproic acid (EACA), methyl prednisolone sodium succinate (MP), and a combination of EACA and MP after similar trauma. The biogenic amines were measured in three 1 cm segments of the cord, rostral, middle, and caudal, one hour after trauma. There was no change in NE concentration in any of the

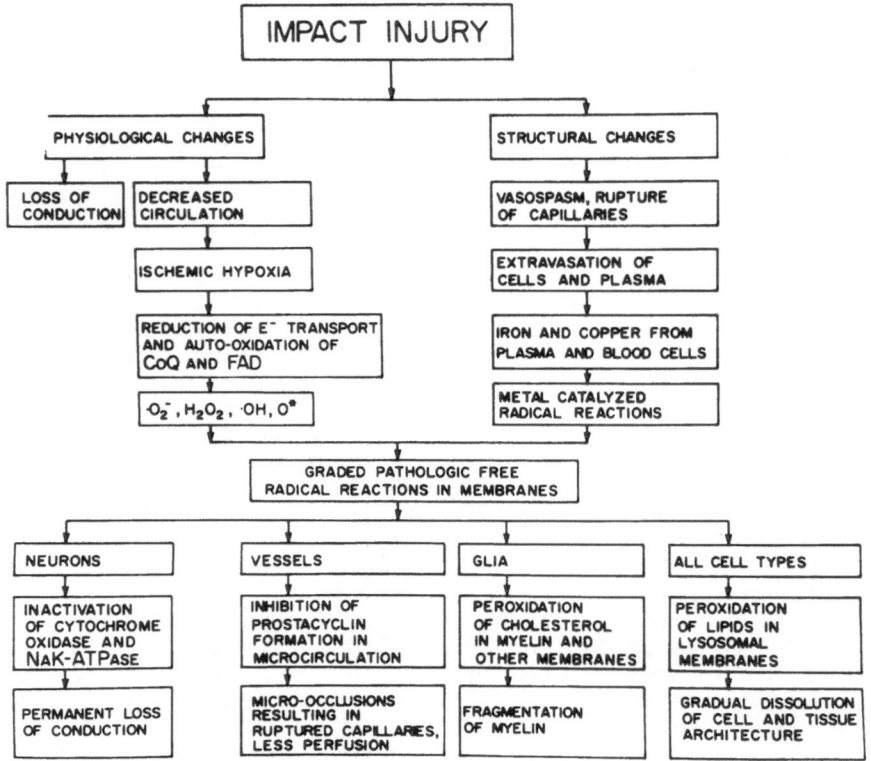

Fig. 7. Schematic diagram representing the pathophysiological changes in the spinal cord after traumatic injury.*

three segments after impact, compared with laminectomized controls, nor was the NE concentration in the impacted (middle) area higher than that in the rostral or caudal sites. Although the NE content of the cord in treated animals decreased, compared with that of laminectomized controls, the decrease was not significant. The concentration of DA, however, significantly increased after impact and sharply decreased after treatment with EACA and EACA plus MP. There was no significant change in 5-HT levels, but the level of histamine increased significantly after impact and was lowered by treatment with EACA and EACA plus MP. In this sense, EACA, in addition to its antifibrinolytic activity, either blocks the release of neuronal or mastal histamine, or both. This action of EACA will contribute to the reduction of inflammatory processes.

Three other groups of cats were injected with L-tyrosine (2,6-^{3}H). All control cats underwent laminectomy. One hour after intravenous injection of tyrosine, each experimental animal received a 400 gm-cm impact to the exposed dura. The animals were sacrificed one, two, and three hours after contusion of the spinal cord. The disappearance rate of dopamine decreased one hour and reached a plateau two hours after contusion, but that of norepinephrine leveled off within one hour. The results demonstrate that *there is a decrease in the activity of tyrosine hydroxylase as evidenced by a sharp increase in the specific activity of dopamine* (Figure 5). The activity of the membrane-bound enzymes dopamine-β-hydroxylase and mitochondrial monoamine

* Reprinted from Advances in Experimental Medicine: A Centenary Tribute to Claude Bernard, H. Parvez and S. Parvez, eds. Copyright 1980 Elsevier/North Holland Biomedical Press.

oxidase is curtailed, probably due to circulatory stasis, hypoxia, and disruption of the membrane integrity. Although tyrosine hydroxylase activity is low, a reduction in the MAO and DBH activities, result in accumulation of dopamine and no change in norepinephrine concentration.

A traumatic injury to the spinal cord leads to the immediate cessation of the propagation of action potential that is accompanied by progressive vascular changes, including ischemic focal hemorrhages and collapsed vessels, which in turn cause pathological alternations in the membrane lipids that are termed free radical reactions. The latter reactions adversely affect the lipid-dependent enzymes and disturb the endothelium, causing hemorrhagic necrosis of the central gray matter. Microvascular endothelial pathology, which is studied by scanning electron microscopy, correlates with the reduction in blood flow, progressive tissue degeneration, and free radical damage.

Epsilon aminocaproic acid, by virtue of its antiproteolytic activity, neutralizes lysosomal enzymes and, with the anti-inflammatory agent, MP, synergistically preserves membrane integrity. The reestablishment of deteriorated histological and biochemical variables as well as motor preservation when animals are treated with a combination of both drugs support this tenet. Two hours after impact, MAO activity *in vitro* is significantly reduced, but the activities of L-AAD and DBH, although lower, are not significantly different from those of the control (Table II). The *in vivo* concentration of molecular oxygen, a primary substrate for tyrosine hydroxylase, DBH, and MAO, is sharply reduced, owing to local circulatory stasis and hypoxia or anoxia. *In vitro*, provided with all cofactors including oxygen, DBH activity in the spinal cord two hours after impact remains relatively unchanged; within this time interval, little denaturation takes place in DBH protein.

The restoration of impaired histologic and physiologic parameters by membrane stabilizing drugs such as EACA and MP further suggests that the changes seen after trauma may be secondary to a more diffuse process of membrane dysfunction. Membrane pathology is evidenced by the changes in the phospholipid-dependent, membrane-bound enzymes.

Our neurochemical, pharmacologic (Naftchi et al., 1974; Naftchi et al., 1976; Flamm et al., 1976), histologic, and scanning electron microscopic studies on the effect of traumatic injuries in the CNS as well as those of others (Raisman, 1977; Raisman and Field, 1973) strongly suggest plasticity of the CNS. It has long been known that the cells of origin of the cut axons do not degenerate and that the proximal ends of the cut CNS axons possess considerable regenerative capacity to form axon sprouts. Furthermore, the axons that originate from the hippocampus and pass through the ipsilateral fimbria to innervate postsynaptic targets in the septal nuclei, when transected, form presynaptic terminals that are capable of reinnervating the postsynaptic targets (Raisman and Field, 1973). If an appropriate combination of pharmacologic agents can be employed to prevent phospholipid free radical reactions and can make the lesion site penetrable to the axons sprouts by allowing them to elongate and form contacts with their postsynaptic targets, spinal cord regeneration may be realized.

REFERENCES

Cajal, S., and Ramon, Y. *Degeneration and Regeneration of the Nervous System*, Hafner, New York (1928).
Coyle, J.T., and Axelrod, J. *J. Neurochem.* 19:449-459 (1972).

de la Torre, J.C., Johnson, C.M., Harris, L.H., Kajihara, K. and
Mullan, S. *Surg. Neurol. 2:* 5-11 (1974).

Flamm, E.W., Viau, A.T., Ransohoff, J., and Naftchi, N.E. *Neurology
26:* 664-666.

Griffiths, I.R. *J. Neurol. Sci. 27:* 529-544 (1976).

Hedeman, L.S., Shellenberger, M.K., and Gordon, J.H. *J. Neurosurg.
40:* 37-51 (1974).

Jarrot, B. *J. Neurochem. 18:* 7-16 (1971).

Lamprecht, F., and Coyle, J.T. *Brain Res. 41:* 503-506 (1972).

Levitt, M., Spector, S., Sjoerdsma, A., and Udenfriend, S. *J. Pharm.
Exper. Therap. 148:* 1-8 (1965).

Molinoff, P.B., Weinshilboum, R., and Axelrod, J. *J. Pharmacol. Exp.
Therap. 178:* 425-431 (1971).

Naftchi, N.E., Lowman, E.W., Sell, G.H., and Rusk, H.A. *Arch. Phys.
Med. Rehabil. 53:* 357-362 (1972).

Naftchi, N.E., Wooten, G.F., Lowman, E.W., and Axelrod, J. *Circ.
Res. 35:* 850-861 (1974).

Naftchi, N.E., Demeny, M., Lowman, E.W., and Tuckman, J. *Circ.
57 (No. 2):* 336-341 (1978).

Naftchi, N.E., Demeny, M., DeCrescito, V., Tomasula, J.J., Flamm,
E.S., and Campbell, J.B. *J. Neurosurg. 40:* 52-57 (1974).

Naftchi, N.E., and Tuckman, J. *Am. Heart J. 97 (No. 4):* 536-538
(1979).

Naftchi, N.E., Demeny, M., Flamm, E.S., and Lowman, E.W.
Catecholamines and Stress, Pergamon Press, Great Britain, p. 367-375
(1976).

Osterholm, J.L. and Mathews, G.J. *J. Neurosurg. 36:* 386-394 (1972).

Osterholm, J.L., and Mathews, G.J. *J. Neurosurg. 36:* 395-401 (1972).

Raisman, G. *Philos. Trans. R. Soc (Biol) 278:* 349-359 (1977).

Raisman, G., and Field, P.M. *Brain Res. 50:* 241-264 (1973).

Rothman, J.E., and Engelman, D.M. *Nature 237:* 24-44 (1972).

Schoultz, T.W., and DeLuca, D.C. *Life Sci. 15:* 1485-1495 (1974).

Strittmatter, W.J., Hirata, F., and Axelrod, J. *Science 204:* 1205-1207
(1979).

Vise, W.M., Yashon, W., and Hunt, W.E. *J. Neurosurg. 40:* 76-82
(1974).

Weissman, G. *New Engl. J. Med. 273:* 1084-1090 (1965).

Wurtman, R.J., Chou, C., and Rose, C. *J. Pharmacol. Exp. Therap.
174:* 351-356 (1970).

4

Molecular Pathogenesis of Spinal Cord Degeneration After Traumatic Injury

H.B. DEMOPOULOS, E.S. FLAMM, M.L. SELIGMAN,
J. RANSOHOFF, and N.E. NAFTCHI

INTRODUCTION

The sequence of morphologic changes that result from impact injuries to the spinal cord in experimental animal models have been described in morphologic (Campbell et al., 1973; Ducker et al., 1971; Dohrmann et al., 1972) and biochemical parameters (Molvy et al., 1973; Demopoulous et al., 1977; Seligman et al., 1977). It is evident, from comparative pathologic studies, that the same changes take place in most human spinal cord injuries. Therefore, the animal models are valid subjects for study. The post-impact alterations are not immediate but instead occur over a period of hours and are responsible for permanent paraplegia, which often develops. The initial impacting force is actually a minimal one and directly causes few detectable structural changes; other organs and tissues that are injured in an identical manner show very few alterations and no permanent damage. The reasons for the unusual sensitivity of the central nervous system (CNS) to impact injuries that do not permanently damage other tissues is not known. Different pathogenetic mechanisms for the degeneration of the minimally injured spinal cord have been proposed and include mechanical (Kobrine, 1975), vascular (Nelson et al., 1977), and free radical chemical (Milvy et al., 1973; Demopoulous et al., 1977; Seligmann et al., 1977) processes. It may be possible that all three types of processes are responsible to some degree for the irreparable tissue and cellular changes that accompany the development of permanent paraplegia or quadriplegia. Because these pathologic alteratons occur over a period of hours after impact, it would be feasible to intercede if the exact mechanisms and chain of events were known. The ability to walk requires the maintenance of only a small percent of the long tracts of the cord. Hence, if it were possible to intervene and protect, even to a partial degree, it may become possible to decrease the risk of permanent aparalysis after acute spinal cord injuries. In order to understand the possible protective approaches that are now under development, it is necessary to describe the background research. The principal hypothesis underlying the idea that it may be possible to intervene immediately after trauma, to ameliorate the potentially paralytic changes, centers around membrane pathology. The idea is that the cell membranes of neurons, glia, and blood vessels undergo pathologic changes as a result of trauma, and, once the cell membranes are destroyed, the changes are irreversible. In terms of subacute and chronic care, a knowledge of the pathogenetic mechanisms of degeneration assumes importance because the affected level of the spinal cord injury may change segments, up or down. The possible causes and the potential for preventing a more cephalad extension of the level of injury are both based on an exact knowledge of the pathogenetic mechanisms.

The spinal cord and other nervous system componenets, more than other organ systems, have strict requirements for membrane integrity. Barriers, such as the blood-CNS barriers, which maintain a unique environment for the CNS not only by excluding substances but also by markedly enhancing the transport of compounds such as ascorbic acid (Spector, 1977), require that the membrane lipids and proteins be structurally intact; the same is true for the excitable membranes that are involved in conduction and transmission. Even minor perturbations in the configuration of strategic membrane molecules, such as the lipids that help to maintain the active shape of key enzymes, like Na+,K+ ATPase, adenylate cyclase, and prostaglandin synthetase, can have far-reaching consequences, (Brady et al., 1974; Fourcans and Jain, 1974; Shaeffer et al., 1975). Altering the fluidity of the lipids will affect synaptosome formation, while disturbing the plasma membrane of the endothelium can lead to a failure on the part of the endothelial cells to maintain a clear lumen (Moncada et al., 1976).

In spinal cord trauma, experiments have shown that the two major pathologic components of trauma, *ischemia* and *focal hemorrhages*, can lead to a series of pathologic changes in the membrane lipids that are termed free radical reactions; these, in turn, may adversely affect the lipid dependent enzymes and disturb the endothelium, causing a broad spectrum of cellular and tissue changes. The most marked tissue change after impact is the gradual development of hemorrhage in the central gray matter. In the first 15-30 minutes, there are only scattered petechial hemorrhages in the gray, and, by 60 minutes, some of these have enlarged and coalesced (Campbell et al., 1973; Ducker et al., 1971). The long tracts show no evidence of morphologic change at this time except for enlargement of the periaxonal space in a small percentage of the myelinated fibers, as seen ultrastructurally (Dohrmann et al., 1972). The amount of blood extravasated in the gray appears to reach its maximum at the end of three to four hours, and, by this time, there may be petechial hemorrhages in the white matter, in the long tracts (Campbell et al., 1973; Ducker et al., 1971). Approximately 25% of the myelinated fibers show enlargement of the periaxonal space and fraying of the myelin by four hours (Campbell et al., 1973; Ducker et al., 1971). At 24-36 hours, the central gray has undergone hemorrhagic necrosis and the long tracts show extensive structural degeneration.

The vascular aspects of spinal cord damage may be of particular interest because they offer a possibility for relating pathogenic mechanisms as seemingly diverse as mechanical deformation and free radical chemistry (i.e., mechanical deformation → partial breakdown of extravasated blood → initiation and catalysis of free radical damage to membrane lipids by iron as inorganic and organic compounds, as well as other blood-borne metals → further vascular pathology, including vasospasm, occlusion, and rapture of components of the microcirculatory beds). If vascular perturbations are a major mechanism and are part of a self-perpetuating cycle of destructive change, there is a possibility of interrupting the cycle with vaso-active agents (Flamm et al., 1975).

Blood flow to the impacted segment of injured spinal cord models has been shown to be markedly decreased, suggesting that ischemia may be an important pathogenetic mechanism (Nelson et al., 1977; Griffiths, 1976). The diminished blood flow may be due to vasospasm or microvascular occlusions, or both. Morphologic studies by light and transmission electron microscopy have not revealed evidence of occlusions nor damage to the vessel walls, particularly in the first one to two hours after injury, in the white matter; except for petechial hemorrhages in the gray, there is no adequate explanation for the marked decrease in blood flow in the gray matter soon after impact. Others have shown that 30 to 60 minutes of ischemia in large, nonparenchymatous arteries, such as experimentally perfused carotids, results in the development of many endothelial defects, including *craters* and adhesion of cells and noncellular material (Nelson et al., 1977; Nelson et al., 1975; Gertz et al., 1976).

Pathological morphologic changes in the microvascular endothelium, occurring early after spinal cord injury, have not been described and, if present at early time periods after impact, might help to explain progressive tissue degeneration. Free radical damage, leading to lipid peroxide formation in the endothelium, can inhibit the normal synthesis of prostacyclin (PGI$_2$); this substance is produced by endothelial cells from arachidonate-derived prostaglandin endoperoxides and is required to actively prevent platelet adherence and aggregation, which is constantly promoted by thromboxane A$_2$, another product from endo-peroxides (Gryglewski, et al., 1976; Moncada et al., 1976).

A summation of the background of free radical reactions in lipids and a review of the evidence for their occurrence in CNS trauma is presented together with new data, regarding major pathologic changes in the endothelium of the parenchymal microcirculation. These alterations in the vasculature occur early and provide a possible link between the lipid free radical damage that has been chemically documented and the apparent perturbations in spinal cord blood flow which occur after impact injury.

LIPID FREE RADICAL DAMAGE

Membrane phospholipids are the basic skeleton of all cell membranes as shown in Figure 1. The fatty acid tails of the phospholipids are the portions of these molecules that can undergo free radical damage. Unsaturated fatty acids become progressively more susceptible to radical attack as their number of double bonds increases (Demopoulous, 1973). Arachidonic acid (20 carbons long, with four unsaturations) undergoes radical reactions more readily than linolenic (18:3) and linoleic (18:2) acids. This type of radical attack, however, is not always pathological because this is fundamentally how prostaglandins, thromboxane, and prostacyclin are synthesized, i.e., arachidonic acid is subjected to rigidly controlled, normal free radical reactions, to produce endoperoxides, which then serve as the parent compounds (Hamberg and Samuelsson, 1974; Kolata, 1974). It is important to note that these reactions, even when occurring under pathologic circumstances, can be of graded severity and can proceed in irregular steps, with fitful stops and starts, depending on the strength of the *initiating* and *catalyzing* factors, Figures 1 and 2 diagramatically depict, in summary fashion, *all* of the consequences of pathologic, uncontrolled free radical damage to the unsaturated fatty acids of membrane phospholipids. Analogous changes take place in cholesterol as well, adjacent to the unsaturated site in the ring (Lamola et al., 1973). Radical reactions are easily initiated in lipids, particularly unsaturated ones, by molecular oxygen, since it is itself a diradical capable of initiating reactions and

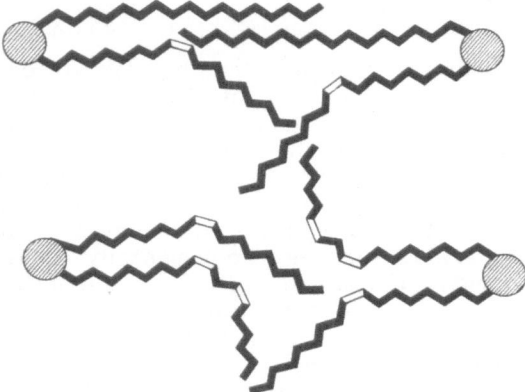

Fig. 1.   Schematic representation of bimolecular leaflet of phospholipid
molecules, forming the skeleton of a plasma membrane.   The circles
are the glycerophosphate head groups, which are polar, while the fatty
acid tails extend into the hydrophobic midzone.   Unsaturated bonds are
bent at an angle of 123°, in the cis isomeric configuration in the fatty
acid tails.   In the normal membrane, there is a saturated carbon sepa-
rating the two carbons that have unsaturated bonds.   This saturated
carbon is partly activated and can lose one of its hydrogens quite
readily.   Note the spaces between the phospholipids.   These are the
archways wherein cholesterol and other sterol-like compounds inter-
calate.*

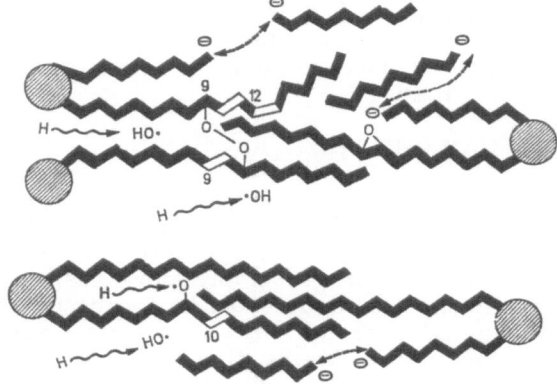

Fig. 2.   Schematic summary representation of free radical peroxidative
damage to fatty acids that formed the hydrophobic midzone seen in
Fig. 1.   The double bonds are now largely in the non-bent, trans-
configuration; a saturated carbon no longer separates the carbons with
unsaturated bonds and this is referred to as conjugation; alkoxy radicals, RO·, are present and react to form peroxides, ROOR, to join
two adjacent fatty acids in an abnormal bond; mobile ·OH radicals are
shown as the result of hydroperoxide schism; hydrogens are shown
being abstracted possibly from adjacent lipid and protein molecules;
abstracted hydrogens react with hydroxyls to form water in the hydrophobic midzone; fragmentation of fatty acid tails is shown with eventual
production of negatively charged carboxylic acid groups, represented
as a minus sign inside an oval mark.   The numerals 9, 10, 12, signify
the carbon atom number in the carbon chain that makes up the fatty
acid.*

Reprinted from Advances in Experimental Medicine: A Centenary Tribute to Claude
Bernard, H. Parvez and S. Parvez, eds. Copyright 1980 Elsevier/North Holland
Biomedical Press.

is also preferentially soluble in nonpolar environments, compared to polar, by a ratio of 7 to 1 (Lawrence et al., 1946).

Simply initiating radical reactions, however, is not sufficient to maintain *ongoing* reactions, especially in biologic membranes, because naturally occurring antioxidants (α-tocopherol, ascorbic acid, glutathione and others) and enzyme defense systems (superoxide dismutase and glutathione peroxidase) quench the radical reactions (Demopoulos, 1973; Kellog and Fridovich, 1977). Even if the antioxidants and protective enzymes were to be exhausted, there are natural termination reactions in free radical chemistry that would limit the degree of spread. Propagation of destructive lipid free radical reactions to the point of irreversible cellular changes requires *catalysts* that will speed the reactions beyond the capacities of the anti-oxidants and protective enzymes, and beyond the reparability rate.

INITIATION AND CATALYSIS OF RADICAL REACTIONS BY CNS TRAUMA

Unfortunately, CNS injury appears capable of providing the means for vigorous initiation and catalysis of lipid free radical damage by virtue of *ischemia* and *focal hemorrhages*.

Ischemia appears to initiate radical reactions in lipids largely because of a sudden decrease in the supply of oxygen to the electron transport chains in mitochondria. The bioenergetically linked transport of electrons and hydrogen to molecular oxygen involves multiple steps through factors that assume free radical configurations; flavin adenine dinucleotide (FAD) and coenzyme Q (CoQ) are key substances that normally have a free radical form (·FAD, ·CoQ) in mitochondrial electron transport and are present in relatively large amounts in the mitochondria rich neurons (Ruzicka et al., 1975). In the presence of adequate O_2, these large concentrations of electron transport factors remain tightly associated, and there is little opportunity for ·FAD or ·CoQ to initiate spurious, destructive lipid free radical reactions along the inner mitochondrial membranes where they are found. However, when O_2 is diminished abruptly, as from the ischemia that usually accompanies trauma, a certain proportion of the mitochondrial electron transport chains will not be provided with sufficient concentrations of molecular oxygen to accept the ongoing flow of electrons and hydrogen. Among the several immediate consequences is the dislocation of electron transport substances with the result that ·FAD and ·CoQ become available for initiating lipid radical reactions. Molecular oxygen is not entirely absent, and sufficient amounts persist in traumatized tissues to support pathologic radical reactions. Analogous reactions from radiobiologic studies indicate that only trace amounts of O_2 are needed to promote the pathologic free radical reactions that are initiated by ionizing radiation (Michael et al., 1973).

Eventually, FAD and CoQ, along with all the other electron transport substances, become reduced. This, however, is potentially dangerous because the reduced FAD and CoQ can then autooxidize in a cyclical manner, even in the presence of small amounts of oxygen, to produce two radicals as follows:

$$\text{(reduced)} \quad CoQ + O_2 \rightarrow \cdot CoQ + \cdot O_2^-$$

The ·CoQ accepts hydrogen and electrons from reducing species that are still being produced and becomes reduced again; in this way, the CoQ cycles and keeps producing the superoxide radical $\cdot O_2^-$ (Fridovich, 1977). If this cycle of reducing and auto-oxidizing the CoQ can be broken, then amelioration of ischemic cell injury may become possible.

Barbiturates have long been known to block electron transport, specifically by preventing the reduction of CoQ (White et al., 1973). Keeping CoQ in the oxidized state would break the pathologic auto-oxidative/reductive cycling of CoQ that has been hypothesized in cerebral ischemia. Recently, by the use of electron paramagnetic resonance (epr) spectrometry, a specific interaction between barbiturates and ·CoQ has been demonstrated (Demopoulos et al., 1977). This interaction is demonstrated in Figure 3. The superoxide radical ($\cdot O_2^-$)

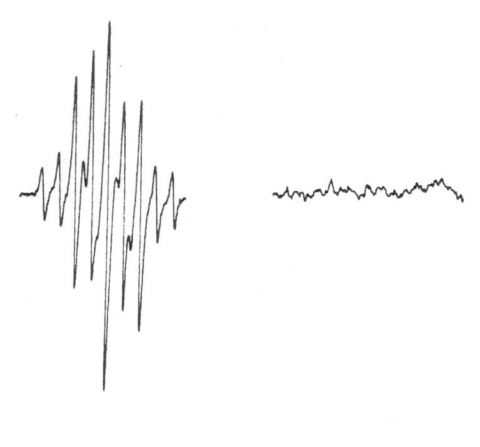

Fig. 3. The electron paramagnetic resonance (epr) spectrum of the coenzyme Q free radical is shown on the left hand sie. Normal decay time in this solution (alkaline ethanol with tetrahydrofuran and DMSO) is 45 minutes. The addition of equimolar methohexital, a highly lipid soluble barbiturate, immediately abolishes the epr signal of CoQ, in a preparation whose remaining decay time was 40 minutes. This is shown on the right.

spontaneously disproportionates to form H_2O_2 and singlet oxygen; the latter is capable of initiating and propagating pathologic lipid radical reactions, but, in addition, the H_2O_2 reacts with other $\cdot O_2^-$ through the Haber Weiss reaction to form the extremely dangerous hydroxyl radical, ·OH (Kellog and Fridovich, 1977). The latter acts as a major *initiator* and *catalyst* of lipid free radical reactions (Demopoulos, 1973). The enzyme, superoxide dismutase (SOD) generally dismutates $\cdot O_2^-$ safely to H_2O_2, without the production of singlet oxygen; further, because it rapidly destroys $\cdot O_2^-$, the concentration of the superoxide radical is kept low, and there is a decreased opportunity for $\cdot O_2^-$ to react with H_2O_2 to form ·OH (Kellog and Fridovich, 1977). Unfortunately, lipid peroxides can inactivate SOD and remove a major protective enzyme (Fridovich, 1977).

Focal hemorrhage may also lead to catalysis of pathologic lipid radical reactions, probably through the metals that are present in blood. Trace quantities of iron or copper as inorganic, or organic, compounds are known to be powerful catalysts of lipid free radical reactions unstable hydroperoxide that is capable of producing a variety of oxygen radicals and is thought to be a mediator of edema in inflammation.

(Demopoulos, 1973). Iron salts are used routinely in experiments to
initiate and catalyze lipid radical reactions in liposomal model membrances,
in vitro (Suwa et al., 1977). Citrate or high concentrations of phosphate
are.excellent inhibitors of destructive lipid radical reactions in liposomal
membrane model systems, because they chelate the trace metals that
catalyze (Demopoulos et al., 1977). In extravasated blood, the metals
available include iron and copper in the serum, as well as the iron
and copper in red blood cells. Lysis, or leakage of small numbers
of extravasated blood cells can add additional metals to those supplied
by the serum. Copper has been shown to increase the rate of radical
oxidation of lipids by three orders of magnitude, and iron, as in hematin
compounds, will accelerate this rate by five orders of magnitude (Tappel,
1961). The other formed elements in extravasated blood, such as
leucocytes and platelets, cannot be dismissed as contributing to initiation
and catalysis of pathologic CNS radical reactions. Polymorphonuclear
leucocytes normally produce large quantitites of $.O_2-$, H_2O_2, and $.OH$;
these are used in killing phagocytosed micro-organisms (Stossel et al.,
1974). Platelets carry high concentrations of prostaglandin (PG)
endoperoxides, derived by controlled free radical oxidation of arachidonic
acid (Hamberg and Samuelsson, 1974); the PG endoperoxides include an

EVIDENCE FOR LIPID RADICAL DAMAGE IN THE CNS

A number of reports have appeared that suggest that pathologic free
radical reactions can take place *in vivo*, in the CNS, as a result of
chemical or physical injuries. The parameters of such reactions, which
have been followed by different research groups, are listed in Table I.
Actually detecting the lipid free radicals themselves (e.g., alkyl,
peroxy) is not possible because they are reactive transients and do not
have a sufficiently high steady state concentration. As a result, the
consequences of free radical damage, which are distinctive, are used.
This includes the loss of susceptible molecules, anti-oxidant consumption,
metastable products, and final products.

Reports indicating that CNS injuries are accompanied by lipid free
radical damage are listed in Table II. The earliest free radical changes
that have been detected thus far involve the consumption of the CNS
antioxidant, ascorbic acid. It has been found to be significantly
decreased as early as one hour after a 400 gm-cm (20 gm x 20 cm)
impact injury of feline spinal cords, and at one hour following regional
cerebral ischemia (Demopoulos et al., 1977).

CONSEQUENCES OF LIPID FREE RADICAL DAMAGE

Damage to membrane lipids would be of potentially less importance
were it not for the fact that a number of major proteins derive their
active configurational shape as a result of intimate interactions between
the hydrophobic portions of the proteins and the fatty acid tails of
specific membrane phospholipids. A list of major intrinsic membrane
proteins that are phospholipid dependent is presented in Table III
(Fourcans and Jain, 1974). Because of the susceptibility of the phospholipid fatty acids to radical damage, such proteins might be viewed as
having a liability in depending on phospholipid integrity. One of these
enzymes, Na+,K+ ATPase, has been shown by several workers to be
inhibited by free radical mechanisms. Brody et al. (1974) has demonstrated that the chlorpromazine free radical, and related free
radicals, can significantly inhibit Na+,K+ ATPase. Schaefer et al (1975)
has shown that Na+,K+ ATPase activity in rat brain microsomes can be
inhibited when the membrane lipids undergo free radical damage; the

TABLE I

Parameters of Lipid Free Radical Damage

EARLY, OR MODERATE FREE RADICAL DAMAGE TO MEMBRANE PHOSPHOLIPIDS

. diene conjugation in fatty acids
. cis → trans isomerization in fatty acids
. hindered rotation of nitroxide spin probes placed within liposome membrane systems that are composed of lipids from the damaged membrane system
. minor losses in polyunsaturated acids such as arachidonic acid, 20:4, with quantitation by gas chromatography/mass spectrometry (GC/MS)
. prevention of the above with lipophilic or amphipathic antioxidants

LATE, OR SEVERE FREE RADICAL DAMAGE TO MEMBRANE PHOSPHOLIPIDS

. malonaldehyde production
. lipid soluble fluorescence due to malonadlehyde additions
. production of short chain and sometimes branched chain, fatty acids of lengths that are not normally present
. decreased hinderance of rotation of nitroxide spin probes within liposome membrane systems that are composed of lipid from the damaged membrane system
. major losses in polyunsaturated fatty acids such as arachidonic acid, 20:4, *plus* minor losses in mono-unsaturated and saturated fatty acids
. prevention of the above with lipophilic or amphipathic antioxidants

FREE RADICAL DAMAGE TO CHOLESTEROL

. decrease in extractable cholesterol and measurement by gas chromatography
. appearance of several cholesterol oxidation products in polar solvents

CONSUMPTION OF TISSUE ANTIOXIDANTS

. ascorbic acid (reduced) by epr spectrometry
. alpha tocopherol
. glutathione
. cysteine

ALTERATIONS IN PROTECTIVE ENZYMES

. superoxide dismutase
. glutathione peroxidase

LIPOSOMES FROM CNS LIPID EXTRACT FROM DIFFERENT ANIMAL MODELS

. rates of free radical damage under conditions of auto-oxidation
. spin probe analyses of fluidity by epr spectrometry
. permeability rates of solutes in aqueous channels

TABLE II

Free Radical Lipid Damage in CNS

SPINAL CORD IMPACT INJURY MODELS IN CATS HAVE SHOWN
- potentiation of trauma by ethanol
- appearance of increased levels of malonaldehyde
- apperaance of increasing levels of lipid soluble fluorescence, representing addition products of malonaldehyde
- loss of extractable cholesterol
- consumption of a major CNS antioxidant, ascorbic acid

FOCAL CNS COLD TRAUMA IN CATS AND RATS HAS SHOWN
- amelioration of cerebral edema with DPPD, an antioxidant
- loss of polyunsaturated fatty acids from gray and white matter
- loss of extractable cholesterol from gray and white matter
- consumption of a major CNS antioxidant, ascorbic acid, from gray and white matter
- amelioration of all free radical pathology parameters with synthetic corticosteroids, which have been shown to also have antioxidant properties in model membrane systems undergoing free radical damage
- increased production of malonaldehyde
- loss of thiols

REGIONAL CNS ISCHEMIA IN CATS HAS SHOWN
- loss of polyunsaturated fatty acids from the gray matter
- loss of extractable cholesterol from the white matter
- consumption of a major CNS antioxidant, ascorbic acid, from gray and white matter
- amelioration of all of the above with barbiturates, which were shown to have lipid antioxidant properties in model membrane systems undergoing free radical damage

HYPOXIA, BRAIN
- loss of thiols

BIOGENIC AMINES
- 6-OH dopamine is concentrated in sympathetic fibers and destroys them by free radical mechanism

DEFICIENCY STATES
- alpha tocopherol deficiency leads to encephalomalacia

---

radical reactions were initiated by *low* concentrations of ascorbic acid, possibly by an indirect route involving auto-oxidation of ascorbic acid with the formation of $\cdot O_2^-$, and then H_2O_2 and $\cdot OH$ (Fridovich, 1977). High concentrations of ascorbic acid, as are normally found in the CNS, do *not* initiate these pathologic radical reactions (Shaeffer et al., 1975). Acetylcholinesterase, a membrane protein that is *not* intrinsic and *not* dependent on phospholipids, is *not* inhibited by the lipid radical reactions that has decreased the Na+,K+ ATPase activity (Shaeffer et al., 1975).

Because cytochrome oxidase and succinic dehydrogenase are phospholipid dependent enzymes, they could be specifically inhibited by pathologic free radical reactions following trauma. Recent work has shown that cytochrome oxidase activity is decreased within 15 minutes, after impact injury to the spinal cord (Terifumi et al., 1978). Part of the reason for decreased oxidative respiration, and the accompanying increase in glycolysis that is seen after trauma (Nilsson et al., 1977), may lie in decreases in the activity of cytochrome oxidase, brought about perhaps by pathologic lipid free radical reactions in the inner mitochondrial membrane.

Another potential consequence of membrane lipid free radical reactions involves the endothelial cells. Arachidonic acid (four unsaturations) is present in large quantities in platelets, and their microsomes oxidize and cyclo-oxygenate arachidonic acid into prostaglandin (PG) endoperoxides, which are unstable intermediates (Hamberg and Samuelsson, 1974). There are three major classes of compounds produced from the PG endoperoxides: (1) prostaglandins E and F; (2) thromboxane A_2 (TxA_2); and (3) prostacyclin (PGI_2). The latter two are directly antagonistic and far more powerful than the PG's (*The Lancet, 1977*). Thromboxane A_2 is an extremely potent platelet aggregator, whereas prostacyclin prevents, as well as disaggregates, platelets (*The Lancet, 1977*). The balance between TxA_2 and PGI_2 is critical for homeostasis. Recent work has shown that lipid peroxides will selectively inhibit the formation of PGI_2 and result in the unopposed action of TxA_2 (Moncada et al., 1976). Since previous work has demonstrated that ischemia or trauma lead to lipid free radical damage and the production of lipid peroxides, this may serve to explain why ischemia or injured endothelium allows platelets and other coagulable material to adhere. The normal absence of adherent material on normal endothelium is the result of continual activity on the part of the endothelial cells to produce PGI_2, which serves to keep the lumenal surfaces clear (Gryglewski et al., 1976).

Accordingly, the present study was performed, utilizing high-resolution, topologic scanning electron microscopy to examine the microvasculature within the parenchyma of the cord at early time periods following experimental injuries and specifically to study the endothelial lining. The topologic examination of the endothelium of small parenchymatous vessels became possible by using a particularly low-angle, obliquely cut section through the cord.

SCANNING ELECTRON MICROSCOPY METHODS

Mature cats were impact injured as described in previous studies (Campbell et al., 1973; Ducker et al., 1971). A total of six cats were used for this study: two were sacrificed at one hour after injury, two were sacrificed at two hours after injury, and two served as noninjured controls. Warmed (37°C) glutaraldehyde in phosphate buffer, prepared as in previous work (Sjostrand, 1967), was instilled through the left ventricle by cannula into the ascending aorta by using gravity from a

TABLE III
Phospholipid Dependent Proteins   (11)

MICROSOMES	PLASMA MEMBRANE	MITOCHONDRIA
prostaglandin-synthetase system	NaK-ATPase	cytochrome oxidase
	adenylate cyclase	succinic dehydrogenase
hydroxylase system with cytochrome p450	lectin binding glycoproteins & surface glycolipids	monoamine oxidase
NADH-cytochrome b5 reductase	5'-nucleotidase	NADH cytochrome c/NADH-ubiquinone reductase
steroid-glucuronyl transferase	RBC acetyl cholin-esterase	succinate-cytochrome reductase
UDP-glucuronyl transferase		ATP synthetase system
		hexokinase
phosphatidic acid phosphatase		citric acid cycle enzymes
phosphoryl choline transferase		NADPH$_2$':NAD oxido-reductase
glucose-t-phsopho-hydrolase		GTP-dependent acyl CoA synthetase
		deoxycorticosterone 11-β-hydroxylase
		D-β-hydroxybutyrate dehydrogenase

reservoir that was six feet above the cat's heart. The trachea was intubated and positive pressure ventilation of the lungs was instituted prior to the perfusion; ventilation was maintained throughout the perfusion for oxygenation and to provide sufficient negative pressure to facilitate return through the veins. When the perfusion was started, the right atrium was cut open to permit the blood to wash out. The perfusion continued for 15 minutes and consumed approximately three liters of fixative. Following this procedure, virtually the entire cord was removed, the dura was peeled off, and the cord was placed in glutaraldehyde for additional fixation by immersion for 12 hours. The cord was then cut obliquely at a low angle, approximately 10-15°, using a fresh, disposable metal microtome blade; each cut was made freehandedly in one motion. Obliquely cut slices were taken through the impacted area, as well as 3 cm distal and 3 cm proximal to the injury. The tissues were then washed in running distilled water for 12 hours and slowly dehydrated through graded ethanol over a period of six hours to 100% alcohol. The tissues were critical-point dried and then coated with 100-150 Å of gold-palladium, using rotation and continuous tilt of the specimen for uniformity (DeEstable-Puig and Estable-Puig, 1975).

The slices of cord tissue (one hour post injury; two hours post injury; noninjured, obliquely, horizontally, and longitudinally cut sections; impact area, as well as distal and proximal segments) were examined in AMR scanning electron microscopes; one of which had a tungsten filament to which an accelerating voltage of 20 Kv was applied, and one that was equipped with a lanthanum-hexaboride crystal to which either 20 or 30 Kv were applied.

Semiquantitative analyses were conducted of the pathologic changes that were observed on the endothelium after examining the entire area that was exposed by the section.

SCANNING ELECTRON MICROSCOPY RESULTS

The oblique sections, cut at a very small angle with the oblique plane studied *en face* (Figure 4), greatly facilitated the examination of the vascular components in the parenchyma of the spinal cord. The gray and white matter were readily distinguished in the noninjured controls, and Figure 4 also shows the central canal, which is patent in cats.

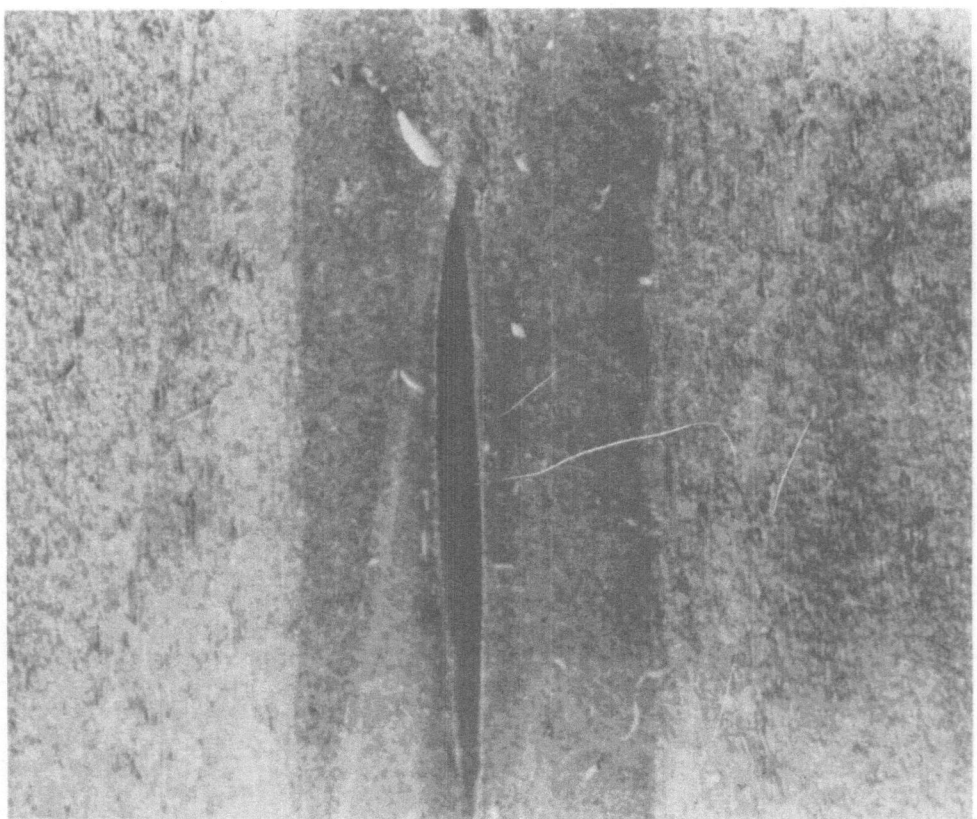

Fig. 4. Very low magnification of an obliquely cut, normal cat spinal cord showing the central canal (patent in cats), surrounding gray matter, and the long tracts in the white matter. Magnification 40X.*

Reprinted from Advances in Experimental Medicine: A Centenary Tribute to Claude Bernard, H. Parvez and S. Parvez, eds. Copyright 1980 Elsevier/North Holland Biomedical Press.

In the noninjured controls, the central gray matter provided large numbers of opened vessels of the microcirculation for study, as can be seen in a representative area from a noninjured cord in Figure 5.

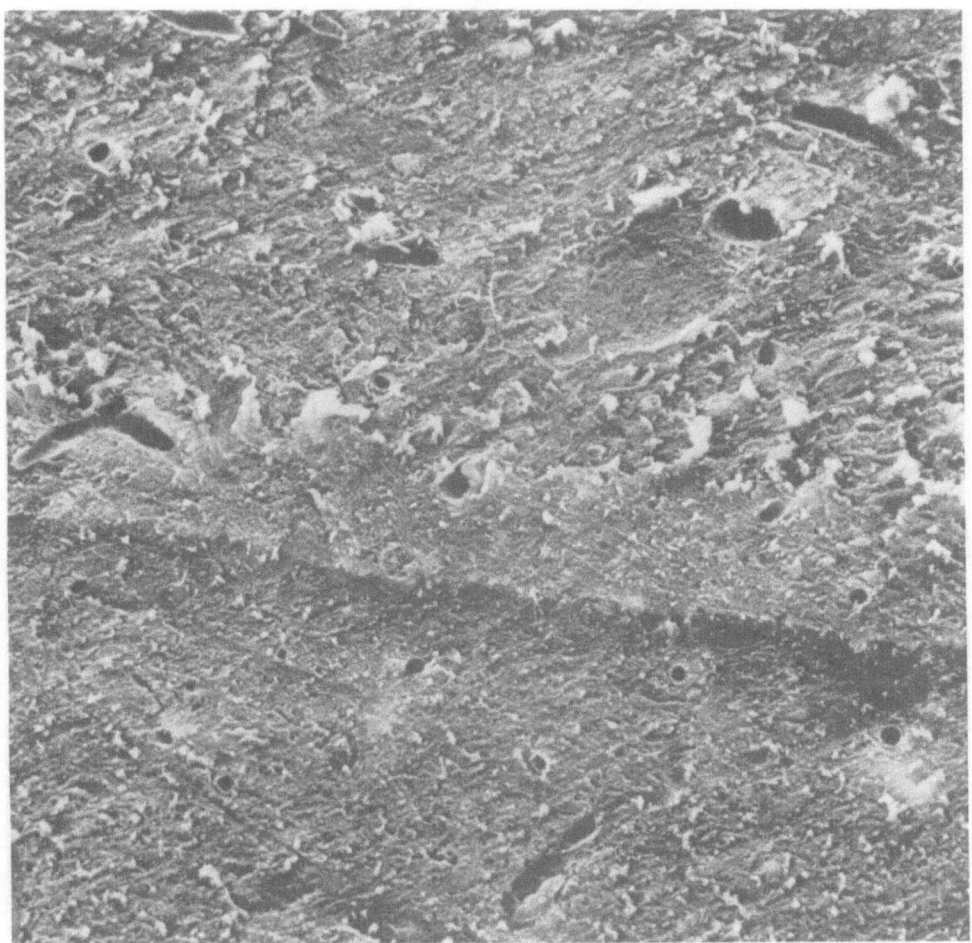

Fig. 5. Slightly higher magnification of gray matter in Fig. 4. Numerous capillaries are present and have been opened by the oblique cut. Magnification 530X.

Most of the vessels seen in this figure are capillaries. At higher magnification of the border of white and gray matter, the number of capillaries seen per unit area decreased, but the vessels presented similar features. Figure 6 shows a capillary in the white matter. Figure 7 is a higher magnification of a capillary in the white matter and demonstrates micro-villi and pinocytic vesicle orifices. The junctions of the normal endothelial cells in all the examined vessels were flat and did not override. The lumena of the normal vessels were free of adherent or occlusive material and/or cells.

In the impacted spinal cords within the injured segment, several types of changes were noted in the endothelial lining; they seemed to

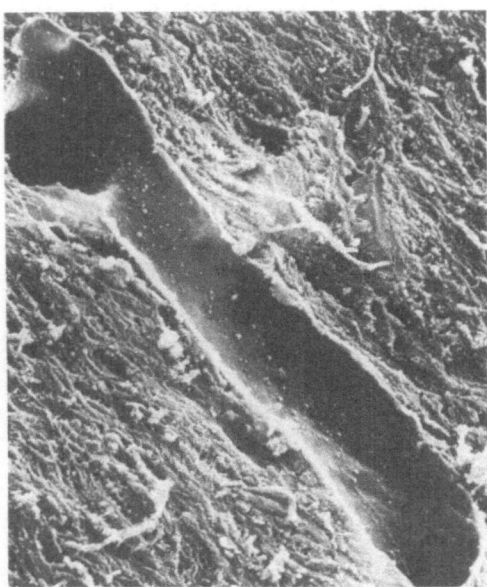

Fig. 6. Higher magnification of a white matter capillary, from a section similar to that in Figs. 4 and 5. The lumen and its endothelial lining are readily observed. The vessel lumen is devoid of adherent material, and has a smooth surface marked only by the presence of normal microvilli. Control cat. Magnification 5000X.

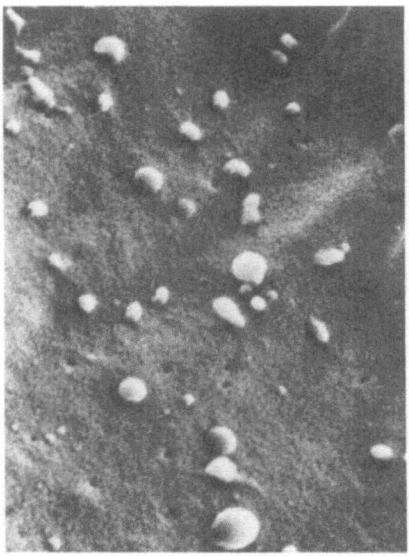

Fig. 7. A still greater magnification of the endothelial lining of a white matter capillary from a normal cat. The microvilli and pinocytotic vesicle openings of the endothelial cells' plasma membrane are visible. Magnification 45,000X.

progress from one hour to two hours after injury and were seen in a
majority of the vessels of the parenchymal micro-circulation, in gray
and in white matter.   The changes described were observed in approximately 30% of the capillaries; in each prepartion of a spinal cord
segment, a minimum of 200 capillaries were examined.   The endothelial
cell changes, per se, included: craters (Figure 8), adherent noncellular
material (Figure 8 and 10), overriding of endothelial cell junctions
(Figure 9), and micro-globular formations at cell junctions as well as
away from cell junctions (Figure 10).   The latter might represent platelet
fragments or a substance from the endothelial cell.

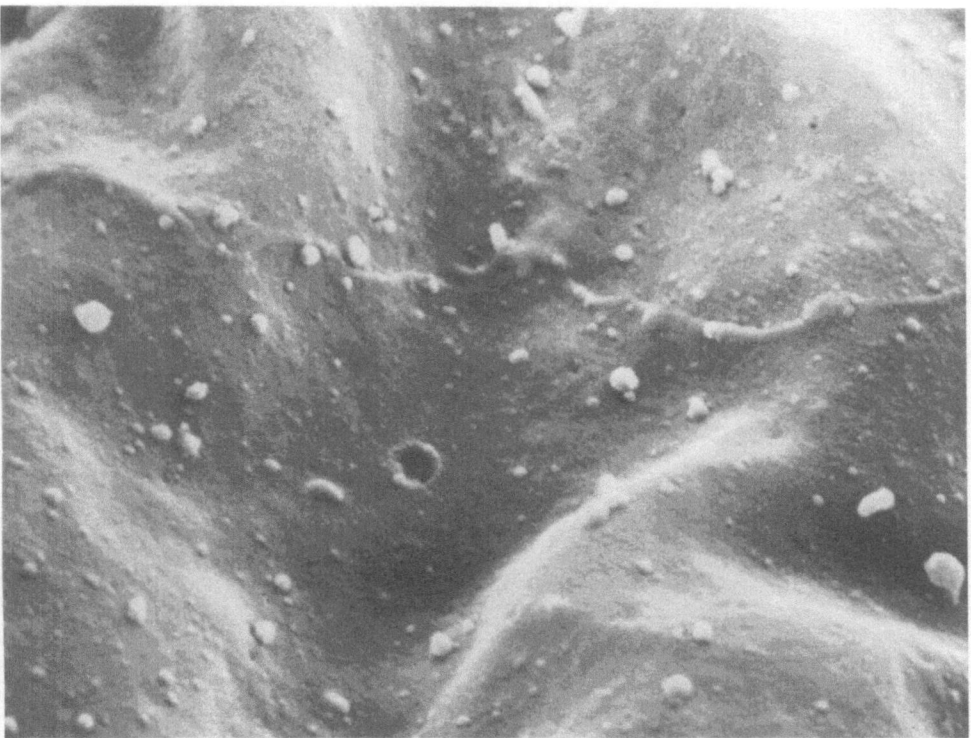

Fig. 8.   One hour after impact injury, the endothelium of a white
matter arteriole shows a crater and adherent non-cellular material.
The undulation of the surface is due to contraction of elastic and
muscle elements in the arteriolar wall, secondary to the spasm that
accompanies perfusion-fixation.   Magnification 32,000X.

In the spinal cords that were examined two hours after impact,
there were changes in the micro-circulation in the distal and proximal
segments, approximately 3 cm from the point of impact.   The most
frequently encountered change was adherent noncellular material
(Figure 11).   The changes were more severe distally than proximally
but did not approach the degree seen at the impact site.

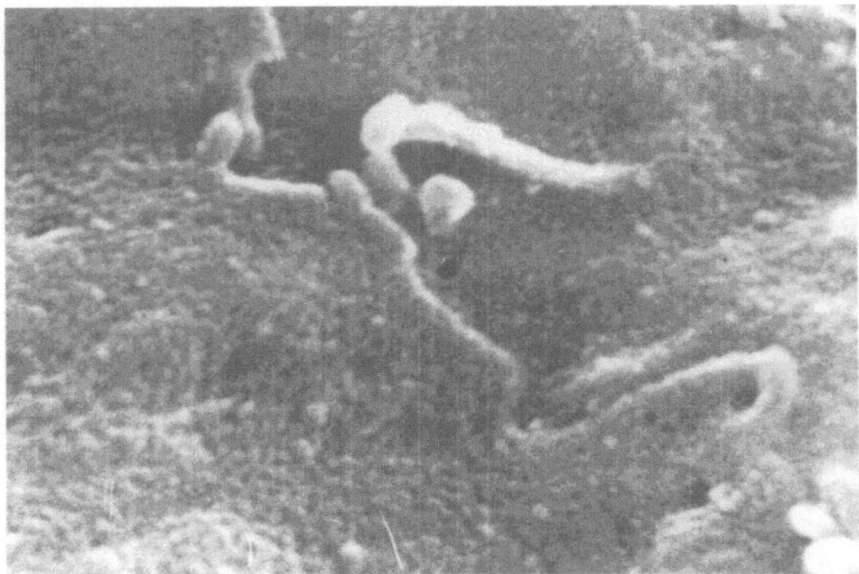

Fig. 9. One hour after impact injury, the junction of two endothelial cells in a white matter capillary show over-riding. Magnification 87,000X.

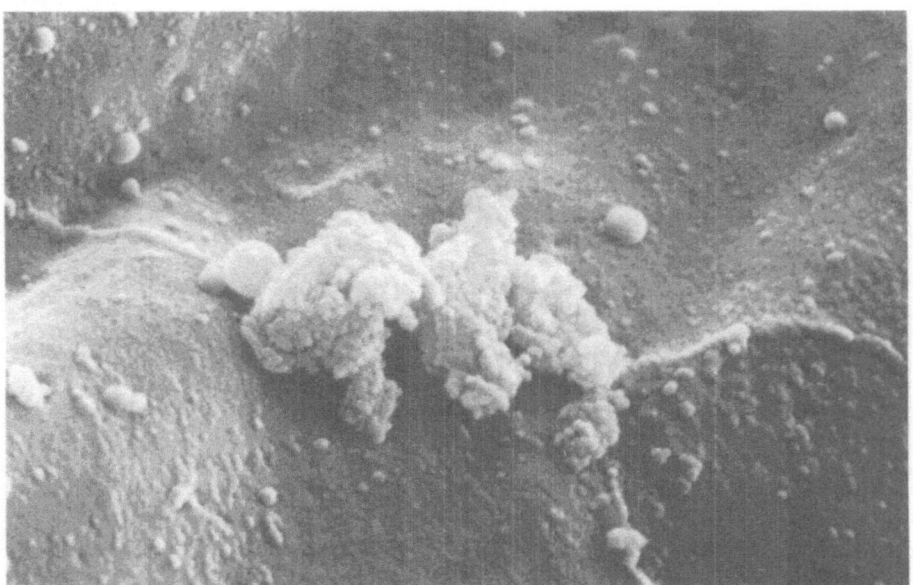

Fig. 10. One hour after injury, the endothelium of a white matter vessel (undulation of background is due to contraction of elastic and contractile elements in vessel wall) displays a micro-globular formation whose greatest diameter is approximately two microns. The multiple micro-globules comprising the formation are about 0.1 micron in diameter each; adherent non-cellular material is present on the adjacent surfaces. Magnification 45,000X.

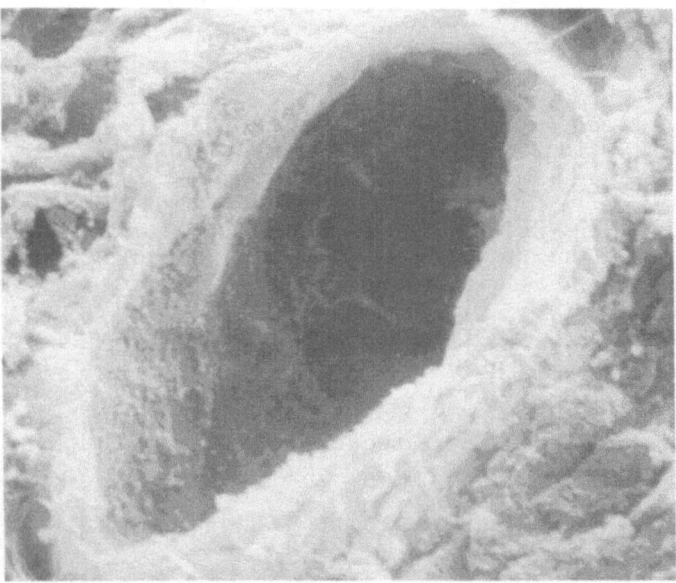

Fig. 11. Two hours after injury, a white matter vessel, 3 cm distal to the point of impact, contains adherent non-cellular material on its endothelial lining. Magnification 8,700X.

CONCLUSIONS

There is *chemical* evidence that pathologic free radical reactions occur in the spinal cord as early as one hour after impact injury and progress so as to lead to the destruction of the membrane lipids, phospholipids, and cholesterol. *Biochemical* enzyme assays have shown that a variety of membrane enzymes have decreased activity following CNS trauma. *Scanning electron microscopy* confirms that one important group of cells, i.e., the endothelium of the spinal cord parenchymal microcirculation, show early injury to the plasma membranes that line the capillaries and other small vessels. This occurs at the impact site as early as one hour after injury, with a suggestion that some of the changes become progressively more severe two hours following the impact and extend proximally and distally.

These three parameters of degeneration, i.e., free radical damage to lipids, enzyme inhibitions, and microcirculatory damage, all have a potential for spreading above and below the actual impact site. This appears to be particularly true for the endothelial damage in the micro-circulatory bed. Therefore, these changes may be responsible for alterations in the level, several days after the acute injury, e.g., in a high thoracic injury, a cephalad extension into the cervical region would produce greater clinical losses. If the free radical damage to the cell membranes can be brought under control and if the blood supply can be kept normal, it may become possible to minimize the clinical losses.

REFERENCES

Brody, T.M., Akera, T., Bashink, S.I., Gubitz, R., and Lee, C.Y. Interaction of NaK-ATPase with chlorpromazine free radical compounds. *Ann. N.Y. Acad. Sci. 242:*527 (1974).

Campbell, J.B., DeCrescito, V., Tomasula, J.J., Demopoulos, H.B., Flamm, E.S., and Ransohoff, J. Experimental treatment of spinal cord contusion in the cat. *Surg. Neurol. 1:*102 (1973).

Cohen, G., and Heikkila, R.E. The generation of hydrogen peroxide, superoxide radical and hydroxy radical by β-hydroxy-dopamine, dialuric acid, and related cytotoxic agents. *J. Biol. Chem. 249:* 2447 (1974).

DeEstable-Puig, R.F., and Estable-Puig, J.F.: Brain cyst formation. A technique for SEM study of the central nervous system. Scanning Electron Microscopy/1975, IIT, Chicago, 1975, p. 282.

Demopoulos, H.B., Flamm, E.S., Seligman, M.L., Poser, R., Pietronigro, D.D., and Ransohoff, J. Molecular pathology of lipids in CNS membranes. In *Oxygen and Physiological Function*, ed. F.F Jöbsis, P.I.L., Dallas, 491 (1977).

Demopoulos, H.B. The basis of free radical pathology. *Fed. Proc. 32:* 1859 (1973).

Demopoulos, H.B. Control of free radicals in biologic systems. *Fed. Proc. 32:*1903 (1973).

Demopoulos, H.B., Flamm, E.S., Seligman, M.L., Jorgensen, E., and Ransohoff, J. Antioxidant effect of barbiturates in model membranes undergoing free radical damage. *Acta Neurol. Scand., Suppl. 64, 56:*152 (1977).

Demopoulos, H.B., Flamm, E.S., Seligman, M.L., Mitamura, J., and Ransohoff, J. Membrane perturbations in CNS injury. In *Third Chicago Symposium on Neural Trauma*, Bourke, R., ed., Raven Press, New York, 1978 (in Press).

Dohrmann, G.J., Wagner, F.C., Jr., and Bucy, P.C. Transitory traumatic paraplegia. Electron microscopy of early alterations in myelinated nerve fibers. *J. Neurosurg. 36:*407 (1972).

Ducker, T.B., Kindt, G.W., and Kempe, L.G. Pathological findings in acute experimental spinal cord trauma. *J. Neurosurg. 35:*700 (1971).

Editorial: The prevention of thrombosis. *The Lancet*, p. 127, January 15, 1977.

Fischer, V.W., and Nelson, J.S. Cerebrovascular changes in tocopherol-depleted chicks fed linoleic acid. *J. Neuropath. Exp. Neurol. 32:* 474 (1973).

Flamm, E.S., Kim, J., Lin, J., and Ransohoff, J. Phosphodiesterase inhibitors and cerebral vasospasm. *Arch. Neurol. 32:*569 (1975).

Flamm, E.S., Demopoulos, H.B., Seligman, M.L., Tomasula, J.J., DeCrescito, V., and Ransohoff, J. Ethanol potentiation of central nervous system trauma. *J. Neurosurg. 46:*328 (1977).

Flamm, E.S., Demopoulos, H.B., Seligman, M.L., and Ransohoff, J. Possible mechanisms of barbiturate-mediated protection in regional cerebral ischemia. *Acta Neurol. Scand., Suppl. 64, 56:*150 (1977).

Fourcans, B., and Jain, M.H. Role of phospholipids in transport and enzymic reactions. *Adv. Lipid Res. 147* (1974).

Fridovich, I. Duke University, personal communication, 1977.

Gertz, S.D., Rennels, M.L., Forbes, M.S., Kawamura, J., Sunaga, T., and Nelson, E. Endothelial cell damage by temporary arterial occlusion with surgical slips: Study of the clip site by scanning and transmission electron microscopy. *J. Neurosurg. 45:*514 (1976).

Griffiths, I.R.   Spinal cord blood flow after acute experimental cord injury in dogs.   *J. Neurol. Sci. 27:*247 (1976).

Gryglewski, R.J., Bunting, S., Moncada, S., Flower, R.J., and Vane, J.R.   Arterial walls are protected against deposition of platelet thrombi by a substance (prostaglandin X) which they make from prostaglandin endoperoxides.   *Prostaglandins 12:*685 (1976).

Hamberg, M., and Samuelsson, B.   Prostaglandin endoperoxides. Novel transformation of arachidonic acid in human platelets.   *Proc. Nat. Acad. Sci. 71:*3400 (1974).

Kellog, E.W., and Fridovich, I.   Liposome oxidation and erythrocyte lysis by enzymatically generated superoxide radical and hydrogen peroxide.   *J. Biol. Chem. 252:*6721 (1977).

Kobrine, A.I.   The neuronal theory of experimental traumatic spinal cord dysfunction.   *Surg. Neurol. 3:*261 (1975).

Kolata, G.B.   Thromboxanes: The power behind the prostaglandins?   *Science 190:*770 (1975).

Lamola, A.A., Yamane, T., and Trozzola, A.M.   Cholesterol hydroperoxide formation in red blood cell membranes and photohemolysis in erythropoietic protoporphyria.   *Science 179:*1131 (1973).

Lawrence, J.H., Loomis, W.F., Tobias, C.A., and Turpin, F.H. Preliminary observations on the narcotic effects of xenon with a review of values for solubilities of gases in water and oils.   *J. Physiol. 105:*197 (1946).

Michael, B.D., Adams, G.E., Hewitt, H.B., Jones, W.B.G., and Watts, M.E.   A post effect of oxygen in irradiated bacteria: A submillisecond fast mixing study.   *Rad. Res. 54:*239 (1973).

Milvy, P., Kakari, S., Campbell, J.B., and Demopoulos, H.B.   Paramagnetic species and radical products in cat spinal cord.   *Ann. N.Y. Acad. Sci. 222:*1102 (1973).

Milvy, P., Kakari, S., Campbell, J.B., and Demopoulos, H.B.   Paramagnetic species and radical products in cat spinal cord.   *Ann. N.Y. Acad. Sci. 222:*1102 (1973).

Mitamura, J.A., Seligman, M.L., Flamm, E.S., Ioppolo, A., and Demopoulos, H.B.   Loss of cholesterol and ascorbic acid in rat brain following cold trauma and protection by methylprednisolone. Presented at the Annual Meeting of the American Association of Neurological Surgeons, Toronto, Canada, 1977, and submitted to *Brain Research*.

Moncada, S., Gryglewski, R.J., Bunting, S., and Vane, J.R.   A lipid peroxide inhibits the enzyme in blood vessel microsomes that generates from prostaglandin endoperoxides the substance (prostaglandin X) which prevents platelet aggregation.   *Prostaglandins 12:*715 (1976).

Moncada, S., Gryglewski, R.J., Bunting, S., and Vane, J.R.   A lipid peroxide inhibits the enzyme in blood vessel microsomes that generates from prostaglandin endoperoxides the substance (prostaglandin X) which prevents platelet aggregation.   *Prostaglandins 12:*715 (1976).

Nelson, E., Gertz, S.D., Rennels, M.L., Ducker, T.B., and Blaumanis, O.R.   Spinal cord injury: The role of vascular damage in the pathogenesis of central hemorrhagic necrosis.   *Arch. Neurol. 34:*332 (1977).

Nelson, E., Sunager, T., Shimamoto, T., Kawamura, J., Rennels, M.L., and Hebel, R.   Ischemic aortid endothelium.   *Arch. Path. 99:*125 (1975).

Nilsson, B., Astrup, J., Blennow, G., and Siesjo, B.K.   Cerebral function and energy metabolism at critical thresholds of oxygen availability: A study in rats during status epilepticus induced by bicuculline. *Acta Neurol. Scand.*, *Suppl. 64, 56:* 112 (1977).

Ortega, B.D., Demopoulos, H.B., and Ransohoff, J. Effects of antioxidants on experimental cold-induced cerebral edema. In *Steroids and Brain Edema*, Reulen, H.J., and Schürmann, K., eds., Springer-Verlag, New York, 1972, p. 167.

Rap, Z.M., and Wideman, J. Changes in sulfhydryl group level and influence of exogenous glutathione on dynamics of vasogenic brain edema. In *Dynamics of Brain Edema*, Pappius, H.M., and Feindel, W., eds., Springer-Verlag, New York, 1976, p. 164.

Ruzicka, F.J., Beinert, H., Schepler, K.L., Dunham, W.R., and Sands, R.H. Interaction of ubisemiquinone with a paramagnetic component in heart tissue. *Proc. Nat. Acad. Sci. 72:* 2886 (1975).

Schaefer, A., Komlos, M., and Seregi, A. Lipid peroxidation as the cause of the ascorbic acid induced decrease of ATPase activities of rat brain microsomes and its inhibition by biogenic amines and psychotropic drugs. *Biochem. Pharmacol. 24:* 1781 (1975).

Seligman, M.L., Flamm, E.S., Goldstein, B., Poser, R., Demopoulos, H.B., and Ransohoff, J. Spectrofluorescent detection of malonaldehyde as a measure of lipid free radical damage in response to ethanol potentiation of spinal cord trauma. *Lipids 12:* 945 (1977).

Seligman, M.L., Flamm, E.S., Goldstein, B., Poser, R., Demopoulos, H.B., and Ransohoff, J. Spectrofluorescent detection of malonaldehyde as a measure of lipid free radical damage in response to ethanol potentiation of spinal cord trauma. *Lipids 12:* 945 (1977).

Spector, R. Vitamin homeostasis in the central nervous system. *New Eng. J. Med. 296:* 1393 (1977).

Sjostrand, F.S. *Electron Microscopy of Cells and Tissues. Vol. I.* Academic Press, New York, 1967, p. 155.

Stossel, T.P., Mason, R.J., and Smith, A.L. Lipid peroxidation by human blood phagocytes. *J. Clin. Invest. 54:* 638 (1974).

Suwa, K., Kimura, T., and Schaap, P.A.P. *Biochem. Biophys. Res. Comm. 75:* 785 (1977).

Suzuki, O., and Yagi, K. Formation of lipoperozide in brain edema induced by cold injury. *Experienta 30:* 248 (1974).

Tappel, A.L. Biocatalysis: Lipoxidase and hematic compounds. In *Autoxidation and Antioxidants*, W.O. Lundberg, ed. Interscience, New York, 1961, p. 325.

Terifumi, I., Allen, N., and Yashon, D. A mitochondrial lesion in experimental spinal cord trauma. *J. Neurosurg. 48:* 434 (1978).

Wideman, J., and Domanska-Janik, K. Regulation of thiols in the brain. 1. Concentration of thiols and glutathione reductase activity in different parts of the rat brain during hypoxia. *Resuscitation 3:* 27 (1974).

White, A., Handler, P., and Smith, E.L. *Principles of Biochemistry.* McGraw-Hill, New York, 1973, p. 356.

SECTION TWO

Sequelae of Spinal Cord Injury: Possible Mechanisms of Spasticity and Pain Perception

5

Changes in the CNS Biogenic Amines and Tyrosine Hydroxylase Activity After Spinal Cord Transection in the Rat

N.E. NAFTCHI, A.K. KIRSCHNER, M. DEMENY, and A. VIAU

ABSTRACT

In 134 male Wistar rats weighing 250-350g, the spinal cord was transected between the fifth and sixth thoracic vertebra. In the spinal cord above the lesion, concentrations of norepinephrine and serotonin increased three and twofold, respectively, compared with control levels. Below the lesion, however, the levels of these amines decreased significantly, and, after seven to twelve days, their concentrations were undetectable. In the brain stem, starting at seven days after transection, norepinephrine, serotonin, and histamine concentrations were sharply higher than those of controls. In the brain, during the first 24 hours, there were sharp fluctuations in serotonin, norepinephrine, and histamine concentrations; after which time, serotonin and histamine reached the control levels. Norepinephrine levels, however, dropped sharply at seven days and returned to normal levels thereafter. In the heart, the concentrations of serotonin dropped significantly to less than 40%, and those of norepinephrine and histamine dropped to less than 70% of the control. In the brain stem and adrenals, tyrosine hydroxylase activity reached a peak (two and fourfold increase, respectively) five days after spinal cord transection. The activity in the brain, however, reached a maximum (twofold above control) seven days after transection. Adrenal enzyme activity was still twice that of control, seven to thirty days after transection. In the spinal cord, changes in the enzyme activity were negligible at all times. Fluctuations in cyclic adenosine 3',5'-monophosphate levels were similar to those of tyrosine hydroxylase activity except that in the adrenals, there was a tenfold increase in its concentration five minutes following spinal cord transection.

The increase in tyrosine hydroxylase activity in the brain and brain stem may be partly due to curtailed end-product feedback inhibition and partly to reduced receptor activation. The sustained induction of the adrenal medullary tyrosine hydroxylase is probably a consequence of a continual stimulation of splanchnic nerve, resulting in de novo enzyme synthesis as indicated by the marked increase in c-AMP concentrations in the adrenals.

INTRODUCTION

Our work in spinal cord injured subjects demonstrated a faulty regulation of catecholamine metabolism. Furthermore, during hypertensive crises in quadriplegic subjects, there was an increased excretion of catecholamine metabolites and enhanced serum dopamine-β-hydroxylase (DPH) activity (Naftchi et al., 1972; Naftchi et al., 1973; Naftchi et al., 1974; Naftchi et al., 1978). In order to elucidate the biochemical events underlying some of the pathophysiologic manifestations after spinal cord injury, a study of monoaminergic dysfunctions in an animal model was undertaken.

Several models of spinal cord injury have been used in order to assess the short-term acute effects of trauma to the spinal cord (Naftchi et al., 1974; Doppman and Zivin, 1976; Osterholm and Mathews, 1972). Severe trauma to the spinal cord in humans and animals leads to immediate curtailment of propagation of action potential and the so-called neurologic transection of the spinal cord and, ultimately, to scar formation. Therefore, the complete neurologic transection depends on the adequacy of traumatic force to produce irreversible damage. To avoid possible criticism associated with such models and to assure reproducibility of the results over a long-term longitudinal study of the biochemical sequelae of transverse myelopathy, after laminectomy, the spinal cord was raised and transected.

Tyrosine hydroxylase (tyrosine 3-monoxygenase, EC1.10.3.1) activity in adrenergic neurons and in the adrenal medulla is modulated by the activity of sympathetic nerves. The mechanism of control of the activity of this enzyme involves release of neurotransmitter, activation of adenylate cyclase, and synthesis of molecular structural components of the enzyme. This study was intended, therefore, to determine the effect of spinal cord transection on the activity of tyrosine hydroxylase and the fate of the putative neurotransmitters, norepinephrine, serotonin, and histamine, and the changes in cyclic adenosine 3',5'-monophosphate (c-AMP) concentration in the central nervous system and other vital organs.

METHODS

One hundred and thirty-four male Wistar rats[1] weighing 250-350g were anesthetized with 30-40mg/kg Nembutal (Sodium Pentobarbitol).[2] After laminectomy, the spinal cord was gently raised by means of a glass probe and transected at the level of thoracic fifth vertebra. After the operation, each animal, including the sham-operated controls, received 15,000 i.u. of penicillin[3] for three days. The urinary bladder was expressed twice daily for approximately a week until automatic voiding was resumed. Animals were sacrificed by decapitation; all organs (spinal cord, brain, brain stem, heart, and adrenals) were removed in a temperature-controlled room (4°C) and stored at -20°C, if not used immediately.

---

[1] Charles River, 251 Ballard Vale Street, Wilmington, Massachusetts, 01887.

[2] Abbott Laboratories, North Chicago, Illinois, 60064

[3] Squibb, Lawrenceville-Princeton Road, P.O. Box 4000, Princeton, New Jersey, 08540

Analysis of the Biogenic Amines

Methods for determination of biogenic amines were based on several fluorometric techniques described previously (Naftchi et al., 1974; Doppman and Zivin, 1976; Osterholm and Mathews, 1972). The frozen tissue samples were homogenized on ice in acidified butanol. After centrifugation, norepinephrine (NE), dopamine (DA), serotonin (5-HT), and histamine were extracted from the organic phase into water phase and quantitated by fluorometry.

Determination of Tyrosine Hydroxylase (TH) Activity

The tissue was homogenized in 10 volumes of double distilled water and centrifuged at 2,500g for 30 minutes. The supernatant was recentrifuged at 11,000g for one hour. The new supernatant was used for the enzyme assay.

Tyrosine Hydroxylase activity was measured by the modification (Musacchio and Wurzburger) of the methods of Nagatsu and Udenfriend (1964) and Ikeda (1966). The substrate L-tyrosine (3',5'-H[3]; ^{3}H-tyr, specific activity 50 Ci mM)[e] was purified before each procedure. Measurement of adenosine 3',5'-cyclic monophosphate (c-AMP): Tissue samples were rapidly excised, homogenized in 1ml of ice cold 5% trichloracetic acid and centrifuged for 15 minutes at 1,500 g and $0°C$. The supernatants were extracted with ether, dried, dissolved in 50mM sodium acetate/acetic acid buffer pH 4.5, and analyzed for c-AMP, using the protein binding radioassay of Gilman (1970). The only modification consisted of using sodium acetate/acetic acid buffer pH 4.5 instead of pH 4.0 (Brastom and Kon, 1974). A standard binding curve ranging from 0.4 to 8.0 pmoles of c-AMP was determined with every experiment. The linear portion of the standard curve was between 0.6 and 7.0 pmoles of c-AMP. All the samples were assayed in duplicate. Inter- and intra-assay variations for this method in 10 samples were 5.9% and 7.2%, respectively.

Protein content in the samples was determined on the trichloracetic acid precipitate that was dissolved in 1N sodium hydroxide, using the method of Lowry (1951).

All general chemicals were purchased from Fisher Scientific Co.[4], c-AMP from Sigma,[5] and tritiated c-AMP (22 c/mM) from New England Nuclear.[6] Statistical Analysis: The Students's "t" test was used for comparison of the results obtained from experimental and sham-operated animals. Only the probability values that were less than 5% (p<0.05) were considered significant.

RESULTS

Fate of Biogenic Amines in the Spinal Cord

Norepinephrine

One half hour after transection of the spinal cord, the concentration of NE increased sharply in the segment above the level of transection (Figure 1A). One hour after transection it decreased to almost control

---

[4] Fisher Scientific Company, 52 Fadem Road, Springfield, New Jersey.

[5] Sigma Chemical, PO Box 14508, St. Louis, Missouri.

[6] New England Nuclear, 549 Albany Street, Boston, Massachusetts.

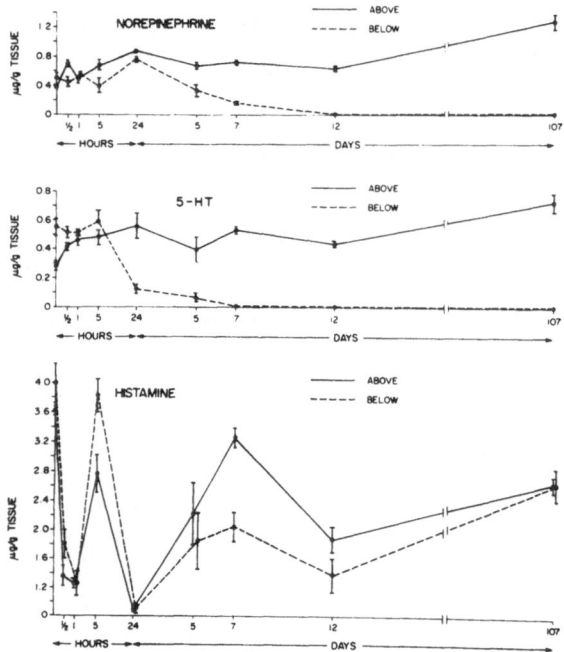

CONCENTRATIONS OF NOREPINEPHRINE ,5-HT, AND HISTAMINE
IN THE SPINAL CORD ABOVE AND BELOW THE LEVEL OF
TRANSECTION AT THE 5TH THORACIC DERMATOME IN RAT.

Fig. 1. Concentration of Norepinephrine, 5-HT and Histamine in the spinal cord above and below the level of transaction at the fifth thoracic vertebra rat. Each point represents the mean ± SEM of four to six samples. Figures 1A and 1B are good illustrations of axoplasmic transport of norepinephrine and 5-HT in the spinal cord. Both these substances accumulate in the spinal cord above the level of transection and decrease in the portion below the transection, indicating a disruption of axoplasmic transport. Histamine (Figure 1C), however, is not only neuronal in origin but also mast cell in origin; therefore, it does not behave the same.

values but increased gradually thereafter, reaching the concentration three times higher than that of the controls 107 days later.

At 24 hours after transection, the NE content of the spinal cord below the level of transection had increased twofold to a concentration approximately equal to that above the level of transection. Norepinephrine levels decreased significantly thereafter and were undetectable 12 days following the transection of the spinal cord.

Serotonin

Twenty-four hours after transection of the spinal cord, 5-HT concentration above the level of transection had sharply increased and was three times greater than that of controls 107 days later (Figure 1B). Below the lesion, 5-HT concentration remained relatively unchanged within the first five hours but dropped sharply to one-fourth of the control value 24 hours after transection. Seven days after transection,

5-HT was not detectable in the distal stump of the spinal cord.

Histamine

Unlike NE and 5-HT, concentrations of histamine in the spinal
cord above and below the transection followed a similar pattern (Figure
1C). There was an approximate threefold decrease in histamine content
one-half to one hour after spinal cord transection, followed by a return
to control levels five hours after transection and by a fourfold decrease
24 hours after transection. Histamine content of the rostral and caudal
portions of the spinal cord reached a peak on the seventh day. Although
histamine content of the caudal segment was higher than that of the
rostral at five hours after spinal cord lesion, the content of the latter
segment was significantly greater than that of the former at the seventh
and twelfth days after the transection. Both segments contained
approximately equal amounts of histamine 107 days after the lesion.

Fate of NE in brain, brain stem, and heart

One hour after transection, brain NE dropped sharply and reached
its lowest level seven days after transection (approximately 45% of
control concentrations). Between 12 and 107 days after the transection,
NE concentration remained markedly low and was 40% below that of the
controls (Figure 2).

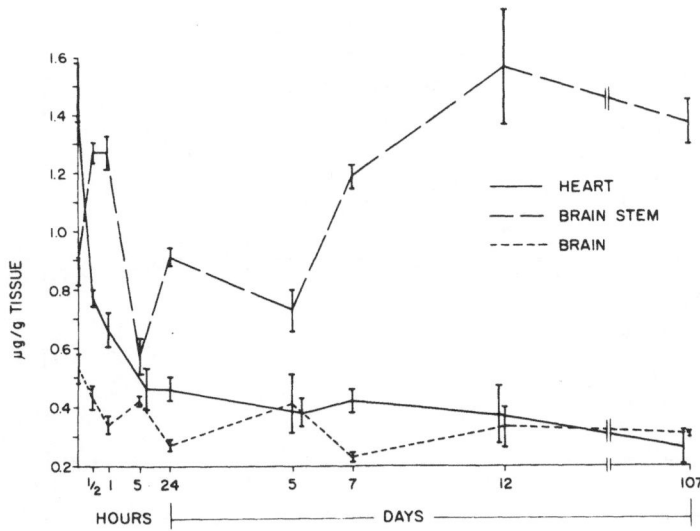

Fig. 2. Norepinephrine concentration in the brain, brain stem, and
heart after spinal cord transection at the fifth thoracic vertebra in rat.
Each point represents the mean ± SEM of four to six samples. Brain
tissue includes the two cerebral hemispheres and the cerebellum, while
the brain stem included diencephalon, midbrain, pons, and medulla.

Concentrations of NE in brain stem rose sharply one-half hour after
transection, decreasing to below control levels five hours after transection.

Norepinephrine concentration increased thereafter and was significantly higher at seven days after transection. At 12 and 107 days after transection, it was approximately 40% above that of controls (Figure 2).

The NE concentration in the heart was about 50% of that in controls, one-half hour after transection (Figure 2). Five hours after transection, only 30% of the original concentration was detectable. At 107 days after transection, myecardial NE concentration had further decreased to less than 20% of the control levels (Figure 2).

Fate of Serotonin in brain, brain stem, and heart

Concentration of 5-HT in the brain and brain stem followed a similar pattern (Figure 3). After one-half hour, 5-HT in the brain and brain stem increased, and, at five hours, it decreased sharply. Thereafter, the concentration of 5-HT increased in both tissues, reaching control levels in the brain. In the brain stem, however, 5-HT continued to increase, and, at 107 days after transection, its concentration was twice that of controls. Serotonin concentration in the heart fell almost immediately after transection. At seven and 12 days after transection, 5-HT level was 40% below the control and had decreased to 50% of control 107 days after transection (Figure 3).

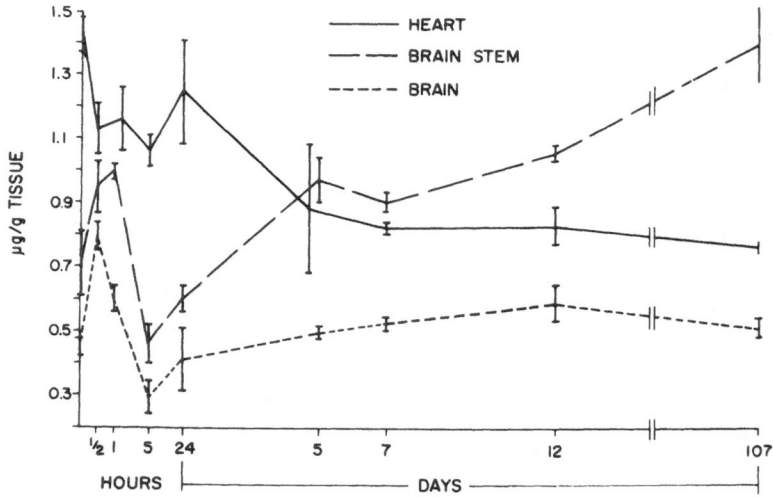

SEROTONIN (5 HT) CONCENTRATION IN BRAIN, BRAIN STEM AND HEART AFTER SPINAL CORD TRANSECTION AT THE 5th THORACIC DERMATOME IN RAT.

Fig. 3. Serotonin (5-HT) concentration in the brain, brain stem, and heart after spinal cord transection at the fifth thoracic vertebra in the rat. Each point represents the mean ± SEM of four to five samples. Brain tissue includes the two cerebral hemispheres and the cerebellum, while the brain stem includes the diencephalon, midbrain, pons, and medulla.

Fate of Histamine in brain, brain stem, and heart

The concentration of histamine in the brain decreased by 50% one hour after transection but within the control range 24 hours after transection.   There was no significant change between 24 hours and seven days, after which time the levels decreased.   Histamine concentrations were less than 40% of those of controls 107 days after transection (Figure 4).

Brain stem concentrations of histamine did not change appreciably during the first five days after transection.   The concentrations, at 12 and 107 days, were significantly higher than those of the controls.

Myocardial histamine concentrations, similar to those of NE and 5-HT, dropped sharply from control values; 12 and 107 days after transection they were about 35% and 30%, respectively, of the control levels, (Figure 4).

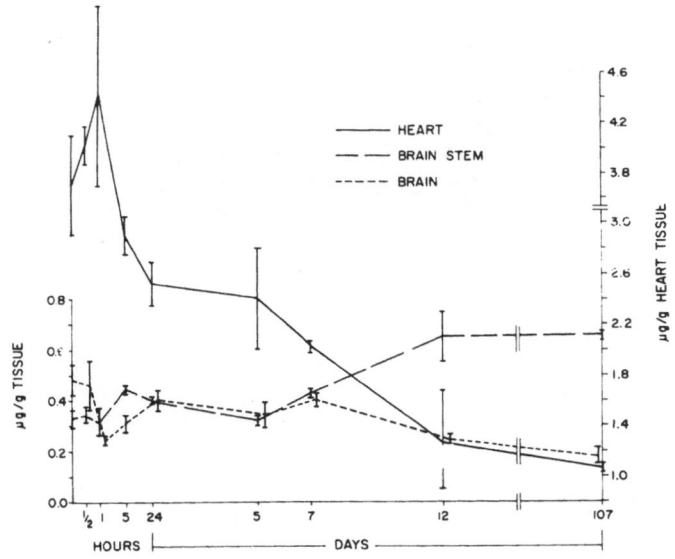

Fig. 4. Histamine concentration in the brain, brain stem, and heart after spinal cord transection at the fifth thoracic vertebra in the rat. Each point represents the mean ± SEM of four to six samples. Brain tissue includes the two cerebral hemispheres and the cerebellum, while the brain stem includes the diencephalon, midbrain, pons, and medulla.

Tyrosine Hydroxylase activity in brain, brain stem, and adrenals

Tyrosine hydroxylase (TH) activity in the brain, brain stem, and adrenals was elevated as early as 24 hours after transection of the spinal cord.   Enzyme activity maxima in brain stem and adrenals were reached at five days.   The increase in TH activity was greater than twofold in brain stem and fourfold in the adrenal glands, compared with the control levels (Figure 5).   Brain TH activity peaked five to seven days after transection when it was twofold higher than that of controls.   Thereafter, brain and brain stem TH activity dropped. Twelve and 20 days after transection, the activity was still 40% greater than that of controls, but, 30 days after transection, it had decreased to approximately control levels. Following maximum activity on the fifth day, adrenal TH activity dropped sharply, and, at seven days after transection, it reached a plateau at a level twice that of the control and remained unchanged 20 and 30 days after transection (Figure 5).

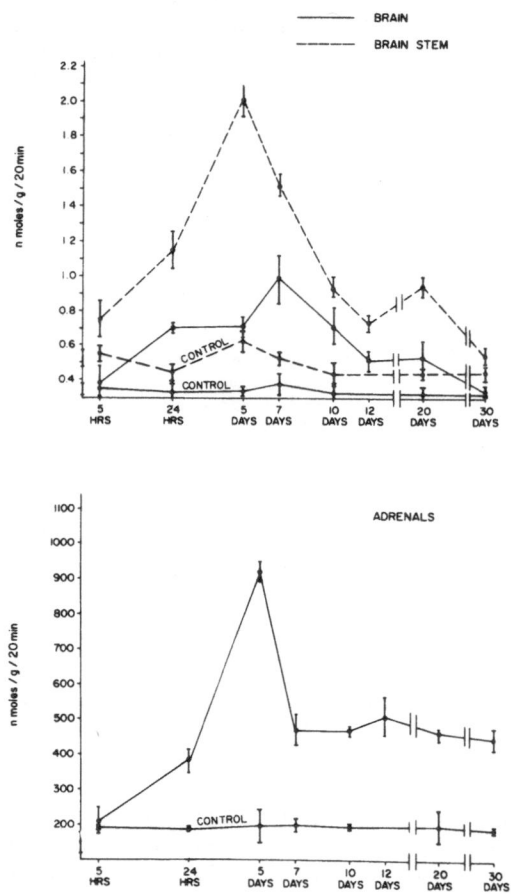

Fig. 5. Tyrosine hydroxylase activity in the brain, brain stem, and adrenals after spinal cord transection at the fifth thoracic vertebra in the rat. Each point represents the mean ± SEM of four to ten samples. All assays were performed immediately after sacrificing the animals without freezing the tissue. Tyrosine hydroxylase activity in the spinal cord was undetectable using this assay.

Cyclic AMP concentrations in the brain, brain stem, spinal cord, heart, and adrenals

Within five minutes after the transection of the spinal cord, c-AMP levels in the brain and brain stem increased by more than twofold, and those of adrenal glands rose by tenfold (Figure 6).   The levels decreased markedly in the brain two days after transection of the spinal cord and in brain stem and adrenals one day after transection.   In all three tissues, there was an increase in c-AMP concentration five days after spinal cord transection.   Seven days after transection of the spinal cord, however, c-AMP concentrations returned to control levels.   The concentration of c-AMP in the spinal cord and the heart did not change appreciable after spinal cord lesion (Figure 6).

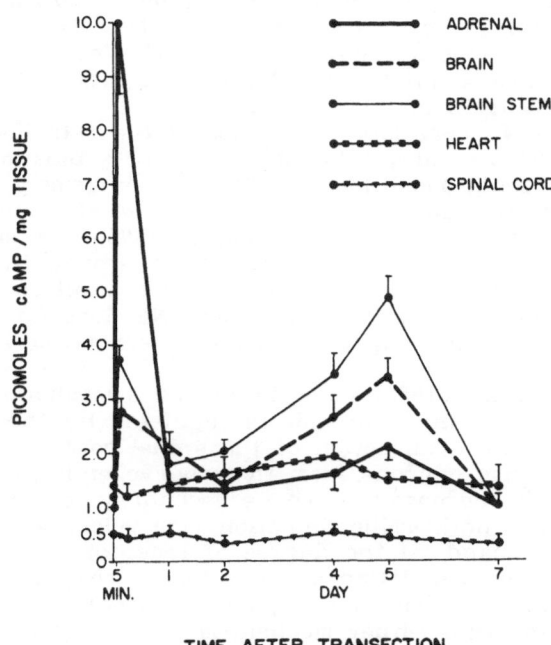

Fig. 6.   Cyclic AMP concentrations after transection of the spinal cord at the fifth thoracic vertebra.   Each point represents the mean ± SEM of four to six samples.   Note the dramatic increase in c-AMP levels in the adrenals five minutes after transection.

DISCUSSION

Most monoaminergic neuronal pathways in the spinal cord are descending (Andeu et al., 1964; Carlsson et al., 1964; Carlsson et al., 1972; Carlisson et al., 1973).   Therefore, transection of the spinal cord will interrupt communication between cell bodies in the brain and the nerve terminals that are located below the level of the lesion.

In the present study, serotonin and norepinephrine concentrations in the spinal cord decreased to undetectable amounts below the level of transection.   Norepinephrine concentrations underwent a few changes during the first 24 hours and thereafter declined sharply (Figure 1A).   In the distal stump, concentrations of serotonin, however, fell more sharply than those of norepinephrine, especially from five to 24 hours after transection (Figure 1B).   The time course of disappearance of

5-HT in this study is in agreement with that of Anden (1964) and Carlsson (1973), who reported a sharp fall in 5-HT three days after transection and undetectable levels five days after. Our results of the changes in NE concentrations were also similar to those found by these investigators.

In contrast, the concentrations of 5-HT and NE increased in the spinal cord above the level of transection. Synthesis of these amines originates in the brain stem neurons. Therefore, their accumulation in the rostral portion of the spinal cord and disappearance in the caudal stump is due to the disruption of proximo-distal axoplasmic transport. However, since histamine in the spinal cord is partly neuronal and partly mast cell in origin, the changes in its concentrations in the spinal cord were the same both above and below the level of transection. The loss of 30% of histamine in the spinal cord may reflect the loss of neuronal histamine (Figure 1 and Figure 4).

Do the changes in NE correlate with those of the rate-limiting enzyme (Levitt et al., 1965; Sato et al., 1967) involved in its biosynthesis? The amount of free cytoplasmic NE in the brain is extremely small due to the high activity of monoamine oxidase and to the efficiency of the granular uptake and storage mechanism (Weiner, 1975). A small chemically undetectable compartment of free intraneuronal NE is critical in the regulation of NE biosynthesis, however, this small compartment is depleted during nerve stimulation; therefore, NE does not exert any feedback inhibition during prolonged adrenergic nervous activity (Alousi and Weiner, 1966).

Carlsson and Lindqvist (1963) have suggested a mechanism of feedback control by which catecholamine synthesis is regulated by the degree of receptor activation. After transection of the spinal cord, owing to isolation of the brain stem neurons from their nerve endings, nerve stimulation frequency is increased, perhaps secondary to carotid sinus activation, which causes both amine depletion (via release) and TH induction. On the other hand, if the degree of receptor activation is partly responsible for the regulation of tyrosine hydroxylase activity, the sustained elevation of NE may be in part a consequence of decreased receptor activation and, thus either mechanism may regulate tyrosine hydroxylase activity or both.

Our results show that soon after transection of the spinal cord, norepinephrine levels in the brain and brain stem decreased, whereas tyrosine hydroxylase activity began to increase. When norepinephrine concentration was very low, tyrosine hydroxylase activity reached a peak. Norepinephrine levels continued to rise until levels greater than control were reached, while tyrosine hydroxylase activity in the brain stem returned to and remained at control levels. In addition, the high levels of norephinephrine were maintained in the spinal cord above the lesion and in the brain stem 107 days after transection (Figure 1 and Figure 2). The increase in NE in the spinal cord and brain stem at the time when tyrosine hydroxylase activity in the brain stem was normal may be explained on the basis of normal NE synthesis and transport by axoplasmic flow and its continual accumulation in the rostral stump.

Administration of drugs that interfere with post-ganglionic sympathetic transmission is believed to produce an increase in pre-ganglionic sympathetic impulse frequency. The latter would trigger a reflex increase in the activity of the sympatho-adrenal system (Iggo and Vogt, 1960; Dontao and Nickerson, 1957), accompanied by an increased release of neurotransmitter and a quick rise in catecholamine synthesis (Gordon et al., 1966; Dairman et al., 1968). Moreover, any condition which impairs post-ganglionic sympathetic transmission over a prolonged period elicits an increase in tyrosine hydroxylase activity in adrenals, sympathetic ganglia and brain stem of various species (Sedrall and Kopin, 1967; Meuller et al., 1964; Mueller et al., 1969). Since the rise in tyrosine hydroxylase activity is abolished by adrenal denervation, the increase is, therefore, mediated through the augmented activity of the splanchnic nerves and is termed "trans-synaptic" induction (Theonen et al., 1969). The trans-synaptic induction of tyrosine hydroxylase occurs after a time latency from the termination of the inducing stimulus when the intermediate steps, that are involved in the enzyme induction have transformed the increase in sympathetic activity into an increase in protein synthesis (Costa et al., 1974; Kurosawa et al., 1976).

Induction of adrenal tyrosine hydroxylase is preceded by an increase in adrenal medullary adenosine 3',5'-cyclic monophosphate (c-AMP) (Costa et al., 1974; Kurosawa et al., 1976; Waymere et al., 1971; McKay and Iverson, 1972; Kvetnansky et al., 1971). Five minutes after transection of the spinal cord at the level of T5-6 (Figure 6), c-AMP level in the adrenals was increased tenfold, and its concentration in the brain and brain stem was elevated twofold. The immediate rise in c-AMP probably reflects the release of biogenic amines from the CNS and catecholamines from the adrenal medulla as a response to the stress from the spinal cord transection. Five days after the cord lesion, there was a twofold elevation of c-AMP in the brain and a fourfold increase in the brain stem and adrenals. The trans-synaptic induction of tyrosine hydroxylase in the brain stem lasted for 20 days. The peak of enzyme activity in the brain was lowest at 24 hours and seven days and, in the brain stem, was lowest at 24 hours and five days (Figure 2) after spinal cord transection. Tyrosine hydroxylase activity in these tissues peaked at the same times. The latter findings suggest the presence of *in vivo* mechanism for end-product inhibition of tyrosine hydroxylase activity by norepinephrine as an immediate short duration regulatory mechanism for the biosynthesis of NE (Gordon et al., 1966).

Following maximum activity five days after spinal cord transection, the adrenal tyrosine hydroxylase activity reached a plateau seven days after and remained at the same level, twofold above the control enzyme activity, for 30 days after spinal cord lesion. Therefore, transection of the spinal cord at the level of T5 vertebra had elicited a continual increase in splanchnic nerve activity and a sustained transsynaptic induction of the adrenal tyrosine hydroxylase (Figure 5). The increased activity of splanchnic nerve is probably due to curtailed spinal and supraspinal inhibitory influences, causing a facilitation of reflexes below the level of the spinal cord transection. Furthermore, since the splanchnic fibers originate in part from the thoracic nerve roots, it is possible that pre-ganglionic input was not completely interrupted, and thus through adrenals may reflect the enhanced sympathetic activity rostral to the lesion; in order to abolish neurogenic stimulation of the adrenal medulae, Carlsson and Lindqvist (1973) had to transect the spinal cord at C7.

The disappearance of serotonin from the distal stump may also be partially responsible for or synergistically potentiate the induction of the activity of this enzyme in the adrenals, since interference with serotonergic nerve function potentiates trans-synaptic induction of adrenal tyrosine hydroxylase (McKay and Iverson, 1972). Inhibition of serotonin synthesis produces hypertension, implying an inhibitory effect of serotonergic nerves on peripheral sympatho-adrenal function (Ito and Schanberg, 1972). Electrophysiological studies have also demonstrated that intravenous serotonin administration results in a depression of sympathetic reflexes in the spinal cat (Have et al., 1972). Therefore, these nerves may normally suppress peripheral sympathetic nervous activity (Baumgarten et al., 1971; Koe and Weissman, 1966).

Almost immediately after transection, there is a decrease in the activity of tryptophan hydroxylase below the lesion (Carlsson et al., 1973). This reduced enzyme activity was attributed to a loss of impulse flow rather than any enzyme loss resulting from degeneration of the serotonergic fiber system. In our study, the sudden decrease in serotonin content of the distal stump, five to 24 hours after transection of the spinal cord (Figure 1B), coincides with the sharp fall in tryptopha: hydroxylase activity (Carlsson et al., 1973). The continual decrease in the concentration and the eventual disappearance of serotonin seven to nine days after transection probably results from the cessation of the proximo-distal axoplasmic flow, transporting 5-HT from the cell bodies of serotonergic neurons (Dahlstrom, 1971) and/or degeneration of the serotonergic fiber system below the lesion. The decrease in tryptophan hydroxylase activity in the distal stump cannot be due to end-product inhibition since high concentrations of serotonin have not been found to inhibit the enzyme activity *in vitro* (Jequier et al., 1969). The increase in 5-HT concentration above the transection level is probably due to continual synthesis and, to the transport of serotonin from the brain stem and its accumulation in the proximal stump of the spinal cord.

Spinal cord transection resulted in a 70% loss of the heart's norepinephrine content (Figure 2). Adrenal tyrosine hydroxylase activity, however, increased to levels twice those of control. Depletion of cardiac NE that was due to spinal cord transection has not been reported previously. It may represent an increased NE stimulation of spinal cord sympathetic outflow above the lesion. Without turnover studies, however, the significance of this finding will remain unclear.

REFERENCES

Alousi, A., and Weiner, N. The regulation of norepinephrine synthesis in sympathetic nerves. Effect of nerve stimulation, cocaine and calcium releasing agents. *Nat. Acad. Sci. 56:*1491-1496 (1966).

Anden, N.E., Haggendal, J., Magnusson, T., and Rosengrin, E. The time course of disappearance of norepinephrine and 5-hydroxytryptamine in the spinal cord after transection. *Acta. Physiol. Scand. 62:*115-118 (1964).

Baumgarten, H.G., Bjorklund, A., Lachenmayer, L., Nobin, A., and Stenevi, U. Long-lasting selective depletion of brain serotonin by 5,6-dihydroxytryptamine. *Acta. Physiol. Scand. (Suppl.) 373:* 1-15 (1971).

Brostom, C.O., and Kon, C. An improved protein binding assay for cyclic-AMP. *Analytical Biochem. 58:*459-468 (1974).

Carlsson, A., Kehr, W., Lindqvist, M., Magnusson, T., and Atack, C.V. Regulation of monoamine metabolism in the central nervous system. *Pharmac. Rev. 24:*371-383 (1972).

Carlsson, A., and Lindqvist, M. Effect of chlorpromazine or haloperidol on formation of 3-methoxytyramine and normetanephrine in mouse brain. *Acta. Pharmak. Toxicol. 20:*140-144 (1963).

Carlsson, A., Falck, B., Fuxe, K., Hillarp, N.A. Cellular localization of monoamines in the spinal cord. *Acta. Physiol. Scand. 60:*112-119 (1964).

Carlsson, A., Lindqvist, M., Magnusson, T., and Atack, C.V. Effect of acute transection on the synthesis and turnover of 5-HT in the rat spinal cord. Nauyn-Schmiedeberg's *Arch. Pharmacol. 277:*1-12 (19

Costa, E., Guidotti, A., and Hanbauer, I.   Do cyclic nucleotides
    promote trans-synaptic induction of tyrosine hydroxylase?   *Life
    Sciences 14:*1169-1188 (1974).
Dahlstrom, A.   Axoplasmic transport (with particular respect to
    adrenergic neurons).   *Phil. Trans. Roy. Soc. Lond. B. 261:*325-
    358 (1971).
Dairman, W., Gordon, R., Spector, S., Sjoerdsma, A., and Udenfriend,
    S.   Increased synthesis of catecholamines in the intact rat following
    administration of β-adrenergic blocking agents.   *Mol. Pharmac. 4:*
    457-464 (1968).
Dontas, A.S., and Nickerson, M.   Central and peripheral components
    of the action of "ganglionic" blocking agents.   *J. Pharmac. Exp.
    Ther. 12:*147-159 (1957).
Doppman, J.L., Zivin, J.A.   A rapid non-operative technique for
    producing spinal cord injury in animals.   *Inves. Radiol. 11:*150-151
    (1976).
Gilman, A.G.   A protein binding assay for adenosine 3'5'-cyclic mono-
    phosphate.   *Proc. Nat. Acad. Sci. 67:*305-312 (1970).
Gordon, R., Reid, J.V.O., Sjoerdsman, A., and Udenfriend, S.
    Increased synthesis of norepinephrine in rat heart on electrical
    stimulation of stellate ganglia.   *Mol. Pharmac. 2:*610-613 (1966).
Gordon, R., Spector, S., Sjoerdsma, A., and Udenfriend, S.   Increased
    synthesis of norepinephrine and epinephrine in the intact rat
    during exercise and exposure to cold.   *J. Pharmac. Exp. Ther. 153:*
    440-447 (1966).
Have, B.D., Neumayer, R.J., and Franz, D.N.   Opposite effects of
    L-dopa and 5-hydroxytryptamine on spinal sympathetic reflexes.
    *Nature 239:*336-337 (1972).
Iggo, A., and Vogt, M.   Pre-ganglionic sympathetic activity in normal
    and reserpine treated cats.   *J. Physiol. (Lond.) 150:*114-133 (1960).
Ideda, M., Fahien, L.A., and Undenfriend, S.   A kinetic study of
    bovine adrenal tyrosine hydroxylase.   *J. Biol. Chem. 241:*4452-4456
    (1966).
Ito, A., and Schanberg, S.M.   Central nervous system mechanisms
    responsible for blood pressure elevation induced by p-chloropheny-
    lalanine.   *J. Pharmac. Exp. Ther. 181:*65-74 (1972).
Jequier, F., Robinson, D.S., Lovenberg, W., and Sjoerdsma, A.
    Further studies on tryptophan hydroxylase in rat brain stem and
    beef pineal.   *Biochem. Pharmac. 18:*1071-1081 (1969).
Koe, B.K., and Weissman, A.   p-Chlorophenylalanine: A specific
    depletor of brain serotonin.   *J. Pharmac. Exp. Ther. 154:*499-516
    (1966).
Kurosawa, A., Guidotti, A., and Costs, E.   Induction of tyrosine-3-
    monooxygenase in adrenal medulla: role of protein kinase activation
    and translocation.   *Science 193:*691-693 (1976).
Kvetnansky, R., Gewirtz, G.P., Weise, V.K., and Kopin, I.J.   Effect
    of dibutyryl cyclic AMP on adrenal catecholamine synthesizing
    enzymes in repeated immobilized hypophysectomized rats.   *Endocrinology
    89:*50-55 (1971).
Levitt, M., Spector, S., Sjoerdsma, A., and Udenfriend, S.   Elucidation
    of the rate-limiting step in norepinephrine biosynthesis in the
    prefused guinea pig heart.   *J. Pharmac. Exp. Ther. 148:*1-8 (1965).
Lowry, O.H., Rosebrough, N.J., Farr, A.L., and Randall, R.J.
    Protein measurement with the folin phenol reagent.   *J. Biol. Chem.
    193:*265-274 (1951).
McKay, A.V.P., and Iversen, L.L.   Increased tyrosine hydroxylase
    activity of sympathetic ganglia cultured in the presence of dibutyryl

cyclic AMP. *Brain Res. 48:* 424-426 (1972).

Mueller, R.A., Theonen, H., and Axelrod, J. Compensatory increase in adrenal tyrosine hydroxylase activity after chemical sympathectomy *Science 163:* 468-469 (1969).

Mueller, R.A., Theonen, H., Axelrod, J. Increase in tyrosine hydroxylase activity after reserpine administration. *J. Pharmac. Exp. Ther. 169:* 74-79 (1969).

Musacchio, J.M., and Wurzburger, R. Aggregation of beef adrenal tyrosine hydroxylase. *Fed. Proc. 28:* 287.

Naftchi, N.E., Lowman, E.W., Sell, G.H., Rusk, H.A. Peripheral circulation and catecholamine metabolism in paraplegia and quadriplegia. *Arch. Phys. Med. and Rehabil. 53:* 357-362 (1972).

Naftchi, N.E., Wooten, G.F., Lowman, E.W., Axelrod, J. Increased serum dopamine-β-hydroxylase activity during neurogenic hypertension in quadriplegia. In *Frontiers in Catecholamine Research.* G. Britain, Pergamon Press, 1973, pp. 1143-1147.

Naftchi, N.E., Wooten, G.F., Lowman, E.W., Axelrod, J. Relationship between serum dopamine-β-hydroxylase activity, catecholamine metabolism, and hemodynamic change during paroxysmal hypertension in quadriplegia. *Circ. Res. 35:* 850-861 (1974).

Naftchi, N.E., Demeny, M., Lowman, E., Tuckman, J. Hypertensive crises in quadriplegic patients: changes in cardiac output, blood volume, serum dopamine-β-hydroxylase activity, and arterial prostaglandin PGE_2. *Circ. 57:* 336-341 (1978).

Naftchi, N.E., Demeny, M., DeCrescito, V., Tomasula, J., Flamm, S., Campbell, J.B. Biogenic amine concentrations in traumatized spinal cords of cats: effect of drug therapy. *J. Neurosurg. 40:* 52-57 (1974).

Nagatsu, T., and Undenfriend, S. A rapid and simple radioassay for tyrosine hydroxylase activity. *Analytical Biochem. 9:* 122-126 (1964).

Osterholm, J.L., Mathews, G.J. Altered norepinephrine metabolism following experimental spinal cord injury. Part I: Relationship to hemorrhagic necrosis and post-wounding neurological deficits. *J. Neurosurg. 36:* 386-394 (1972).

Sato, T.L., Jequier, E., Lovenberg, W., and Sjoerdsma, A. Characterization of tryptophan hydroxylating enzyme from malignant mouse mast cell. *Eur. J. Pharmacol. 1:* 18-25 (1967).

Sedvall, C.C., and Kopin, I.J. Influence of sympathetic denervation and nerve impulse activity on tyrosine hydroxylase activity in the rat submaxillary gland. *Biochem. Pharmac. 16:* 39-46 (1967).

Theonen, H., Mueller, R.A., and Axelrod, J. Trans-synaptic induction of adrenal tyrosine hydroxylase. *J. Pharmac. Exp. Ther. 169:* 249-254 (1969).

Waymere, J.C., Weiner, N., and Prasad, K.N. Regulation of tyrosine hydroxylase activity in cultured mouse neuroblastoma cells: Elevation induced by analogues of adenosine 3',5'-cyclic monophosphate. *Proc. Nat. Acad. Sci. (Wash.) 69:* 2241-2245 (1971).

Weiner, N. Factors regulating catecholamine biosynthesis in peripheral and central catecholaminergic neurons. In *The Nervous System, Vol. 1, The Basic Neurosciences,* Raven Press, New York, 1975, pp. 341-354.

6

Brain Catecholamines, Serotonin, and Gamma-Aminobutyric Acid and Adrenal Catecholamines After High Spinal Cord Transection in the Rat

S.R. SNIDER

In this communication, subacute alterations in whole brain concentrations of the putative neurotransmitter substances, dopamine (DA),
norepinephrine (NE), serotonin (5-HT), and gamma-aminobutyric acid
(GABA), and of adrenal medullary catecholamines (CA) as a result
of complete transection of the spinal cord at the C-7 level are described.
A number of new studies have shown changes in neurotransmitter
substances in the spinal cord, both in the area of injury (Naftchi et
al., 1974) and in the spinal cord segments proximal and distal to the
injury (Magnusson, 1973; Naftchi et al., 1972, 1973). The study by
Magnusson showed that over the long term the monoamines decreased
below the level of the transection (mid-thoracic) and increased above.
The latter increase was considered to represent increased metabolic
activity in the remaining proximal portions of the monoamine pathways.
Monoamine decreased metabolic activity distal to spinal cord transection
may also be reflected in decreased CA turnover in the sympathoadrenal
system (Snider and Carlsson, 1972).

The present study was a survey of neurotransmitters in brain and
of the CA neurohormones in the adrenal gland after spinal cord
transection. The purpose was to determine whether spinal cord transection would result in neurotransmitter changes in regions of the
nervous system that was remote from the area of injury.

Male Sprague-Dawley rats weighing about 200g were used. The
spinal cord was transected at the level of the seventh cervical vertebra
under ether anesthesia. Control of animals were sham-operated. After
operation all animals were given a balanced electrolyte solution
subcutaneously and also had free access to food and water. The urinary
bladder was emptied manually.

Eighteen to 24 hours after the operation, animals were killed by
decapitation. The brain and adrenals were rapidly removed and
homogenized in 0.4 N percholoric acid according to a standard extraction
procedure (Fahn et al., 1975). The extract was passed through a
strong cation exchange column and GABA, DA, NE [plus epinephrine
(E)] and 5-HT were sequentially eluted (Fahn et al., 1975). GABA
was assayed by a fluorimetric modification of an enzymatic assay
(Fahn and Cote, 1968). Dopamine, NE, and 5-HT were assayed by
fluorimetric assays (Atack, 1973; Laverty and Taylor, 1968; Korf et al.,
1973).

In adrenal there was a decrease in DA and an increase in NE + E
(Table I). This presumably reflects a reduction in nerve impulse flow

that was due to disconnection of the peripheral sympathetic nervous system from supraspinal influences and has been seen in previous experiments (Snider and Carlsson, 1972; Snider and Waldeck, 1974).

Table I.

Adrenal Catecholamines in Rats with C-7 Spinal Cord Transection

	CONTROL (17)	TRANSECTED (8)
DA (nm/pr)	1.05 ± .06	0.74 ± .17*
NE + E (nm/pr)	110 ± 3	132 ± 5*

Mean ± SEM concentrations of dopamine (DA) and norepinephrine plus epinephrine (NE + E) in nmoles/adrenal pair.

* = p < .05.

In brain there was an increase in the concentration of DA and 5-HT and a decrease in GABA. The slight decrease in NE was not significant (Table II).

Table II.

Brain Neurotransmitters in Rats with C-7 Spinal Cord Transection

	CONTROL	TRANSECTED
DA (nm/g)	4.58 ± .±8 (7)	4.99 ± .16 (9)*
NE (nm/g)	1.76 ± .16 (8)	1.60 ± .11 (7)
5-HT (nm/g)	1.72 ± .10 (7)	1.99 ± .07 (8)*
GABA (μm/g)	3,43 ± .07 (7)	2.73 ± .15 (8)**

Spinal cord transection was performed 18 to 24 hours before death. Shown are the mean ± SEM concentrations of dopamine (DA), norepinephrine (NE), serotonin (5-HT), and GABA in the whole brain of sham-operated control and transected rats. Number of values in parentheses.

* = p < .05
** = p < .01 (Student's t-test).

Magnusson (1973) found in the upper portion of the spinal cord, above the level of the transection, that monoamines increased steadily, starting the first day after surgery. Specific neurochemical data on the effects of spinal cord transection on other central nervous system structures have not been obtained to our knowledge. However, the experiments of Andén and co-workers (1964) on a section of central noradrenergic axon collaterals are relevant. In these studies it was shown that section of the NE collateral fibers resulted in an increase in NE metabolism in other brain regions, innervated by intact axons of the same noradrenergic neurons. This mechanism could explain the present data, i.e., section of descending NE and possibly DA and 5-HT, pathways in the spinal cord (Andén, 1965) may result in increased activity in the cells of origin and in the intact pathways within the brain.

The explanation for the reduction in GABA concentration in the present experiment is not clear. One must consider that GABA has metabolic as well as neurotransmitter functions and that alterations in its level may reflect a general effect of the operation on cerebral amino acid metabolism, a.g. subarachnoid blood or monoamines that are released from the site of injury could alter the blood-brain barrier. Such metabolic changes could also effect the transport of tryptophan, the precursor of 5-HT.

SUMMARY AND ABSTRACT

This study on rats shows that C-7 spinal cord transection results in alterations in adrenal catecholamines and in neurotransmitter levels in whole brain when measured 18 to 24 hours after operation. In the adrenal there was a decrease in DA and a increase in NE + E. In the brain, there were 10-15% increases in DA and 5-HT levels and a decrease in GABA. The mechanism may involve altered nerve impulse flow as well as changes in the blood-brain barrier and the availability of substances necessary for neurotransmitter metabolism.

REFERENCES

Anden, N.E. Distribution of monoamines and dihydroxyphenylalanine decarboxylase activity in the spinal cord. *Acta. Physio.. Scand. 64:*197-203 (1965).

Anden, N.E., Haggendal, J., Magnusson, T., and Rosengren, E. The time course of the disappearance of noradrenaline and 5-hydroxytryptamine in the spinal cord after transection. *Acta. Physiol. Scand. 62:*115-118 (1964).

Atack, C.V. The determination of dopamine by a modification of the dihydroxyindole fluorimetric assay. *Br. J. Pharmacol. 48:*699-714 (1973).

Fahn, S., and Côte, L. Regional distribution of gamma-aminobutyric acid (GABA) in the brain of Rhesus monkey. *J. Neurochem. 15:* 209-213 (1968).

Fahn, S., Snider, S., Prasad, A.L.N., Lane, E., and Makadon, H. Normalization of brain serotonin by L-tryptophan in levodopa-treated rats. *Neurology (Minneap.) 25:*861-865 (1975).

Korf, J., Schutte, H., and Venema, K. A semiautomated fluorometric determination of 5-hydroxyindoles in the nanogram range. *Anal. Biochem. 53:*146-153 (1973).

Laverty, R., and Taylor, K.M. The fluorometric assay of catecholamines and related compounds: Improvement and extensions to the hydroxyindole technique. *Anal. Biochem. 22:*269-279 (1968).

Magnusson, T. Effect of chronic transection on dopamine, noradrenaline and 5-hydroxytryptamine in the rat spinal cord. *Naunyn-Schmiedeberg's Arch. Pharmacol. 278:*13-22 (1973).

Naftchi, N.E., Demeny, M., DeCrescito, V., Tomasula, John J., Flamm, E.S., and Campbell, J.B. Biogenic amine concentrations in traumatized spinal cords of cats: Effect of drug therapy. *J. Neurosurg. 40:*52-57 (1974).

Naftchi, N.E., Demeny, M., Kertesz, A., and Lowman, E.W. The CNS and adrenal tyrosine hydroxylase activity and norepinephrine, serotonin, and histamine in the spinal cord after transection. *Fed. Proc. 31:*832 (1972).

Naftchi, N.E., Demeny, M., Viau, A.T., and Lowman, E.W. Changes in central and peripheral biogenic amines and cyclic AMP in spinal cord injury. *Proc. Inter. Soc. Neurochem. 4:*367 (1973).

Snider, S.R., and Carlsson, A. The adrenal dopamine as an indicator of adrenomedullary hormone synthesis. Naunyn-Schmiedeberg's *Arch. Pharmacol. 275:*347-357 (1972).

Snider, S.R., and Waldeck, B. Increased synthesis of adrenomedullary catecholamines induced by caffeine and theophylline. Naunyn-Schmiedeberg's *Arch. Pharmacol. 281:*257-260 (1974).

ACKNOWLEDGEMENTS

The skilled technical assistance of Mr. Carl Miller and the assistance and advice of Dr. Roger Brown, Professor Arvid Carlsson and Dr. Tor Magnusson are gratefully acknowledged. This investigation was supported by NIMH grant 30129.

7

Substance P and Leucine-Enkephalin Changes in Spinal Cord of Paraplegic Rats and Cats

N.E. NAFTCHI, S.J. ABRAHAMS, H.M. ST. PAUL, and L.L. VACCA

INTRODUCTION

It has long been known that the perception of pain in the central nervous system (CNS) is first integrated in the spinal cord, in the narrow band of gray matter at the apex of the dorsal horns that is known as the substantia gelatinosa. Primary afferent neurons terminate in the substantia gelatinosa and interact with many small interneurons found in this region. High concentrations of the peptides substance P, leucine-enkephalin, and methionine-enkephalin have been found in the substantia gelatinosa, comprising Rexed's lamina II and III and Rexed's lamina I (Abrahams et al., 1978, Brownstein et al., 1976; Elde et al., 1976; Hokfelt et al., 1975; Hokfelt et al., 1975; Hokfelt et al., 1977; Kanazawa and Jessel, 1976; Naftchi et al., 1978). In addition, a dense population of opiate receptors have been demonstrated in the substantia gelatinosa (Atweh and Kuhar, 1977). Thus, these three neuropeptides have been implicated in the mediation of pain and analgesia. Substance P was extracted in 1931 from equine brain and intestine by Von Euler and Gaddum (1931). It was found to possess a vasodilatory effect and to stimulate smooth muscle. It was not until 1970, however, that Chang and Leeman (1970) isolated a sialogogic peptide from bovine hypothalamus, which was purified, characterized as substance P, and synthesized. It was found to be an undecapeptide (Chang et al., 1971). Subsequently, antibodies to substance P were prepared, and, using radioimmunoassay, it was found that substance P had an uneven distribution in the CNS (Powell et al., 1973). Its highest concentrations occurred in the substantia nigra, hypothalamus, pineal gland, and the dorsal gray matter of the spinal cord (Brownstein et al., 1976). These results have been confirmed by immunofluorescence and immunoperoxidase methods in a variety of animals: human, cat, rat and monkey (Hokfelt et al., 1975; Hokfelt et al., 1975; Naftchi et al., 1978; Cuello et al., 1976). In the substantia gelatinosa, the immunoreactivity seems to occur within thin unmyelinated fibers, which are classically known to carry thermal and pain stimuli. This finding suggests that substance P is the first chemical signal of exteroceptive perception in the spinal cord (Cuello et al., 1976). Physiological evidence indicates that substance P can produce slow, long-lasting excitation in spinal neurons when it is applied iontophoretically. These neurons include motoneurons, Renshaw cells, and dorsal horn interneurons in the substantia gelatinosa and Rexed's lamina V (Henry, 1976; Henry et al., 1975). The data support the view that substance P may be a transmitter or modulator that is involved in the perception of pain.

In 1973, binding of radioactive opiates, including morphine, to brain synaptosomal membranes was independently reported by three groups (Pert and Synder, 1973; Simon et al., 1973; Terenius, 1973). The binding could be blocked stereospecifically by the opiate antagonists naloxone and naltrexone, It was postulated, therefore, that opiates must bind to selective sites, or receptors, that are located on the surface of nerve cells in the CNS before they can produce their characteristic pharmacological responses: analgesia, euphoria, sleep, relaxation. The antagonists, which may also possess some agonist effect, would then bind to these specific sites first and, thereby, prevent opiate (agonist) binding (Simon, 1976).

Accordingly, opiate receptors have been reported in various regions of the brain, in especially high amounts in the limbic system (except the hippocampus), in the spinal cord (especially the dorsal gray matter), and in the intestine (Simon, 1976; Kuhar et al., 1975). In addition, opiate receptor binding sites have been demonstrated by radiobinding assay and by autoradiography in brain and spinal cord (Atweh and Kuhar, 1977; Pert et al., 1976; Hiller et al., 1973).

The presence of the opiate receptors in the CNS led to the belief that a biological ligand(s) for opiate receptors might exist in the CNS and might be a naturally occurring endogenous morphine-like substance(s). Several studies reported that electrical stimulation of certain parts of the brain could cause analgesia, which was prevented by injections of naloxone (Liebeskind et al., 1974; Mayer and Hayes, 1975; Mayer and Liebeskind, 1974). These studies suggested a release of an endogenous opiate-like substance. In a search for a substance with morphine-like effects on smooth muscle that could be blocked by naloxone, Hughes and Kosterlitz (1975) screened pig brain extracts. After extensive purification, two such morphine-like substances were characterized as pentapeptides and were called "enkephalins". These compounds were also isolated by Simantov and Snyder (1976) from calf brain. One of the enkephalins was found to have the amino acid sequence (Tyr-Gly-Gly-Phe-Met) and was called methionine-enkephalin. The other had the amino acid sequence (Tyr-Gly-Gly-Phe-Leu) and was named leucine-enkephalin. β-endorphin, a fragment of β-lipoprotein (which is a pituitary peptide), also has a very potent opiate-like effect. The name endorphins was proposed by Simon to denote endogenous morphine-like substances.

The roles of endorphine, leu- and met-enkephalin have not yet been elucidated. At present they are thought to be neurotransmitters or neuromodulators that are probably involved in pain pathways as well as pathways involving higher mental processes.

These peptides have been demonstrated in rat CNS by immuno-fluorescence (Elde et al., 1976; Hokfelt et al., 1975; Simantov and Snyder, 1976). In the brain, fluorescence was confined to neurons, as opposed to glia, and was found most intensely in nerve endings where it would be expected to be concentrated if the peptides were acting as neurotransmitters. In our laboratory, we have investigated the changes in substance P and leu-enkephalin in spinal cord transected rats, cats, and monkeys, using a sensitive and specific peroxidase-antiperoxidase immunocytochemical method (Abrahams et al., 1978; Naftchi et al., 1978). At varying intervals of time after transection, the distribution and changes of substance P and leu-enkephalin were studied in the spinal cord, both above and below the lesion.

In order to further assess the roles of the opiate receptor, substance

P, and the enkephalins in spinal pain pathways, we have studied the effects of chronic morphine treatment *in vivo*. Stereospecific opiate receptor binding is reduced in the substantia gelatinosa after dorsal rhizotomy (LaMotte et al., 1976). Conceivably the opiate receptors are associated presynaptically with substance P-containing primary afferent fibers in the substantia gelatinosa. There is further evidence that opiate receptor sites interact with the enkephalins in this region (LaMotte et al., 1976). We have been exploring the neural circuits between these substances to elucidate the interaction between these peptides and their involvement in pre- and post-synaptic and inter-neuronal events.

MATERIALS AND METHODS

Transection of the Spinal Cord

Rats, cats, or monkeys were anesthetized with Ketamine or Nembutal. A dorsal laminectomy was performed, and the spinal cord was exposed and transected at mid to low thoracic levels. Small pieces of sterile gelfoam were placed between the cut ends of the cord, which immediately stopped any bleeding that had occurred. The gelfoam was left in place and the animals were sutured. Animals were not fed or watered for oen day following surgery but were allowed to eat and drink *ad libitum* thereafter; their bladders were expressed three times daily.

Tissue Preparation

At varying time intervals after transection, tissue from paraplegic and normal control animals was processed for immunocytochemistry. The animals were anesthetized with Nembutal and sacrificed by perfusion through the ascending aorta with 4% paraformaldehyde in 0.1 M phosphate buffer, pH 7.2 for 10 minutes. Sections of spinal cord were removed from above and below the lesion and were immediately immersed in picric acid-formaldehyde fixative for about six hours, after which time they were cut into smaller pieces. The tissues were then rinsed in phosphate buffered saline for two hours to overnight, dehydrated through a graded series of ethanol solutions, put through several changes of xylene and paraffin, and finally embedded in paraffin. Sections were cut at a thickness of 4-5 um and affixed to albumin-coated glass slides. Once prepared, these slides could be incubated for immunoreactivity at any future time.

Antisera

Rabbit antiserum to substance P was generously supplied by Dr. Susan Leeman. Prior to incubation of the tissue, the antiserum was diluted 1:100 with 0.5 M Tris-Saline (pH 7.6) and incubated for two hours at 37°C with rat liver acetone powder (20 mg liver powder per milliliter of diluted serum). This was stored overnight at 4°C and was filtered the next morning through a 0.2 um millipore filter. It was then further diluted with 0.5 M Tris-Saline. Final dilutions that were used in this series of experiments ranged from 1:400 to 1:1000. Antiserum to leu-enkephalin was prepared by the method of Moore et al. (1977). This was diluted with 0.5 M Tris-Saline and used in the dilution range of 1:200 to 1:500.

Immunohistochemical Staining

The peroxidase-anti-peroxidase immunohistochemical method, as first described by Sternberger (1974) and modified by Pickel et al. (1977), was performed on 5 µm tissue sections for localization of substance P and leu-enkephalin in tissues (Naftchi et al., 1978). In some cases, a "double bridge" modification was used which amplified staining (Vacca et al., 1975; Vacca et al., 1980).

Nonspecific protein binding was reduced by incubating the sections with 3% goat serum in Tris-Saline before they were incubated with anti-substance P or antileu-enkephalin antisera for one hour or overnight. Goat anti-rabbit immunoglobulin (Miles Labs) was applied for 30 minutes after two brief rinses with Tris-Saline. Following two more rinses, the PAP reagent (Dako Accurate Chemicals) was applied in 1:25 to 1:50 dilution for 30 minutes. The slides were then incubated for 15 to 30 minutes with 0.05% 3,3'-diaminobenzidine (Sigma) and 0.01% hydrogen peroxide solution in Tris buffer (pH 7.6). A brown precipitate was formed characteristic of polymerized diaminobenzidine. The reaction involves the donation of electrons by peroxidase to hydrogen peroxide. The oxidized enzyme is then reduced by diaminobenzidine and, thus, converted to the active form. The oxidative intermediate of diamino-benzidine is polymerized to an insoluble brown precipitate. After several washes in distilled water, the slides were dehydrated and mounted with coverslips.

Sham-operated animals served as controls for paraplegic animals. Tissues from these animals were processed in the same manner as above.

Morphine-Treated Animals

Rats were chronically exposed to morphine sulfate (10 mg/kg, i.p.) for 10 days and sacrificed by perfusion. Their spinal cords were removed and the tissues were processed as above. Saline-injected animals served as controls.

Immunohistochemical Controls

In order to control for immunohistochemical specificity, normal rabbit serum was routinely substituted for specific rabbit antibody to substance P or leu-enkephalin in all experiments.

The degree of cross-reactivity between the peptide, methionine-enkephalin with antibody to leucine-enkephalin, was assessed by first incubating leu-enkephalin antibody with serial dilutions of either leu-or met-enkephlin antigen prior to application to the slides. It was possible to totally erase the immunoreactive staining when leu-enkephalin was added to the antibody. In the same dilution range, however, negligible staining persisted when met-enkephlin was added to the antibody, indicating the presence of slight cross reactivity.

All the sections were examined with a Jena light microscope at magnifications of 25X to 630X.

RESULTS

Substance P

Tissue from normal and sham-operated cats and rats (Figures 1A and 1B) displayed peroxide-positive staining that appeared as a band of nerve terminals in the dorsal horn at the junction between the white

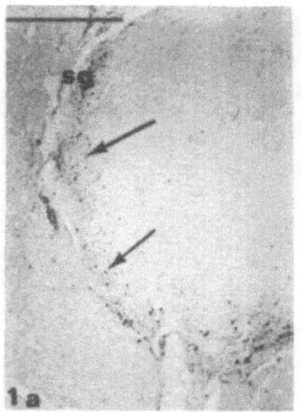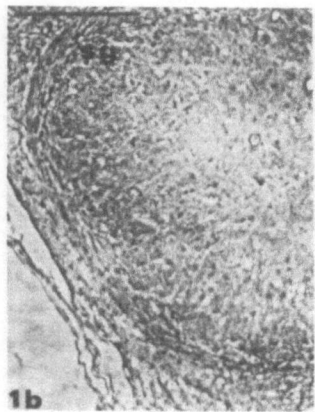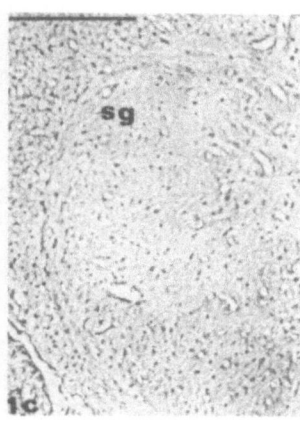

Fig. 1A. Section from T 11-12 region of the spinal cord of a sham-operated
    cat.   Arrow points to immunoreactive substance P (SP) specific
    bodies in dorsal horn (area of substantia gelatinosa, SG).   X 200

    1B. Phase contrast micrograph of the same dorsal horn region seen
    in A.   The section was incubated for SP immunoreactivity.   Note
    the presence of a dark ring in the SG region, indicating the area
    of immunoreactivity. X 200

    1C. Phase contrast micrograph of the same dorsal horn region
    seen in A.   The section was incubated with normal rabbit serum.
    Compared with B, the absence of any SP-specific staining is evident.
    X 200*

and gray matters, the substantia gelatinosa that corresponds to laminae
II and III of Rexed (1954).   Substance P specific staining was also
found in Rexed's lamina I.
    Two and five days after transection of the spinal cord of the rats
and cats, respectively, there was a sharp increase in the amount of
substance P below the lesion that had outlined both dorsal horns and
bridged the two together.   Above the lesion, in the region of the
substantia gelatinosa, the number of punctate bodies was fewer, and
the intensity of staining around the dorsal horn was less than that
in sections that were obtained from below the lesion.   This pattern
was repeated in sections from chronic cats that were sacrificed one to
12 weeks following spinal cord transection and chronic rats one to three
weeks following transection.   Substance P specific immunoreactive
staining in sections that were cut from above the lesion (Figures 2A
and 3A) was little, compared with the great amount of staining found
in sections that were cut from below the lesion (Figures 2B and 3B).
In addition to punctate bodies, long fibers and varicosities were present
in sections that were taken from below the lesion (Figure 2C).   A
network of fibers located centrally within each dorsal horn (Rexed
laminae IV and V) from rats and cats that were sacrificed three and
12 weeks, respectively, after transection were found to be immunoreactive
for substance P (Figures 3B and 3C).   Some staining was often seen
in the ventral horn in the form of small, dense punctate bodies that
were scattered randomly throughout the horn (Figure 4A).   It was
difficult to assess whether the amount of staining in the ventral horn
changed with time either above or below the lesion.   In chronically

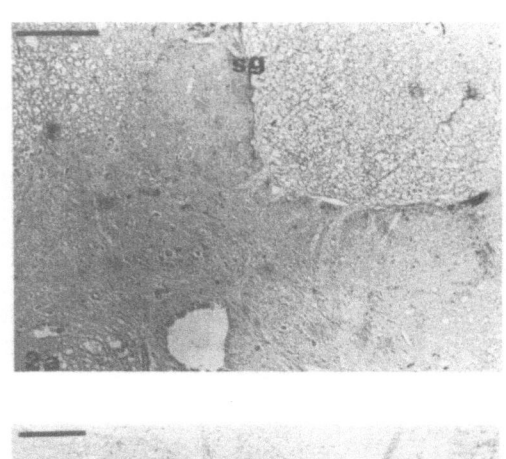

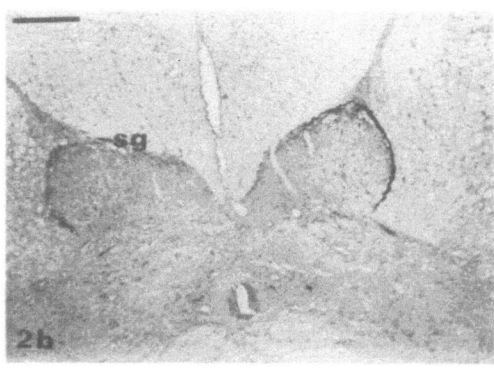

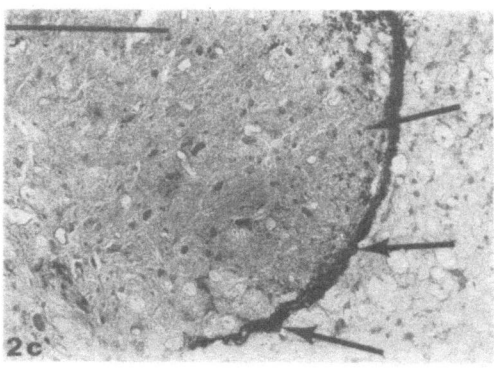

Fig. 2A. Field showing dorsal horns *above* the lesion from a cat transected 5 weeks before perfusion. SG shows slight staining. X 125

2B. Tissue from the same cat as in Figure 2A sectioned *below* the lesion. Note the intense reaction product delineating both dorsal horns. X 100

2C. The detail of the SG seen in Figure 2B. Arrows point to darkly stained SP-immunoreactive punctate bodies and an intense band of bead-like varicosities delineating the entire SG. X 250 *

lesioned monkeys (six months or longer after spinal cord transection), ventral horn and central canal region staining was more prominent,

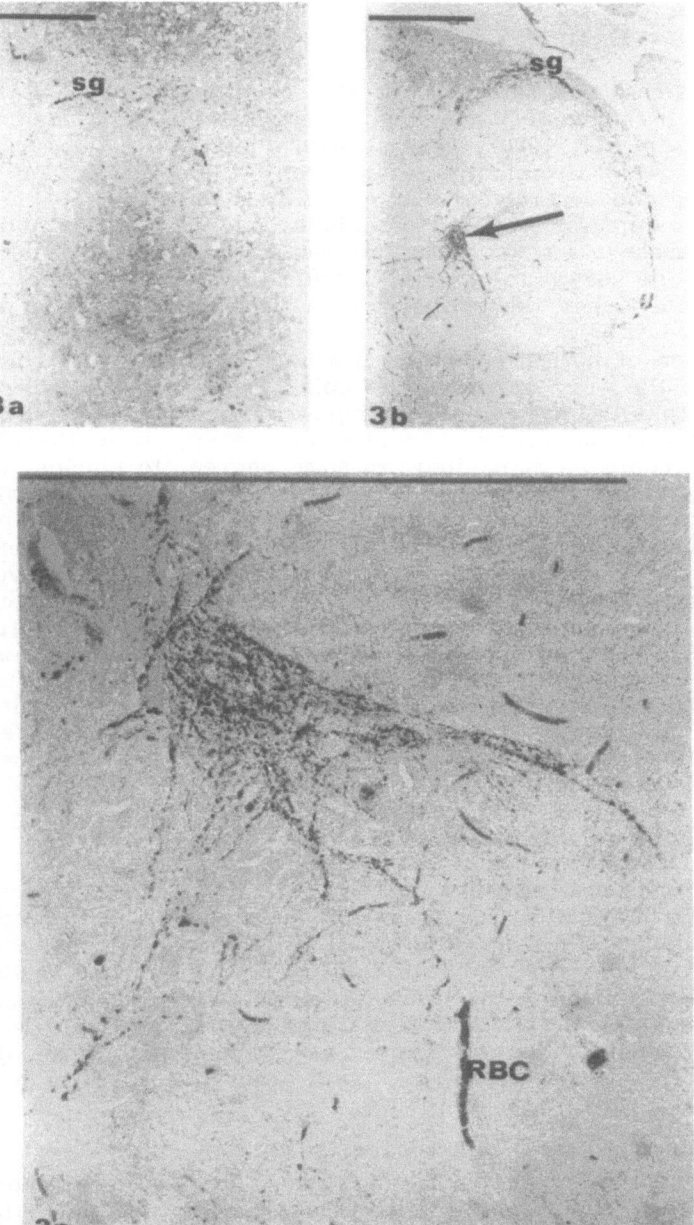

Fig. 3A. Section from *above* the lesion of a cat transected 12 weeks
before sacrifice. Note sparse staining surrounding the dorsal
horn in the SG.   X 160

  3B. Tissue from the same cat as in Figure 3A, sectioned *below*
the lesion. The staining of the band of nerve terminals in the SG
is much more intense in this section than that in the section *above*
the lesion. Note the appearance of the nerve plexus (arrow) near
the center (lamina V) of the dorsal horn. X 160

  3C. A detail of the nerve plexus from Figure 3B. Immunoreactive
substance P appars in bead-like, fibrillar varicosities, which may be
nerve terminals originating from dorsal roots and entering the
spinal cord. RBC = red blood cells present in small capillaries. X 960

compared with cats and rats (Figure 4B). Using a modified PAP method that amplifies immunological staining, especially in sparsly innervated regions (Vacca et al., 1980), ventral horn staining became more prominent in the rat around the motoneurons and other ventral horn cells and along the ventrolateral fringe of the ventral horn (Figure 4C). Additionally, using this modified technique, punctate bodies and subependymal processes can sometimes be seen in the central canal region (Figure 4D). In normal rat tissue, sometimes laminae IV and V appear stained, but only when the double bridge amplification method was applied (Figure 4E).

Substitution of normal serum for immune serum as a control showed no staining in the gray matter of the spinal cord with the exception of red blood cells, which contain endogenous peroxidase (Figure 1C). In some specimens, immunoreactive staining did appear in the white matter, which could be attributed, to some degree, to nonspecific affinity of the rabbit serum for the membranes in the regions where the myelin had leached out since the same type of light-brown background staining appeared in control sections where normal rabbit serum was substituted for the specific antiserum. There were, however, some small, immunoreactive, substance P-specific, dark punctate bodies present in the myelinated axons of the white matter in the ventrolateral and dorsolateral parts of the spinal cord. This may suggest rostral axonal flow of substance P within myelinated fibers possibly belonging to lateral spinothalamic tracts or to shorter tracts concerned with segmental transmission. In monkey tissue additional white matter was bilaterally stained in a uniform, symmetrical pattern that was extended to the ventrolateral white region (Figure 4F).

Effect of Morphine on Substance P Immunoreactivity

Immunocytochemical examination of the rats that were treated chronically (10 days) with morphine sulfate revealed a nonuniform increase in substance P in certain regions of the spinal cord, compared with tissue from saline-treated rats (Figure 5). Substance P was increased in the substantia gelatinosa, Rexed's laminae I, IV, and V, and the ventral horn around the medial and lateral groups of motoneurons and traveling along the ventral roots. Substance P, however, did not increase within processes that were found around the central canal.

Leucine-Enkephalin

Spinal cord sections from sham-operated cats that were taken from the T5 region displayed a pattern of immunoreactive bodies in the substantia gelatinosa (Figure 6A), a fairly dense region lateral and dorsal to the central canal (Figure 6C), and a substantial scattering of immunoreactive bodies throughout the entire ventral horn (Figure 7A). In the substantia gelatinosa of the cat spinal cord, specific leu-enkephalin immunoreactivity in the sections from below the level of the lesion was never as great as that found in comparable tissue sections reacted for substance P.

In contrast to substance P, there was no apparent difference in the amount or distribution of staining with time after spinal cord transection, nor was there any difference in immunoreactivity above or below the level of the lesion (Figure 6B).

The immunoreactive substance was mostly in the shape of punctate bodies, many of which were present in the substantia gelatinosa. Stained varicosities were often seen extending for short distances into

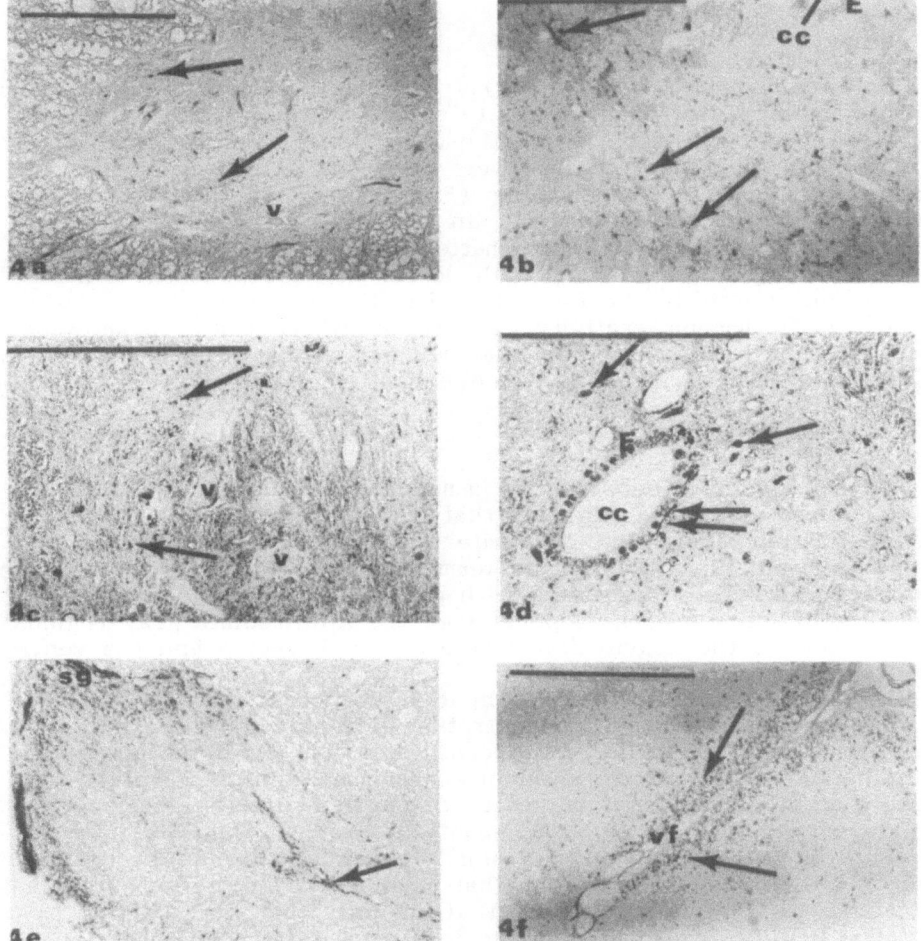

Fig. 4A. Section of the ventral horn from *below* the lesion of a cat transected five weeks before sacrifice. Ventral horn cells (V) are present. Arrows point to immunopositive bodies that are scattered throughout. X 250

4B. Section of the area lateral and ventral to the central canal (CC) of a sham-operated monkey. Arrows point to a few of the large number of immunopositive bodies present. Endothelial cells (E) surround the CC. X 300

4C. Section of normal rat ventral horn to which the double bridge PAP method was applied. Arrows point to immunopositive punctate bodies. Ventral horn cells (V) are present. X 400

4D. Section of normal rat central canal area to which the double bridge PAP method was applied. A fiber (double arrow) that abuts on the ependymal cells (E) appears positively stained. Many stained punctate bodies are present (arrows). X 400

4E. Section from a normal rat dorsal horn area stained by the double bridge PAP method showing SP localization in lamina V (arrow) as well as in the SG. X 200

4F. Area showing the ventral fissure (VF) of the spinal cord of a four week transected monkey. Small bodies (arrows) that appear positively stained for SP bilaterally ring the fissure in the ventral white matter. X 300

Reprinted with permission of Peptides, 2 (Suppl 1): 65, 1981.

the dorsal white matter (Figure 6B). In the ventral horn, long fibrous elements were present that seemed to extend to the ventral horn cells after stretching a distance within the gray matter (Figure 7A). Some long bead-like fibrillar processes were also seen extending a long distance from gray to white matters (Figure 7B). In some instances immunoreactive fibers appeared to run for some distance along the ventral root fibers into the white matter (Figure 7C). A great deal of immunoreactivity was visualized both dorsal and lateral to the central canal region, mostly in the form of varicosities (Figures 6C and 6D).

No specific immunoreactivity was present when normal serum was substituted for immunoserum or when leu-enkephalin antiserum was preincubated with the peptide leu-enkephalin.

DISCUSSION

The abundance of substance P immunoreactive nerve terminals in the substantia gelatinosa suggests that substance P is contained in the primary afferent fibers that penetrate the substantia gelatinosa and dorsolateral funiculus radially and terminate in the dorsal horn. These regions are classically associated with pain transmission. In addition, some SP-containing processes penetrated the intermediate gray regions and extended to the heavily innervated lamina V region and the ventral horn.

Otsuka and co-workers (1975) ligated the dorsal roots of the cat and found that substance P concentration increased on the ganglion side of the ligature and decreased centrally. The findings suggested that substance P was synthesized in dorsal root ganglia and its presence in afferent fibers suggested a role in neurotransmission. Iontophoretic application of substance P to spinal neurons by Henry et al. (1975, 1976) produced a strong but slow and prolonged excitatory action on nearly half the neurons that were tested in the lumbar spinal cord of the cat. It is noteworthy that all units that were excited by substance P were also excited by noxious thermal stimulation of the skin. The highest number of units that were excited by substance P was found in lamina VI and the lowest in lamina IV. In two cases, treatment with substance P led to a response to noxious heat by units that had previously been unresponsive to thermal stimulation. Therefore, Henry suggested, that substance P may be involved specifically in afferent units that are associated with pain sensation. Hokfelt also observed that substance P-containing fibers in peripheral afferent nerves are unmyelinated and that in the skin these fibers terminate in free nerve ending that are usually associated with pain transmission (Hokfelt et al., 1975; Hokfelt et al., 1975).

Using immunohistochemical techniques for localization of substance P, our finding of extensive staining of the nerve plexus in lamina V below the lesion (Figures 3B and 3C) shows the presence of a network of varicosities in the nerve endings in the area classically known to be concerned with noxious transmission. Lamina V networks were never observed in the sections above the lesion. The results demonstrate accumulation of substance P below the lesion and suggest its rostral direction by axoplasmic flow in the spinal cord.

The slow time course of substance P action by Henry et al. (1975) was incompatible with a role as the main excitatory transmitter of primary afferent terminals, but its strong excitatory action might have functional significance as sensitizer or modulator over a long period. Recently, Pickel et al (1977), using immunocytochemical techniques, reported that within axon terminals substance P appeared to be

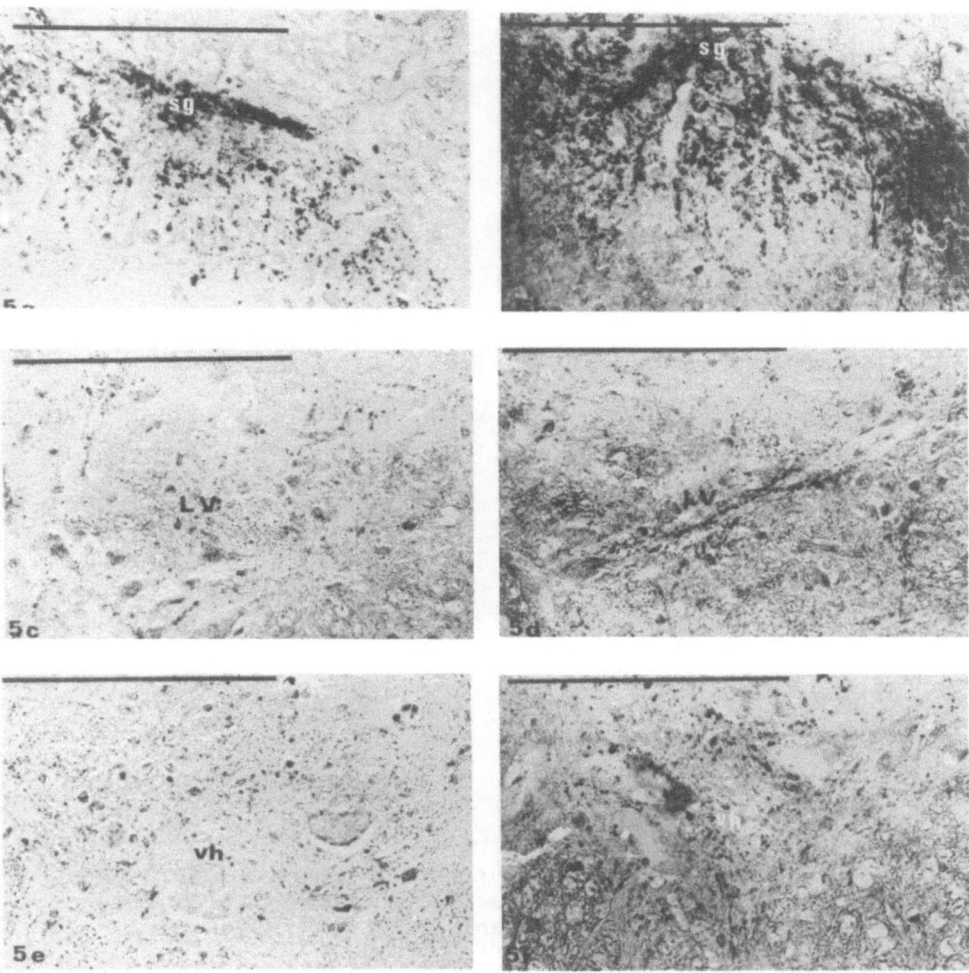

Fig. 5. Tissue from rats chronically injected with morphine, 10 mg/kg for 10 days, compared with saline-injected controls. The double bridge PAP method was used. Figure 5A is a section of the SG region of the dorsal horn of a saline control; 5B is a comparable section from a morphine-treated animal. Fibure 5C is a section through lamina V (LV) of the dorsal horn of a saline control; 5D is a comparable section from a morphine-treated animal. 5E is a section of the ventral horn (VH) from a saline control, 5F is a comparable section from a morphine-treated animal. At each of these levels (dorsal horn, lamina V, ventral horn) there is more immunoreactivity in the morphine-treated animal than in the saline control. X 500

associated with one type of organelle, a large, round vesicle 60-80 nm in diameter. In addition, in the same axon terminal, small unlabeled vesicles were also present. It is generally accepted that such small

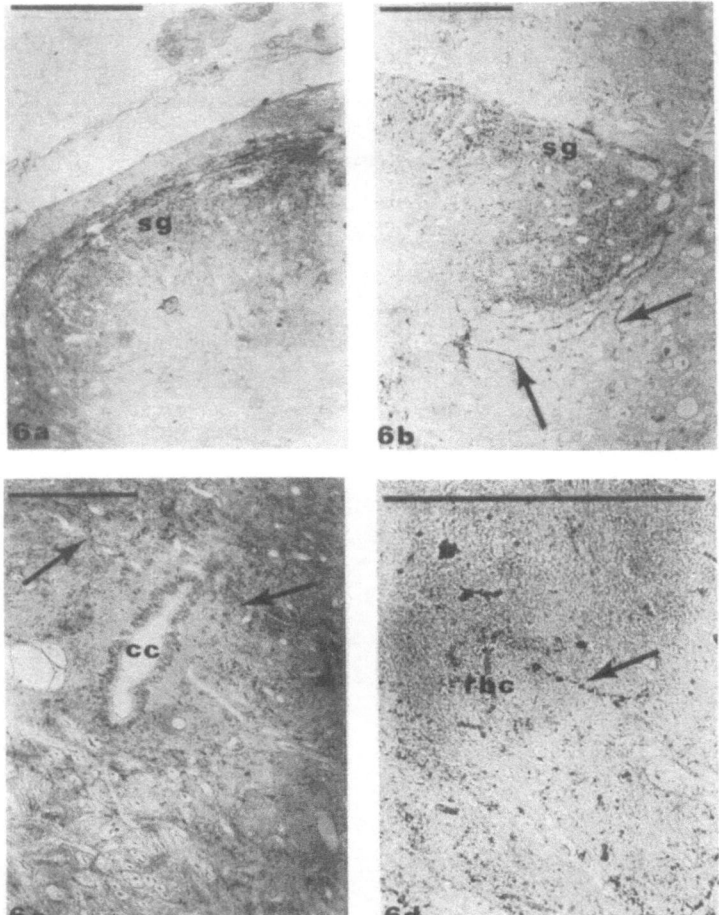

Fig. 6A. Section showing part of the dorsal horn region of the spinal
cord at T 11-12 of a sham-operated cat. Immunoreactive leucine-
enkephalin (LE) specific bodies outline the SG. X 200

6B. Section showing the SG from *below* the lesion of a cat transected
two weeks before sacrifice. The amount of immunoreactive LE-
specific bodies in comparable to Figure 3A. Immunoreactivity is
also present in fibers (arrows) extending into the white matter. X 200

6C. Region around the central canal (CC) area of a sham-operated
cat. Many immunoreactive bodies (arrows) are seen in the region.
X 200

6D. Region lateral to the central canal in a sham-operated cat.
LE positive punctate bodies as well as a beaded fiber (arrow) are
seen. Red blood cells (RBC) in a small vessel are present. X 500

Reprinted with permission of Peptides, 2 (Suppl 1): 67, 1981

vesicles serve as storage sites for most neurotransmitters. This finding
further supports the suggestion that substance P may act as a modulator
rather than the neurotransmitter initiating synaptic events.
    Konishi and Otsuka (1971) showed that on the isolated frog spinal
cord preparation, substance P was about 200 times more active on a
molar basis than L-Glutamate in depolarizing spinal motoneurons. The

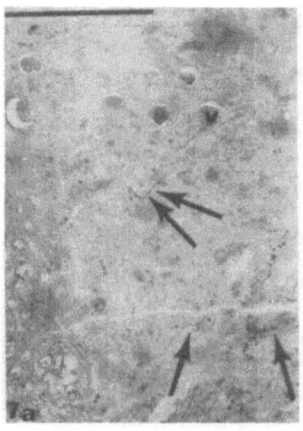 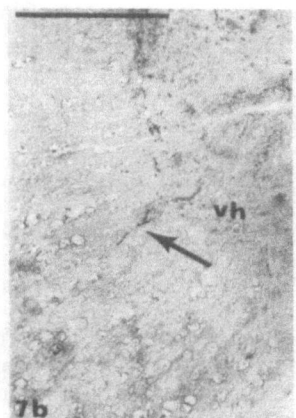 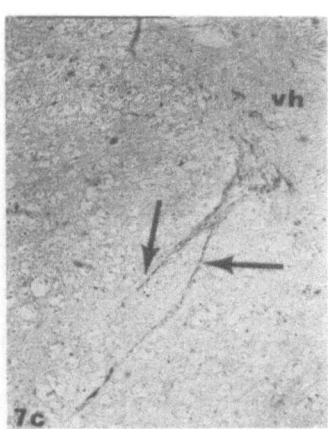

Fig. 7A. Field from the ventral horn of a sham-operated cat. Ventral
horn cells (V) are present. LE positive fibers (arrows) can be
noted and at one point (double arrow) seem to surround one of
the ventral horn cells. X 250

7B. Field showing LE immunopositive bodies at the edge of the
ventral horn (VH) in a sham-operated cat. Arrow points to a
stained branching fiber extending into the white matter. X 250

7C. Long distinct LE immunopositive fibers (arrows), extending
well into the white matter, appear to travel along with the ventral
root fibers that exit from the ventral horn (VH) in this section
taken from a sham-operated cat. X 250

Reprinted with permission of Peptides, 2 (Suppl 1): 68, 1981.

depolarizing action persisted after synaptic transmission was blocked
by Ca++ deficient Ringer's solution or by tetrodotoxin. Therefore,
they concluded, that substance P exerted a transsynaptic action on
motoneurons and was probably a candidate for the excitatory transmitter
of primary sensory neurons. In our work, immunoreactive substance
P endings could often be seen in close association with motoneurons.
    Our data concur with those of other investigators, suggesting a
pathway for substance P starting from the dorsal root ganglion via
primary afferent fibers toward their terminals in the dorsal horn of the
spinal cord. It further extends the work by demonstrating that
substance P accumulates in the dorsolateral part of the dorsal horn
below the level of the lesion, indicating an upward flow of this peptide
in the spinal cord in contrast to the downward movement from the
brain stem of monoamine transmitters by axoplasmic flow (Dahlstrom
1971; Naftchi et al., 1974). Although our data indicate an anterograde
direction of substance P in the spinal cord, it does not elucidate
whether it arises in the collaterals of primary afferent fibers or in
second order fibers.
    It was of interest to note the presence of some fibers that were
stained for substance P in the ventral horn. The amount of immunoreactive product appeared to remain constant both above and below
transection, suggesting that the substance P fibers in the ventral horn
are involved in spinal segmental transmission. The cellular origin of
these fibers is not known at present, nor is the relationship between
these processes in the ventral gray matter and those that appear more
dorsally understood. However, there are indications that they may

derive from the processes that enter the intermediate gray regions
(Vacca et al., 1980). Such considerations, while speculative, may
implicate substance P in mechanisms of visceral pain. The fact that
other substance P fibers cross in the dorsal gray commissure, a
region that also contains sympathetic innervation, lends credence to
this idea.

The immunocytochemical findings from morphine-treated rats
demonstrate that the concentration of intraneuronal substance P increased
in three regions of the spinal cord: the substantia gelatinosa, plus
Rexed's lamina I, Rexed's lamina IV and V, and the ventral horn.
The data suggest that morphine analgesia inhibits the release of intraneuronal substance P. Inhibition of substance P release has been
demonstrated in slices of trigeminal nucleus in vitro (Jessel and Iverson,
1977). Furthermore, by immunocytochemistry, we have shown that
morphine blocks the release of substance P in certain regions of the
spinal cord that are specifically associated with pain transmission: the
substantia gelatinosa and lamina V. Similarly, these regions accumulate
substance P below the level of spinal cord transection. Yaksh (1978)
has shown that lamina V neurons in the dorsal horn are discharged
by the application of noxious stimuli to their receptive fields and by
Aδ and C fiber activation. Administration of narcotics in doses that
are sufficient to produce analgesia will depress these discharges.
Previously LaMotte et al. (1976) demonstrated that opiate binding,
which is high in the substantia gelatinosa, was reduced when the dorsal
roots were cut. This finding implies that opiate receptors that bind
morphine occur on primary afferent fibers (from the dorsal root
ganglion), some of which contain substance P. Thus, they hypothesized
that their data indicated that the opiate receptors are presynaptic and
can thereby block the release of a pain transmitter such as substance P.

In addition to causing an accumulation of substance P in the
substantia gelatinosa and in lamina V, morphine treatment also resulted
in a buildup of substance P in the ventral horn. This phenomenon
raises questions concerning the relationship of the ventral horn fibers
with pain transmission. After morphine treatment, however, certain
other substance P containing processes that appeared around the
central canal, crossing in the dorsal gray commissure and subependymally,
did not differ from those in the controls.

Such differential effects may reflect regional differences in numbers
and types of opiate receptors, or in their pre- and post-synaptic
locations. More detailed dose response and opiate binding studies are
in progress.

Work by Hokfelt et al. has correlated enkephalin-positive nerve
terminals in areas where morphine is known to produce behavioral
analgesia (Hokfelt et al., 1977). In the spinal cord, these regions
also contain high concentrations of substance P. In our studies,
spinal cord transection did not produce any changes in the concentration
of leu-enkephalin-positive nerve terminals. These findings confirm
Hokfelt's results, which have demonstrated that enkephalin-containing
cells are probably interneurons within the spinal cord.

These data implicate the mutual involvement of substance P (a
probable pain transmitter) and leu-enkephalin (an endogenous opiate)
in the transmission of pain and control of pain and analgesia, as
illustrated in the following neural circuit (Figure 8). The scheme
depicts enkephalin-containing interneurons, impinging upon primary
afferent neurons that contain substance P. Enkephalin, like morphine,
binds to the pre-synaptic opiate receptors, thereby preventing the
release of the pain transmitter. This mechanism provides a working

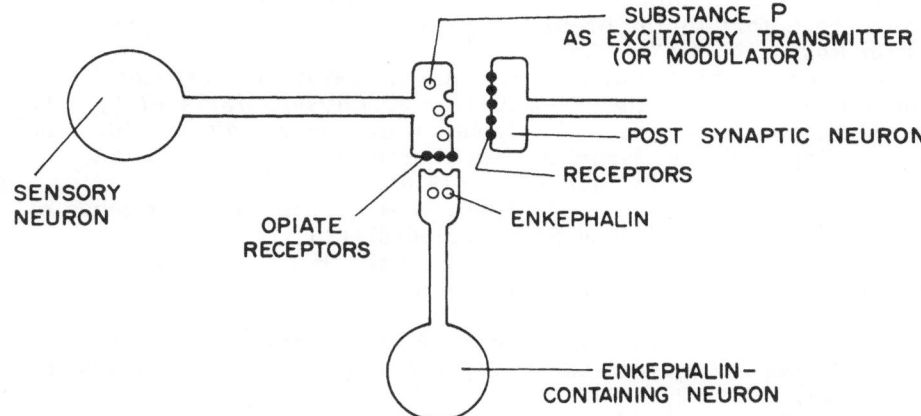

Fig. 8. A hypothetical model of presynaptic inhibition of substance P action by enkephalinergic inhibitory internuerons. Enkephalin released from an interneuron would bind to opiate receptors present on the terminal of a sensory neuron, preventing its release of substance P and thereby disrupting the transmission of pain.

Reprinted with permission of Peptides, 2 (Suppl 1): 68, 1981.

hypothesis for the control of pain by natural physiological substances.

REFERENCES

Abrahams, S.J., Naftchi, N.E., St. Paul, H.M., Lowman, E.W., and Schlosser, W. Localization and changes in substance P and leu-enkephalin in spinal cord of paraplegic cats. *Fed. Proc.* 37:439 (1978).

Brownstein, M.J., Mroz, E.A., Kizer, J.S., Palkovits, M., and Leeman, S.E. Regional distribution of substance P in the brain of the rat. *Brain Res. 116:*229-305 (1976).

Elde, R., Hokfelt, T., Johansson, O., and Terenius, L. Immunohisto-chemical studies using antibodies to leucine-enkephalin: initial observations on the nervous system of the rat. *Neuroscience 1:* 349-351 (1976).

Hokfelt, T., Kellerth, J.O., Nillson, G., and Pernow, B. Substance P: localization in the central nervous system and some primary sensory neurons. *Science 190:*889-890 (1975).

Hokfelt, T., Kellerth, J.O., Nillson, G., and Pernow, B. Experimental immunohistochemical studies on the localization and distribution of substance P in cat primary sensory neurons. *Brain Res. 100:* 235-252 (1975).

Kokfelt, T., Ljungdahl, A., Terenius, L., Elde, R., and Nillson, G. Immunohistochemical analysis of peptide pathways possibly related to pain and analgesia: enkephalin and substance P. *Proc. Nat. Acad. Sci.* 74:3081-3085 (1977).

Kanazawa, I., and Jessel, I. Post mortem changes and regional distribution of substance P in the rat and mouse nervous system; *Brain Res. 117:*362-367 (1976).

Naftchi, N.E., Abrahams, S.J., St. Paul, H., Lowman, E.W., and Schlosser, W. Localization and changes of substance P in spinal cord of paraplegic cats. *Brain Res. 153:*507-513 (1978).

Atweh, S.F., and Huhar, M.J. Autoradiographic localization of opiate receptors in rat brain. I. Spinal cord and lower medulla. *Brain Res. 124:*53-67 (1977).

Von Euler, U.S., and Gaddum, J.H. An unidentified depressor substance in certain tissue extracts. *J. Physiol. 72:*74-87 (1931).

Chang, M.M., and Leeman, S.E. Isolation of a sialogogic peptide from bovine hypothalamic tissue and its characterization as substance P. *J. Biol. Chem. 245:*4787-4790 (1970).

Chang, M.M., Leeman, S.E., and Niall, H.D. Amino acid sequence of substance P. *Nature New Biol. 232:*86-87 (1971).

Powell, D., Leeman, S., Tregear, G.W., Niall, H.D., and Potts, J.T. Radioimmunoassay for substance P. *Nature New Biol. 241:*252-254 (1973).

Cuello, A.C., Polak, J.M., and Pearse, A.G.E. Substance P: a naturally occurring transmitter in human spinal cord. *The Lancet,* 1054-1056, Nov. 12, 1976.

Henry, J.L. Effects of substance P on functionally identified units in cat spinal cord. *Brain Res. 114:*439-451 (1976).

Henry, J.L., Krnjevic, K., and Morris, M.E. Substance P and spinal neurones. *Canad. J. Physiol. Pharmacol. 53:*423-432 (1975).

Pert, C.B., and Snyder, S.H. Opiate receptor: demononstration in nervous tissue. *Science 179:*1011-1014 (1973).

Simon, E.J., Hiller, J.M., and Edelman, I. Stereospecific binding of the potent narcotic analgesic ^{3}H-etorphine to rat brain homogenate. *Proc. Nat. Acad. Sci. 70:*1947-1949 (1973).

Terenius, L. Stereospecific interaction between narcotic analgesics and a synaptic plasma membrane fraction of rat cerebral cortex. *Acta Pharmacol. Toxicol. 32:*317-320 (1973).

Simon, E.J. The opiate receptors. *Neurochem. Res. 1:*3-28 (1976).

Kuhar, M.J., Pert, C.B., and Snyder, S.H. Regional distribution of opiate receptor in rat brain. *Life. Sci. 16:*1849-1854 (1975).

Pert, C.B., Kuhar, M.J., and Snyder, S.H. Opiate receptor: autoradiographic localization in rat brain. *Proc. Nat. Acad. Sci. 73:* 3729-3733 (1976).

Hiller, J.M., Pearson, J., and Simon, E.J. Distribution of stereospecific binding of the potent narcotic analgesic etorphine in the human brain; predominance of the limbic system. *Res. Commun. in Chem. Pathol. and Pharm. 6:*1052-1062 (1973).

Liebeskind, J.C., Mayer, D.J., and Akil, H. Central mechanisms of pain inhibition: studies of analgesia from focal brain stimulation. In *Advances in Neurology,* Vol. 4 (Ed. J.J. Bonica), International Symposium on Pain, Raven press, New York, 1974, pp. 261-268.

Mayer, D.J., and Hayes, R. Stimulation-produced analgesia: development of tolerence and cross-tolerence to morphine. *Science 188:* 941-943 (1975).

Mayer, D.J., and Liebeskind, J.C. Pain reduction by focal electrical stimulation of the brain: an anatomical and behavioral analysis. *Brain Res. 68:*73-93 (1974).

Hughes, J. Isolation of an endogenous compound from the brain with properties similar to morphine. *Brain Res. 88:*295-308 (1975).

Hughes, J., Smith, T., Kosterlitz, H.W., Fothergill, L.A., Morgan, B., and Morris, H.R. Identification of two related pentapeptides from the brain with potent opiate agonist activity. *Nature 258:* 577-579 (1975).

Simantov, R., and Snyder, S.H. Morphine-like peptides in mammalian brain: isolation, structure, elucidation and interaction with the opiate receptor. *Proc. Nat. Acad. Sci. 73:*2515-2519 (1976).

Simantov, R., Kuhar, M.J., Uhl, G.R., and Snyder, S.H.   Opioid
    peptide enkephalin: immunohistochemical mapping in the rat central
    nervous system. *Proc. Nat. Acad. Sci.* *74:*2167-2171 (1977).
LaMotte, C., Pert, C.B., and Snyder, S.H.   Opiate receptor binding
    in primate spinal cord: distribution and changes after dorsal root
    section. *Brain Res.* *112:*407-412 (1976).
Moore, G., Lutterodt, A., Burford, G., and Lederis, K.   A highly
    specific antiserum for arginine vasporessin. *Endocrinology 101:*
    1421-1435 (1977).
Sternberger, L. *Immunocytochemistry,* Prentice-Hall, Englewood
    Cliffs, New Jersey, 1974.
Pickel, V.M., Reis, D.J., and Leeman, S.E.   Ultrastructural
    localization of substance P in neurons of rat spinal cord. *Brain
    Res.* *122:*534-540 (1977).
Vacca, L.L., Rosario, S., Zimmerman, E.A., Tomachefsky, P., Ng,
    P.-Y., and Hsu, K.G.   Application of immunoperoxidase techniques
    to localize horseradish peroxidase tracer in the central nervous
    system. *J. Histochem. Cytochem.* *23:*208 (1975).
Vacca, L.L., Abrahams, S.J., and Naftchi, N.E.   A modified peroxidase
    antiperoxidase procedure for improved localization of tissue
    antigens: localization of substance P in rat spinal cord. *J.
    Histochem. Cytochem.* *28:*297-307 (1980).
Rexed, B.   A cytoarchitectonic atlas of the spinal cord in the cat. *J.
    Comp. Neurol.* *100:*297-379 (1954).
Otsuka, M., Konishi, S., and Takahashi, T.   Hypothalamic substance
    P as a condidate for transmitter of primary afferent neurons. *Fed.
    Proc.* *34:*1922-1928 (1975).
Konishi, S., and Otsuka, M.   The effects of substance P and other
    peptides on spinal neurons of the frog. *Brain Res.* *65:*397-410
    (1974).
Dahlstrom, A.   Axoplasmic transport. *Phil. Trans. B.* *261:*325-358
    (1971).
Naftchi, N.E., Demeny, M., Kertesz, A., Viau, A.T., and Lowman, E.W.
    Effect of spinal cord transection on mammalian biogenic amines,
    c-AMP, and tyrosine hydroxylase activity in CNS, adrenals and
    heart. *Trans. Amer. Soc. Neurochem.* *5:*80 (1974).
Jessel, M.J., and Iverson, L.   Opiate analgesics inhibit substance P
    release from rat trigeminal nucleus. *Nature 268:*549-551 (1977).
Yaksh, T.L.   Opiate receptors for behavioral analgesia resemble
    those related to the depression of spinal nociceptive neurons.
    *Science 199:*1231-1232 (1978).

8

Quarternary and Monoamine Imbalance After Spinal Transection (A Possible Mechanism of Spasticity)

V. SAHGAL, V. SUBARAMI, M. RODRIGUEZ, and C. WURSTER

Imbalance between the major striatal neurotransmitters (monoamines and acetylcholine) has been implicated in the pathogenesis of extrapyramidal disorders such as Parkinson's Disease (McGeer et al., 1961; Barbeau, 1962; Spehlman, 1975; Spehlman and Stahl, 1974 and 1976). Carlsson et al. (1964) demonstrated a presence of monoamine terminals in the rat spinal cord. These amines have been shown to disappear within a week below the level of the transection and are enhanced above the level of the lesion (Carlsson et al., 1964; Magnuson and Rosengren, 1967; Carlsson et al., 1963; Naftchi et al., 1974; Rodriguez et al., 1977). There is a great deal of evidence that acetylcholine is a major transmitter in the spinal cord. There are, however, only scattered reports dealing with the changes in the cholinergic systems following spinal transection. To our knowledge, there are no studies in which the cholinergic and monoamine systems of the spinal cord have been simultaneously studied, and the clinical effects of spinal transection correlated with the alterations in these systems.

In this study we present the distribution of monoamine (norepinephrine, dopamine, and serotonin) terminals, cholinesterase, and choline acetyltransferase activity in the rat spinal cord and a correlation between the clinical and histochemical events following a thoracic transection.

MATERIALS AND METHODS

Female Sprague-Dawley rats weighing 250-300 G were used throughout this study. In all instances a control and an experimental animal run were done together in order to compare the intensity of the reactions and to guard against day-to-day variations. All animals were fed a similar diet (Purina Rat Chow) and kept in single cages.

Experimentals

Rats were anasthetized by intraperitoneal injection of luminal (0.05 ml/100 g) and laminectomy was performed under aspectic conditions. The spinal cord was exposed and transected at the T6 level. Each end was picked up with cotton sutures to insure the completeness of the lesion.

The control animals underwent laminectomy and spinal cord exposure.

Maintenance of the animals

The animals were given appropriate bowel and bladder care. They were examined daily for sensory level, development of spasticity, placing reactions, decubiti, and their bladders and bowels were manually evacuated. When decubiti or infection developed, the animal was excluded from the study. Flexor and extensor reflexes were elicited and quantitiated by the method of Nygren and Olson (1976). Edrophonium hydrochloride 0.25 mg, physostigmine 0.15 mg, and norepinephrine 0.01 mg were injected in the subarachnoid space of spastic rats to see the effects on spasticity.

Sacrifice

The animals were sacrificed by cardiac puncture at 24 hour, three day, five day, two week, and five week intervals. Spinal cords were removed within five to seven minutes and divided into cervical, thoracic, lumbar, and sacral regions. Parts of each region were used for monoamine, choline acetyltransferase and acetyl cholinesterase reactions.

Morphology

The sections were stained by H&E, nissl, or Kluver-Berara stains to observe the morphological changes.

Histochemistry

Monoamines

The spinal cord sections were freeze-dried in a Viritis Model #10-800 Freeze-drier, exposed to formaldehyde vapours equiliberated to 80% water, embedded in paraffin, and cut in serial eight to 10 μ sections. The sections were viewed for fluourescence, using Barrier Filter 530 and excitor filter 1312 (Falck and Hillarp, 1962).

Acetylcholinesterase

This reaction was carried out by using acetylthiocholine as substrate according to the method of Koelle (1956). Preincubation with ISOMPA (10^{-5}M) was carried out to ensure specificity for acetylcholinesterase reaction and eserine sulphate (10^{-6}M) to inhibit all cholinesterase acitivyt. A nonsubstrate control was always run concurrently.

Choline Acetyltransferase

Activity of this enzyme was demonstrated by the method described by Kasa and Morris (1972) using acetyl COA and $Pb(\tilde{N}O3)_2$ as substrate.

RESULTS

Controls: Monoamines

By this treatment, norepinephrine fluoresced green, while serotonin fluoresced yellow. In the adult animals, lipofuscin was always seen in the neurons as yellow-brown fluorescence, and this caused difficulty with the identification of serotonin fluourescence. In order to overcome this, spinal cords from two-day old litters were looked at for fluorescence.

The monoamine terminals throughout the spinal cord varied from 0.3-1.5 µ in size.

Cervical Cord

In this region, both yellow and green fluorescing varicosities were observed. These varicosities were most abundant in the dorsal part of the posterior horn and anterior horn region of the gray matter. The majority of the varicosities in the anterior horn region were seen in the neuropil, and only a few terminals were observed on the anterior horn cell bodies (Figure 1). The varicosities were concentrated in the ventromedial region, corresponding to the Rexed lamina 8, and the ventrolateral rostral region, corresponding to the Rexed lamina 7. Very few varicosities were seen in the region of the Rexed lamina 9. In the white matter, yellow and green fluorescing tracts were only seen in the posterolateral columns. In the posterior horn, the most dorsal part showed a cap of green fluorescing varicosities (Figure 1).

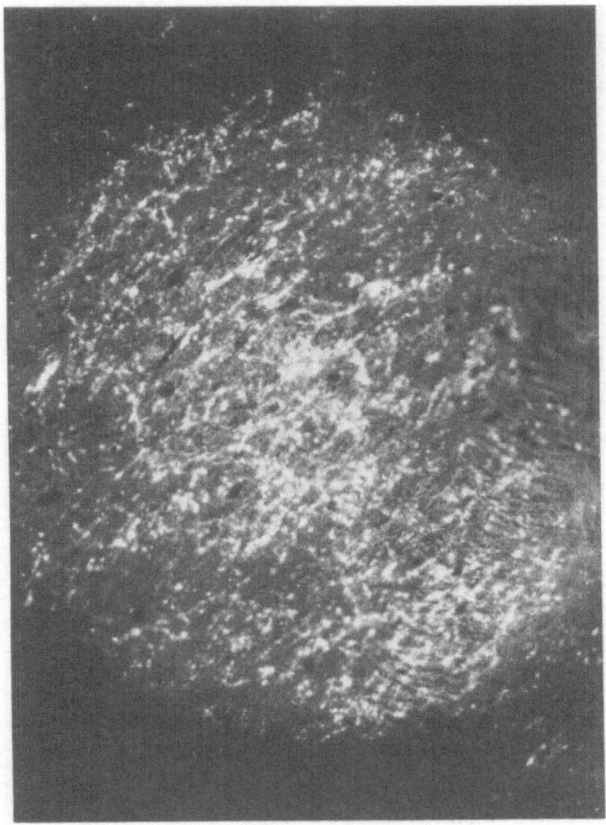

Fig. 1. Anterior horn region at T10 level. Note the intense yellow (serotonin) and yellow-green (norepinephrine) varicosities. Lipofuscin pigments are seen in the neurons.

Thoracic Cord

In this region most of the green and yellow fluorescing varicosities were distributed in the intermedio-lateral gray, internuncial, and the anterior gray region.   In the intermedio-lateral gray zone, there was accumulation of intense green fluorescing terminals (Figure 2).   These terminals seemed to be connected with the other side, as shown by the fluorescent terminals that were observed in the region of the anterior gray commisure (Figure 3).   Many yellow and green terminals were seen in the region corresponding to Rexed laminae 5-6.   In the anterior horn region, the bulk of the terminals again were seen in the neuropil not against the anterior horn cells and were concentrated mainly in the ventrolateral and medial regions, corresponding to the Rexed areas 7 and 8.   In the posterior horn these varicosities were again observed in the dorsal part.

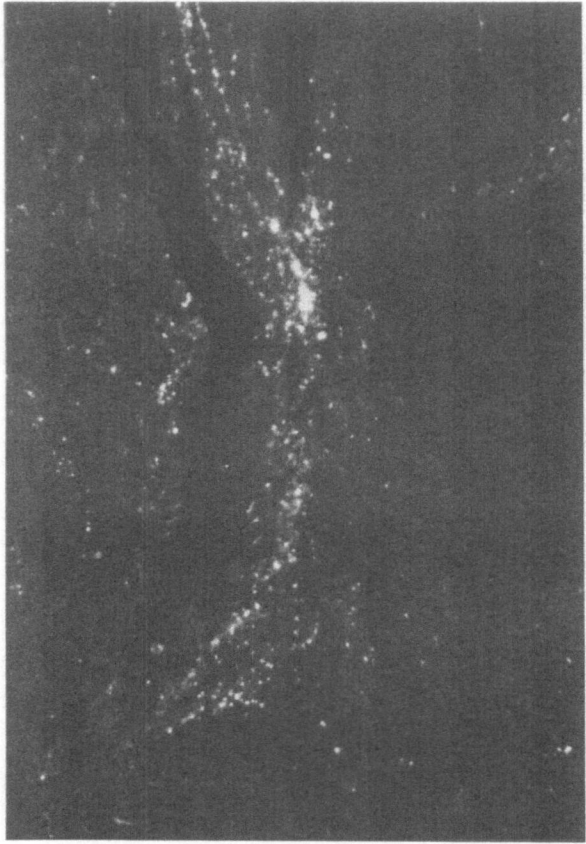

Fig. 2.   Note the fluorescent terminals in the region around the central canal.

Lumbosacral Cord

In this region the distribution of the monoamine terminals was essentially the same as in the thoracic cord; however, their number was far greater and the size was larger.   It was particularly noteworthy that there were more yellow fluorescing terminals in this region.

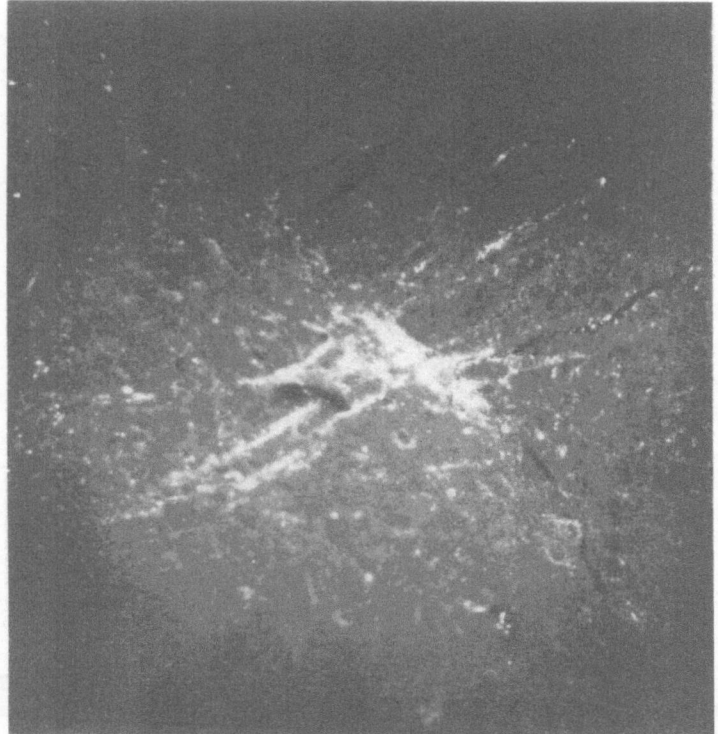

Fig. 3. Intermediolateral cell column showing yellow-green and yellow fluorescence.

Acetylcholinesterase and Choline Acetyltransferase

With these reactions the enzyme activity was demonstrated as brown deposits of lead sulphide. The cholinesterase reaction was completely inhibited by eserine pretreatment while ISOMPA pretreatment had no effect. In general the activity of this enzyme was more definable in the gray than white matter. In the gray matter the enzyme activity was more intense in the neurons than the neuropil.

Cervical Region

In this region the spinal cord showed differential reaction. Dark areas were observed in the dorsal part of the posterior horn, corresponding to the Rexed laminae 1-2. In the laminae 3-4-5 heavy reaction was observed only in the region around the central canal, corresponding to various nuclei. The rest of the areas showed light to intermediate reaction. In the anterior horn, heavy reaction product was observed in the area corresponding to the Rexed lamina 9. In the laminae 7 and 8, there were scattered neurons that showed heavy reaction while the rest of the region showed mixed reaction (Figure 4).

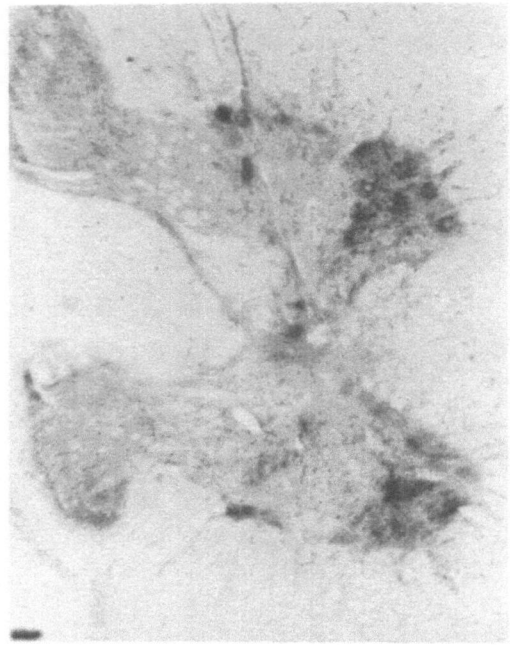

Fig. 4. Choline acetyltransferase activity—thoracic region (T 12)—20 days
after transection. Note the activity in the anterior horn and intermediolateral region.

Thoracic Cord

Throughout the length of the thoracic cord, the distribution of
cholinesterase and choline acetyltransferase activity was quite similar
to the cervical cord except that in this region very heavy reaction
was seen in intermediolateral gray column and the dorsomedial gray
columns. In the lateral part of the ventral horn cells, the neurons
with heavy reaction were 30-60 μ in size (Figure 5).

Lumbosacral Cord

The cholinesterase and choline acetyltransferase distribution was
similar to the thoracic level except for a lateral pool of neurons which
showed heightened activity. The cell diameter in these areas varied
from 15-30 μ.

Spinal Transection

Up to 1-2 days following transection, the animals almost always
showed flaccid motor paralysis, complete loss of sensation below the
level of the lesion, and bladder and bowel incontinence. In all these
animals bowel and bladder needed manual expression for about seven
days. On the fourth post-operative day the animals started showing
evidence of spasticity. In one week, the animals started showing
early placing reaction but still dragged their hind quarter and were
incontinent of bowel and bladder. After 10 days, extensor spasms
were observed and the rats started attempting to stand on their hind

legs. After four weeks, even though the rats had weakness of the
legs, they showed reciprocal leg motion, spasticity, automatic bladder,
and complete anesthesia below the lesion. Atrophy of the legs in
general was constantly observed.

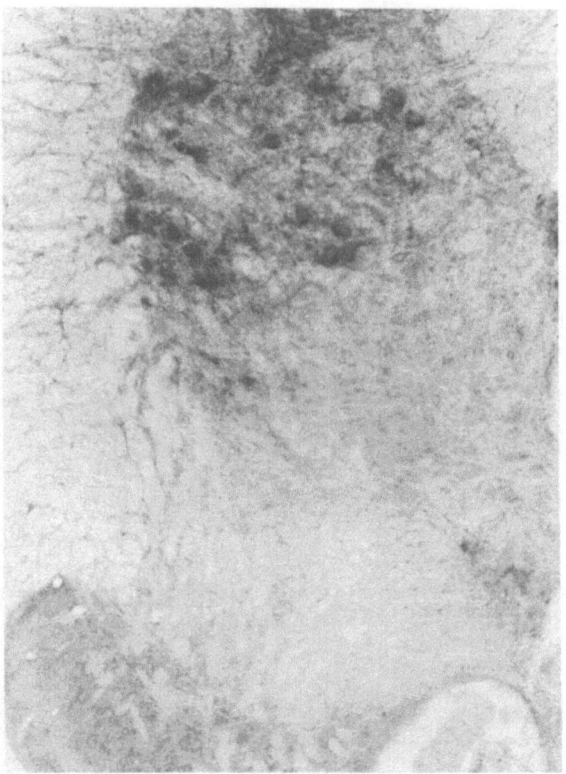

Fig. 5. Choline acetyltransferase activity in the lumbar enlargement.
Note the dark-reacting neurons in the anterior horn region.

Catecholamines

    Above the level of the lesion the green and yellow varicosities
were much more prominent and varied from 1.5-2 μ in size. The
distribution followed the control profile. The large size of the varicosities indicated collection of the transmitter above the lesion
(Figure 6).
    Occasionally, green fluorescing neurons (5-15 μ in size) were
seen in the region of the Rexed laminae 5 and 6. This is the first
time that cell body fluorescence was observed in the spinal cord. On
serial sectioning close to the lesion site, the fluorescent varicosities
became larger and more intense. At the site of the lesion, collections
of intense yellow-green fluorescence were seen as early as eight hours
after the lesion (Figure 6).
    Multiple cavities of varied diameters were seen from the seventh
day onward (Figure 7). This fluorescence corresponded to the regions
where, morphologically, collection of blood was seen. The fluorescence
was stable and had wide spectrum (Figure 7) but decreased significantly

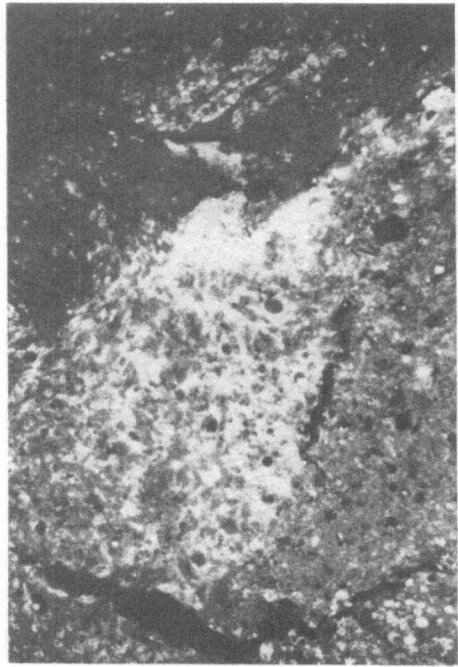

Fig. 6. Two weeks after spinal transection at T6–7 lesion site. Note cavitation and intense yellow fluorescence.

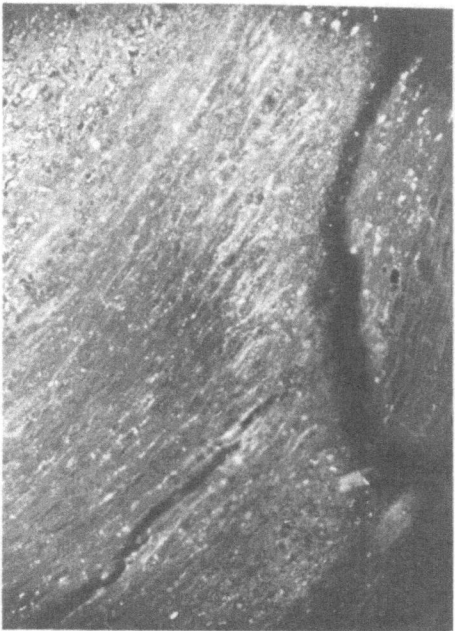

Fig. 7. Above the lesions, four weeks after transection. Note the large size of the varicosities in the gray region. The white matter also shows prominent fluorescent fibers.

over the six week period when gliosis was apparent in the region.
Large green varicosities were also sparingly seen. Below the level of
the lesion, however, green and yellow varicosities could be visualized
only until the fifth day. By one week, no green or yellow fluorescing
varicosities were seen below the lesion, indicating a break in the
continuity of the aminergic fiber system and damming back at the
upper level. The intense green fluorescence that was seen in the
thoracic intermedio-lateral column in the controls was also distinctly
absent (Figure 7). Eight weeks after the transection adjacent to
the lesion site, an irregular network of aminergic tracts could be seen.
Some of the fibers were traced beyond the lesion site. The sympathetic
ganglia maintained the aminergic fluorescence pattern (Figure 8).

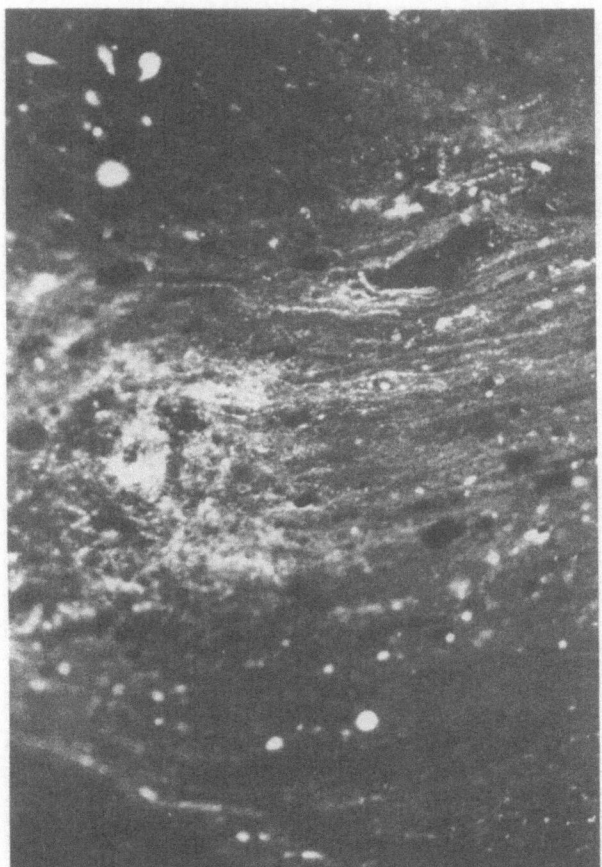

Fig. 8. Lumbar region two weeks after transection. Note the absence
of varicosities and the bare neurons showing lipofuscin pigments.

Cholinesterase and Choline Acetyltransferas.

Above the level of the lesion, the enzyme distribution compared
favorably with the controls. At the site of the lesion, the architecture
of the spinal cord was grossly disrpted and three days after transection,
the enzyme activity was very diffuse. The enzyme activity remained
diffuse and disorganized for about six weeks, at which time a network-
like pattern of activity was seen, indicating sprouting of axon. Below

the lesion, up to six weeks after the transection, enzyme activity
was seen at all levels.   The distribution was mainly at the tip of the
posterior horn and the anterior horn cell region and the intermediolateral
cell column of the thoracic segments.   The neuropil, however, showed
a significant decrease in the intensity of the reaction (Figure 4 and 9).

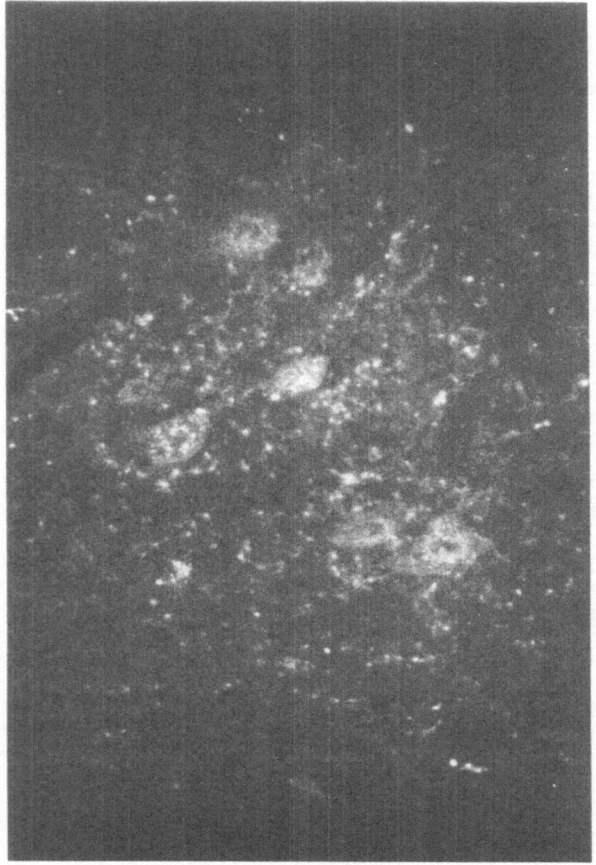

Fig. 9. Below the lesion around T10 lesion, three months after transection,
note the cavitation and large-sized varicosities.   Also, there is a
basketweave pattern of the fluorescent fibers.

Effect of Intrathecal Pharmacologic Agents

Intrathecal administration of edrophonium and physostigmine
elicited extensor spasms and bowel and bladder evacuation.   The injection
of norepinephrine caused dissolution of spasticity and the animals
became flaccid.

DISCUSSION

Our histofluorescence studies show that the amine terminals (5-HT
and NE) are largely distributed in the ventromedial part of the sympathetic column in the thoracic region, the ventral horn, the dorsal horn,
and the central gray zone throughout the spinal cord.   In the ventral

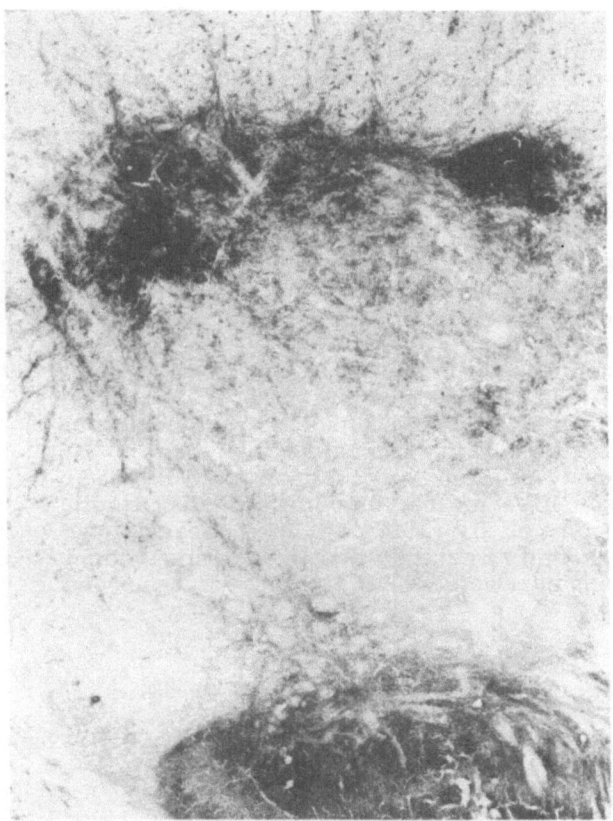

Fig. 10. Choline acetyltransferase activity-seven days after injury. In the lumbar region, note the dark-reacing neurons in the anterior horn region.

gray region, the terminals are most abundant in the ventromedial and ventrolateral areas. Most of these terminals were present in the neuropil. Similar distribution of amines has been observed by Dahlstrom and Fuxe (1965). Unlike these investigators we were able to identify catecholamine cell body fluorescence in the small neurons of the central gray zone. After thoracic transection, terminals above the lesion were swollen, indicating damming back of the transmitters. At the lesion site, there was a collection of intense yellow fluorescence that did not fade on exposure to light and had a very wide emission spectrum, indicating that this was not entirely due to catecholamines. These areas of fluorescence corresponded to the areas of hemorrhagic necrosis. This fluorescence could be observed weeks after the lesion and was later replaced by cavitation. The finding of yellow fluorescence at the site of spinal lesion has been previously observed by Osterholm et al. (1972) and interpreted as solely due to the catecholamines. This led to the use of various agents, like alpha methyl tyrosine, reserpine, and phenoxy benzamine, in the treatment of experimental spinal trauma. However, the efficacy of these agents is very debatable. The wide fluorescent spectrum and the stability of the fluorescence indicate that this yellow fluorescence is not aminergic. The biochemical findings of Naftchi et al., (1974) de la Torre (1974) and Bingham (1975) would agree with our observations.

Of greater significance was the fact that as spasticity developed in the animals and flexor withdrawal reflex gave way to the extensor spasms, there was a gradual decline in the amine fluorescence below the lesion disappearing in seven to 10 days. This observation agrees with the previously described finding of Carlsson et al. (1965). However, they did not correlate their findings with the functional state of the animals. Nygren and Olson, however, have shown that the flexor reflex is dependent on the norepinephrine receptors, which would agree with the clinical transition after spinal injury and the effect of intrathecal clonidine. The extensor spasms, following intrathecal administration of physostigmine, suggest that extensor mechanism may be cholinergic. This contention is further strengthened by the observation of intact choline acetyltransferase and acetyl cholinesterase activity below the lesion. These findings would be in accord with Granit's (1955) theory that cholinergic mechanisms enhance alpha motor activity. Since many of the aminergic terminals are present in relation to the alpha motor neuron, the lack of aminergic neurons make the alpha motor neurons sensitive to acetylcholine. Similar findings have been reported by Galabov et al. (1967). These observations lead us to conclude that spasticity that follows spinal transection is a cholinergic phenomenon, perhaps related to the alpha motor activity.

REFERENCES

Barbeau, A. *Canad. Med. Asso. J. 87:*802 (1962).

Bingham, W.G. *J. Neurosurg. 42:*174 (1975).

Carlsson, A., Falck, B., and Fuxe, K. *Acta Physiol. Scand. 60:*112 (1964).

Dahlstrom, A., and Fuxe, K. *Acta Physiol. Scand. 64:*1 (Supplement 1247 (1965).

De La Torre, J.C. *Surg. Neurology. 5:*11 (1974).

Falck, B., Hillarp, N.A., Thinne, G., and Torp, A. *J. Histochem., Cytochem. 10:*348 (1962).

Galabov, G., Minolov, S., Venkov, L., Nikolov, T., and Itchov, K. *Acta Anat. 18:*432 (1967).

Granit, R. Receptors and Sensory Perception. Yale University Press, New Haven, 1955.

Kasa, P., and Morris, D. *J. Neurochem. 19:*1299 (1972).

Koelle, G.B., and Friedwald, J.S. *Proc. Soc. Exptl. Biol. Med. 70:* 617 (1949).

Magnusson, F., and Rosengreen, E. *Experientia. 19:*223 (1963).

Mc Geer, P.L., Boulding, J.E., Gibson, W.C., and Foulkes, R.G. *JAMA. 177:*665 (1961).

Naftchi, N.E., et al. *J. Neurosurg. 40:*52 (1974).

Nygren, L., and Olson, L. *Brain Research* - In Press, Personal Communication.

Osterholm, J. et al. *J. Neurosurg. 36:*395 (1972).

Rodriguez, M., Sahgal, V., and Subarmani, V. *Arch. PM & R - In Press* (1977).

Spehlman, R., and Stahl, S. *Exp. Neur. 42:*703 (1974).

Spehlman, R. *Brain. 98:*219 (1975).

Spehlman, R., and Stahl, S. The Lancet, p. 724, 1976.

9

Alterations of Various Physiological and Biochemical Parameters During the Development of Spasticity in the Chronic Spinal Cat

W. SCHLOSSER, S. FRANCO, G. BAUTZ,
D.W. HORST, and N.E. NAFTCHI

SUMMARY

In cats that were made paraplegic by total spinal cord transection, a number of changes occur that lead to spasticity. There is a gradual loss of prolonged spinal inhibition (presynaptic inhibition) that is accompanied by a decrease of Km and Vmax values for glutamic acid decarboxylase (GAD), both above and below the lesion. This enzyme is necessary for the conversion of glutamic acid to γ-aminobutyric acid (GABA), the transmitter mediating presynaptic inhibition. Although the Km and Vmax levels for GAD eventually return to the control values, presynaptic inhibition remains depressed. Diazepam enhances presynaptic inhibition in acute and, to a lesser extent, in chronic spinal cats. This increase in presynaptic inhibition is accompanied by a reduction in somatic muscular activity in both acute and chronic spinal animals.

Histochemical fluorescence studies reveal a buildup of catecholamine (norepinephrine) above transection and its disappearance below transection. In the acute spinal cat, inhibition of the monosynaptic response of extensor motoneurons is blocked by a conditioning volley that is applied to cutaneous afferents. As the time interval between conditioning and test stimulus is increased, there is a rapid return of the monosynaptic potential to control values. In contrast, in chronic spinal cats (one week to 12 weeks), the duration of complete blockade of the extensor monosynaptic potential by cutaneous afferents is markedly reduced, followed by a prolonged period when cutaneous nerve stimulation potentiates the monosynaptic discharge. There is a transitional phase of two to five days post-transection, when the conditioning volley to cutaneous afferents only partially inhibits extensor motoneuron monosynaptic responses. It is concluded that spasticity resulting from spinal cord lesion could result from numerous factors, involving changes in various neurotransmitters both above and below the region of transection.

INTRODUCTION

An increased excitability in segmental reflex pathways has been one of the traditional paradigms of positive symptoms that result from the loss of supraspinal control over spinal cord activity. The reason for this phenomenon remains obscure, although a number of explanations have been suggested. Descending pathways exert a marked influence on γ-motoneuron activity. They may either excite or inhibit γ-neurons through a postsynaptic mechanism (Magoun and Rhines, 1946; Magoun, 1950). Indirectly, this mechanism controls α-motoneurons by its action on γ-motoneurons (Granit and Kaada, 1952). This latter system, through the well-known γ-control of muscle spindles, sets the bias for activation of the Ia afferents that form synaptic connection with motoneurons (Granit, 1955). More recent studies have shown the significance of descending noradrenergic and 5-hydroxytrypaminergic pathways as inhibitors of spinal interneurons. These interneurons control transmission from the flexor reflex afferents (cutaneous, joint and high threshold muscle afferents) to motoneurons (Anden et al., 1966a,b; Engberg and Ryall, 1966). Removal of these descending monoaminergic inhibitory structures produces an increased afferent input from the periphery to the motoneuronal pool, thus enhancing the excitability of the system.

At the segmental level, Teasdall and Staraky (1953) suggested that the increase in reflex activity may be in accord with Cannon's law of denervation supersensitivity. Thus, a motoneuron, deprived of a significant portion of its presynaptic input, may respond in an exaggerated fashion when exposed to an excitatory neurotransmitter. Others have suggested that increased neuronal activity may result from sprouting of new excitatory synapses from the dorsal root ganglion to the mononeuronal pool (McCouch et al., 1958).

Clinical studies, in particular those of Burke and Ashby (1972) and Delwaide (1973), suggest a reduction of the presynaptic inhibitory mechanism as one factor in the patholphysiology of spasticity. They have reported that the inhibition of the H-reflex, resulting from vibratory stimulation, is reduced in subjects in a state of spastic hyperreflexia. This methodology for examining presynaptic inhibitory processes in man is based on studies done in the cat, in which the monosynaptic reflex is inhibited by vibration of the intact hindlimb. This suppression of the monosynaptic reflex by vibration was shown to be mediated by presynaptic inhibition since: (1) it correlated with the onset of the dorsal root potential (DRP) evoked by vibration; (2) it was reduced by picrotoxin; and (3) it produced primary afferent depolarization (PAD), as demonstrated by direct stimulation of the afferent fibers (Gillies et al., 1969).

Thus, a number of factors may play a part in the genesis of spasticity: (1) the release from tonic inhibition and excitation by supraspinal structures; (2) supersensitivity of denervated structures; (3) collateral sprouting; and (4) direct changes in segmental spinal inhibitory pathways.

In the present investigation in the chronic spinal cat, we examined spinal reflex activity, neuropharmacological, histochemical, and neurochemical changes during the development of spasticity.

METHODS

Female cats that weigh between 2.1-3.2 kg were selected for this study. Under sterile conditions the animals were anesthesized with 30 mg/kg Ketamine HCl I.M. Supplementary injections were made, if necessary. The spinal cord was exposed by a dorsal laminectomy at T12-L1. The dura was cut and the exposed cord treated with xylocaine, 2 ml of a 1% solution. The local anesthetic properties of the xylocaine served to reduce bleeding when the cord was transected. Complete cord transection was made between T12-L1. Small pieces of gelfoam were then placed into position between the cut ends of the cord. This

aided in reducing the degree of bleeding. The gelfoam was left in
place and each layer, muscle, fascia and skin, was sutured separately.
Terramycin was injected for the next four days. Cats with total
cord transection are unable to urinate. Consequently, their bladder
had to be emptied manually two to three times a day.

Neurophysiological Methods

Animals were selected for study at various times following transection,
from two to ninety-one days. Each animal was anesthetized with
Metofane (Methoxyflurane), the trachea cannulated, and the blood
supply to the head ligated. The spinal cord was transected at
C_1, and the animal placed on a respirator and allowed to recover
from anesthesia. The spinal cord was then exposed from L5-S2. The
most caudal rootlet of L6 dorsal root was dissected free to the level of
its entrance into the cord and placed on recording electrodes for measurement of the DRP. Either L7 or S1 ventral root was placed on recording
electrodes. Three ipsilateral hindlimb nerves, gastrocnemius-soleus
(GS), posterior biceps semitendinosus (PBST), and sural, were
dissected free and placed on stimulating electrodes. Mineral oil maintained at a temperature of $36\pm1°C$ was used to cover exposed tissue.
The end respirator PCO_2 was monitored continuously and maintained
at 3.5-4%. Preparations with blood pressure lower than 90 mm Hg were
not used. Sets of 16 evoked responses were analyzed by a computer
of average transients and displayed on an x-y recorder for later
determination of amplitudes of various potentials. At the end of the
experiment, cord samples from sections above and below transection
were removed for histochemical or biochemical analysis.

Histochemical Methods

Histofluorescent evaluations of spinal cord catecholamines were done
by the method of Falck and Owman (1965). Two cm segments of the
spinal cords above and below transection were removed and placed on
crushed ice, and transverse 1 mm slices were cut. The tissue slabs
were quenched in isopentane, which had been precooled with liquid
nitrogen for thirty seconds, and then freeze-dried in an Edwards-Pearse
tissue dryer. Following freeze-drying for approximately 48 hours,
the samples were placed in a preheated, closed vessel with paraformaldehyde, equilibrated to 65% relative humidity. The reaction vessel was
then placed in an oven at 80°C for one hour, and the tissues were
infiltrated in embedding media for 15 minutes at 60°C in vacuo for
subsequent blocking. Paraffin sections 8 microns thick were cut on a
microtome and were coverslipped with an Entellan-xylene mixture to
remove paraffin. They were then placed on a 56°C warming plate.
In order to rule out nonspecific fluorescence, tissue samples that
served as control were treated exactly as the test samples but were
not exposed to paraformaldehyde.
Fluorescent microscopic examination was done, using an Aus Jena
microscope. During processing, photographs were made from film
that was pushed two full stops to increase the film sensitivity.

Neurochemical Methods

Sample Preparation for Biochemical Measurements

All assays were performed on tissue samples that were homogenized in five volumes of 0.167 M potassium phosphate buffer, pH 6.5.

Glutamic Acid Decarboxylase Kinetic Measurements

Determinations were made on 50 μl portions of the homogenate, according to the method of Bird and Iversen (1974), which involves entrapment and measurement of evolved $C^{14}O_2$. Specific activities of the glutamic acid substrates were so adjusted that each sample contained 0.10 μci of dL[]-^{14}C glutamic acid. Several molarities of nonradioactive 1-glutamic acid (final concentrations = $3.35 \times 10^{-3}M$, $1.03 \times 10^{-3}M$, $3.48 \times 10^{-4}M$, and $1.39 \times 10^{-4}M$) were used and incubated for one hour. Protein was determined by the method of Lowery et al. (1951).

Calculations

Product that was formed per mg protein per hour was analyzed for Km and Vmax, according to the method of Cleland (1967) as modified by Ottaway (1973).

RESULTS

The first signs of spasticity appeared within two to three weeks following transection. The onset was typically seen as a fanning of the toes of the hindlimbs with concomitant twitching of the feet when the cats were raised from the ground. As time progressed, the legs remained in an extended state with spontaneous scissor-like movements and rapid movement of the tail when the preparation was held by the scruff of the neck. During the spastic state, the preparations had an exaggerated flexor reflex. Further, the placement reflex was missing as evidenced by inability of the leg to respond when the dorsal part of the foot came in contact with an object.

Figure 1 illustrates the effect of complete cord transection on prolonged spinal inhibition. A volley of five pulses at two times threshold was delivered through the PBST nerve to condition a test monosynaptic response, evoked by stimulation of the GS nerve. The ordinate shows the amplitude (percent of control) of the monosynaptic discharge that was conditioned by inhibitory impulses at varying time intervals, as shown on the abscissa. The inhibitory curve marked two weeks represents the mean value from eight preparations that were tested two days to two weeks following transection. This curve is similar to that which was observed in the acute spinal preparations. The first sign of a decrease in the prolonged spinal inhibitory mechanism was observed at six weeks, when an apparent reduction in inhibition occurred at the beginning and the end of the curve. The remaining part of the curve does not differ from that of the two week cats. The data for the six week preparations are the mean values from four cats. Two preparations were made at eight weeks. Their curve (not shown) falls between those of six weeks and 12 weeks. At 12 weeks there was a marked attenuation of prolonged spinal inhibition. Note that the duration of inhibition was no more than 50 msec, whereas in the two week cats inhibition lasted over 200 msec.

One of the major effects of diazepam in the acute spinal cat is the

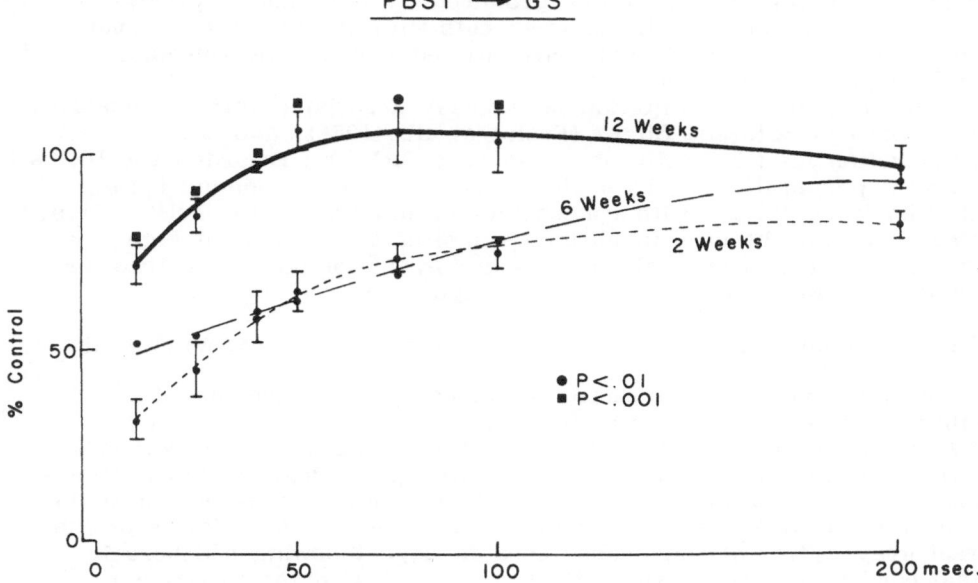

Fig. 1. Effect of complete spinal cord transection on prolonged "pre-synaptic" inhibition of the monosynaptic reflex: the inhibitory curves relate the percent of control of the monosynaptic potential (ordinate) to the interval between conditioning and test volley (abscissae).   The monosynaptic reflex was evoked by two volleys (1.5 msec intervals) in the nerve of the GS.   The first volley produced no reflex but facilitated that which was produced by the second volley.   The mono-synaptic reflex was recorded from either L7 or S1 ventral root.   The GS reflex was inhibited by five volleys (320/sec) in the PBST nerve (2X threshold).   Each point represents the mean value and standard error.   The curve that is marked two weeks represent values from eight preparations studied two days to two weeks after transection and that is marked six weeks is from four animals five to six weeks following transection.   The curve that is labeled 12 weeks is from six preparations ten weeks to 91 days after transection.   The P values compare the two and 12 weeks data.

prolongation and enhancement of presynaptic inhibition (Schmidt et al., 1967; Schlosser, 1971; Stratten and Barnes, 1971). The effect of this drug on presynaptic inhibition in chronic spinal cats is illustrated in Figure 2. The mean values from four preparations that were observed at two days to two weeks following transection and from four preparations that were observed at 10-12 weeks after transection are in Figure 2A. These animals then received 1 mg/kg diazepam i.v. It is evident that diazepam increases the inhibition in each case (Figure 2B). Although the degree of inhibition that was produced by diazepam is greatly reduced when comparing the 12 week cats with the two week animals. Nonetheless, we observed that diazepam reduced somatic muscular spasticity in these chronic animals.

Since presynaptic inhibition is typically associated with a depolarization of primary afferent fibers (Eccles et al., 1964), and this depolarization is most easily observed as a DRP, we recorded the DRP's from most preparations. Typically, a reduction of prolonged spinal inhibition is associated with concomitant attenuation of the DRP. This, however, is not the case in chronic spinal cats as shown in Figure 3. There are little apparent differences in dorsal root potentials recorded from the two week and 12 week cats (Figure 3).

Effect of Spinal Transection on γ-Aminobutyric Acid (GABA) Activity

The putative neurotransmitter involved in prolonged spinal inhibition is GABA. This inhibition is associated with axo-axonic synapses on primary afferent fibers and with axo-dendritic synapses on motoneurons (Curtis et al., 1971). Our physiological data indicates a loss of this inhibitory mechanism as time progresses after transection. Smith et al. (1976) observed an initial decrease in GABA levels of the dorsal gray matter of the lumbar cord in dogs following midthoracic spinal cord transection, which they correlated with the progressive development of spinal spasticity. Twelve weeks after transection, the GABA level was 68% above control. They suggested that the increase in GABA levels may represent diminished release of the neurotransmitter from the interneurons, mediating presynaptic inhibition. Our data on the enzyme 1-glutamate decarboxylase (GAD) activity (Km and Vmax) correlate well with the observations of Smith et al. (1976) on changes in GABA concentration. In the acute spinal cat (Figure 4), in sections below transection, the Vmax for GAD is approximately twice that found above. On the other hand, the Km is essentially the same. Following transection, specimens from both above and below lesion show a gradual decrease in Km and Vmax. Within 84-91 days after transection, the Km and Vmax of the samples taken distal to the lesion return to values similar to those of acute spinal cats. In specimens taken from above transection, there appears to be a tendency for a return to the control (acute) levels, although this return is delayed.

Alterations of Transmission Through the Flexor Reflex Afferents

Carlsson et al. (1964) demonstrated noradrenergic nerve terminals in the spinal cord, which belong to descending spinal pathways. Further work by Anden et al. (1966a,b) suggests that the descending noradrenergic pathways function by inhibiting transmission from flexor reflex afferents (FRA). The FRA system includes high threshold muscle afferents and cutaneous afferents. In the acute spinal cat, the test monosynaptic spike that was evoked by GS stimulation is blocked for a brief time if conditioned by a preceding impulse through the

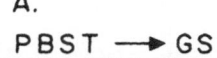

A.

PBST ⟶ GS

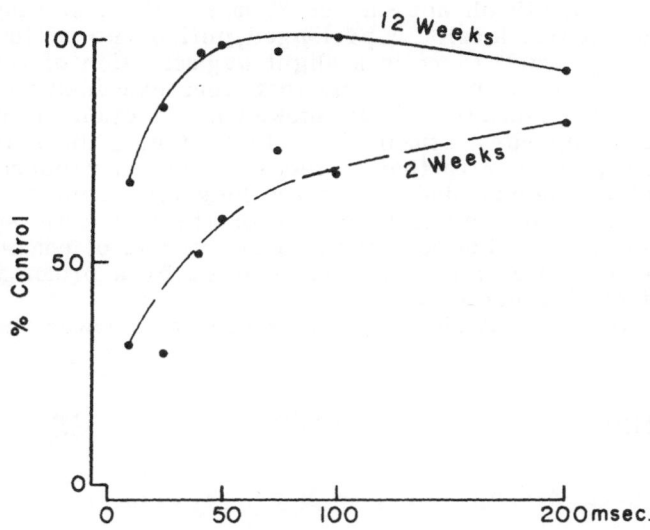

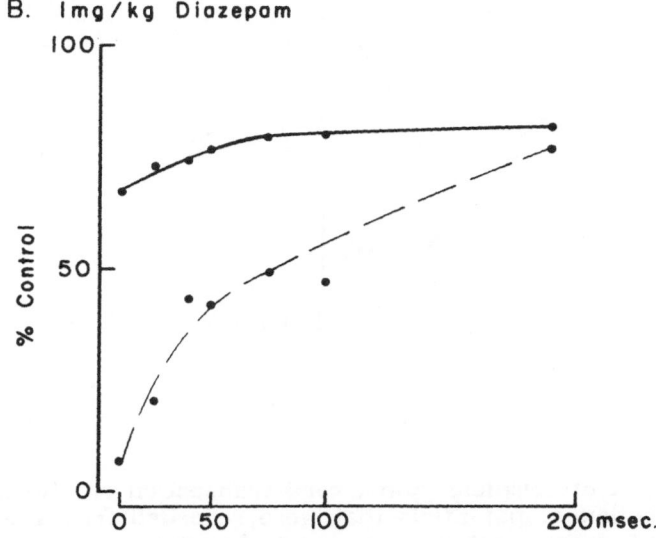

Fig. 2. The effect of diazepam on prolonged spinal inhibition in the chronic spinal cat; the test monosynaptic reflex was evoked by two pulses through the GS nerve; one subthreshold and the other supramaximal for the monosynaptic spike. Inhibition was produced by five volleys (320/sec at 2X threshold) through the PBST nerve. Each point is the mean value determined from four preparations studied approximately two or 12 weeks following transection. A. Control inhibitory curves before diazepam. B. Inhibitory curves determined five minutes after diazepam (1 mg/kg i.v.).

Reprinted from GABA–Biochemistry and CNS Functions, P. Mandel and F.V. DeFeudis, eds. Copyright 1979 Plenum Publishing Corp. , N.Y.

cutaneous sural nerve (Figure 5). When the time interval between
conditioning and test stimuli approaches 25 msec, the test response is
approximately at control level. A prolonged period (up to 100 msec),
then follows during which there is a slight augmentation of the test
response. Of six chronic preparations that were examined two to five
days following cord transection, four showed a reduction of the inhibition
that was produced by sural stimulation. In contrast, the fifth cat had
an inhibitory curve similar to that of the acute spinal preparations,
and the last cat responded similarly to the long-term spinal animals
(one to 12 weeks). The inhibitory curve for the long-term spinal
preparations (Figure 5) showed a very brief interval of complete inhibition of the monosynaptic spike that was followed by a prolonged period
of enhancement of this potential.

The distribution of catecholamine fluorescence in lower thoracic and

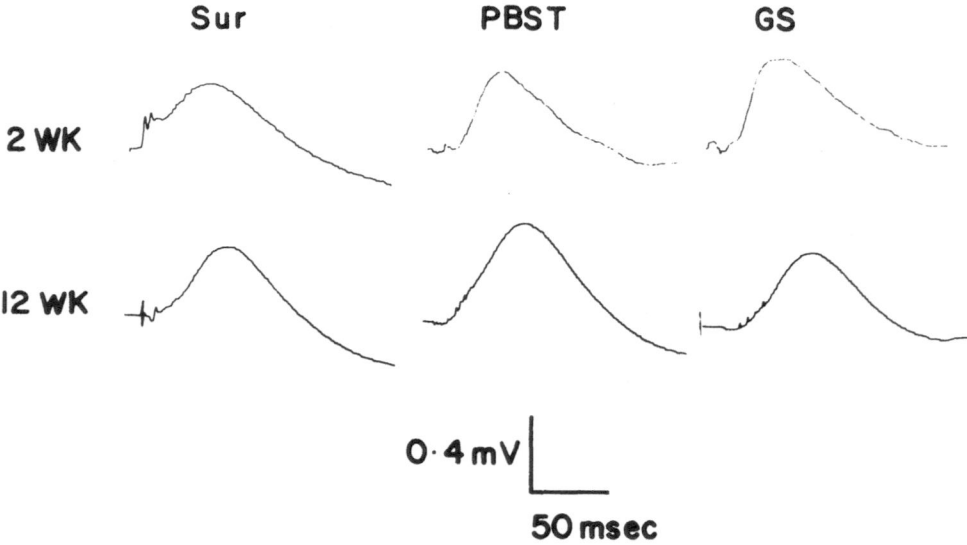

Fig. 3. The effect of complete spinal cord transection on the dorsal root
potentials and reflexes: potentials that were recorded from the caudal
portion of the L6 dorsal root in response to impulses in the sural (Sur),
PBST, and GS nerves. Note the lack of change in dorsal root potential.

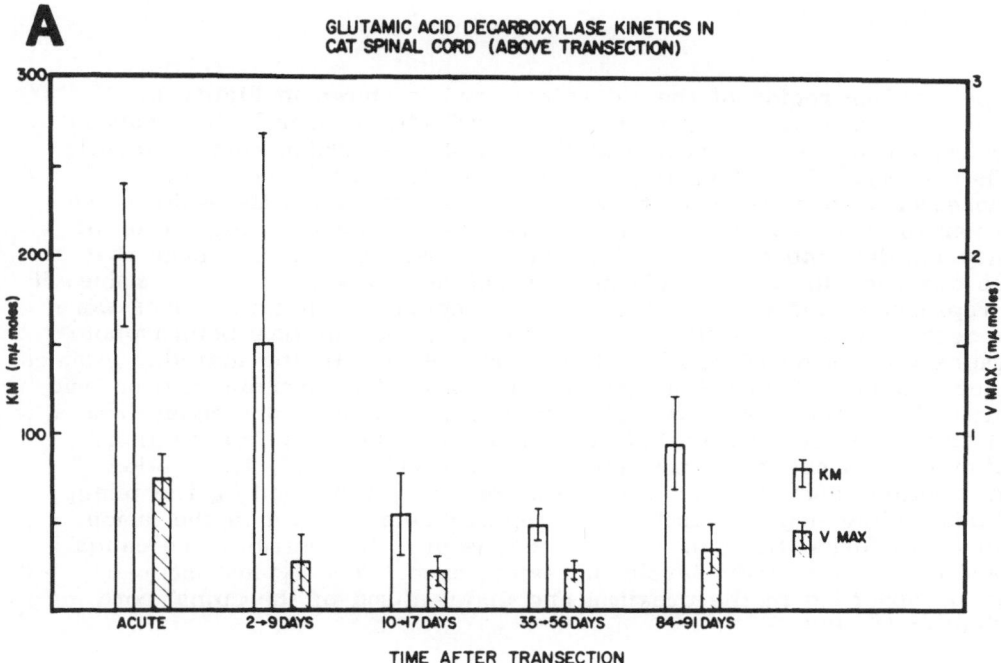

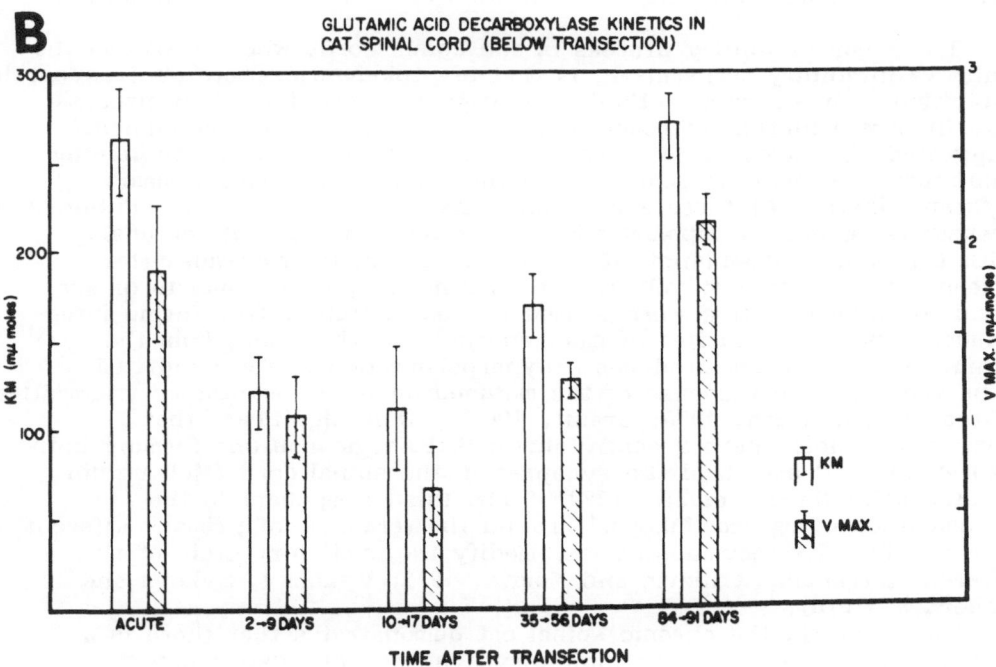

Fig. 4. The effect of complete spinal cord transection on glutamic acid decarboxylase kinetics. A. Data from samples taken above transection (lower thoracic segments). B. Data from samples below transection (lumbosacral region). Standard errors are shown.

upper lumbar region of the cat spinal cord is shown in Figure 6.
Yellowish-green fluorescence was observed within discrete terminals in
the region of the ventral lateral horn in sham-operated control animals
(Figure 6A). Four days following transection (Figure 6B), the
fluorescence in sections that were obtained from above the lesions was
similar to that seen in control. There was, however, a suggestion of
early buildup and diffusion of catecholamines. The fluorescence that
was observed in these specimens was not due to 5-hydroxytryptamine; it
it represents fluorescence due to norepinephrine, since the slides were
exposed to u.v. excitation for a sufficient period of time before photographs were made (Corrodi and Jonsson, 1967). In the four-day samples
taken caudal to transection (Figure 6C), a marked dumping and accumulation of the fluorescent material occurred. Spinal cord samples from a
cat transected five weeks before sacrifice may be seen from sections
obtained from above (Figure 6D) and below (Figure 6E) transection.
The sections show intense yellow fluorescence, representing the pileup
of descending neurotransmitter (norepinephrine) rostral to the lesion
and its diffusion through much of the tissue. In contrast, the caudal
specimen is practically devoid of fluorescence. The typical lacunae
can be observed in the proximal and distal stump of the spinal cord
(Figures 6D and 6E).

DISCUSSION

Effect of Chronic Spinal Cord Transection on GABA Mediated Inhibition

The major inhibitory process in the spinal cord, where GABA is the
putative inhibitory transmitter, is that of prolonged, remote or presynaptic
inhibition. Curtis et al. (1971) suggested that this inhibitory process
may involve a number of components. First, there is the component
suggested by Eccles (1964) involving synapses of the GABA containing
inhibitory interneurons impinging on the axons of incoming primary
afferent fibers. At these axo-axonic synapses, release of the inhibitory
transmitter evokes a depolarization of the primary afferent terminals
with a resultant attenuation of the amount of excitatory transmitter
released by an afferent volley. The second component consists of axo-
dendritic synapses that were formed by the inhibitory GABAergic interneurons and the dendrites of motoneurons. At these junctions the
inhibitory transmitter produces a hyperpolarization of the dendrites,
thus reducing the response of the motoneuron to the excitatory transmitter
(Green and Kellerth, 1966; Granit, 1968). It is significant that
anatomical studies have recently shown GABAergic neurons forming both
axo-axonic and axo-dendritic synapses in the spinal cord (McLaughlin
et al., 1975; Barber et al., 1978). The third component is the
accumulation of extracellular K^+ around the terminals of primary afferent
fibers. This K^+ accumulation may modify the excitatory state of the
afferent terminals (Krnjevic and Morris, 1972; Vyklicky, Sykova and
Mellerova, 1976).

Our study in the chronic spinal cat demonstrates that there is a
gradual loss of this complex inhibitory system. The data support
previous clinical findings in man (Burke and Ashby, 1972; Delwaide,
1973) and observation in cats (Hancock et al., 1973). In conjunction
with the loss of presynaptic inhibition there is alteration of the Km
and Vmax for GAD, the enzyme that converts glutamate to GABA.
Below the level of transection (lumbar region), there is a gradual
reduction of the Km and Vmax, which is followed by an eventual return
to values that are found in acute preparations. A similar reduction in

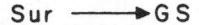

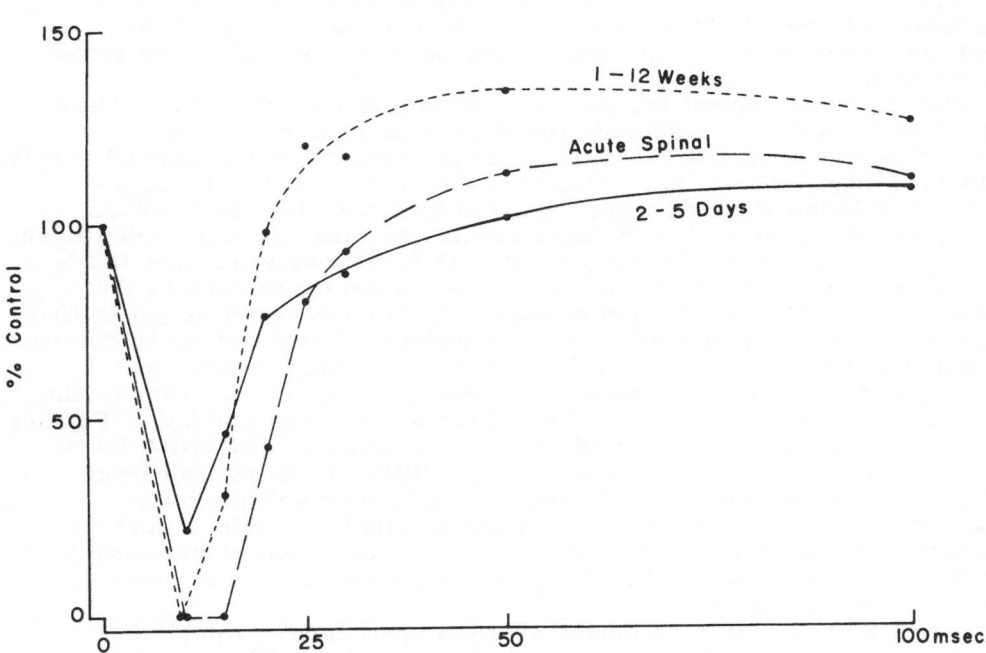

Fig. 5. Inhibition of extensor monosynaptic potentials by flexor-reflex
afferents in acute and chronic spinal preparations: the monosynaptic
spike was evoked by a subthreshold and a supramaximal stimuli to the
GS nerve. This was conditioned by a volley 4X threshold to the sural
nerve. The inhibitory curves relate percent inhibition (ordinate) to the
interval between the inhibitory and testing volley (abscissae). Each
curve represents the mean value from nine acute preparations,
two to five days (four of the six preparations showed this response),
one to 12 weeks (14 preparations).

Km and Vamx occurs in the thoracic segments above the transection.
In samples removed from cats 84 to 91 days after transection, there is
an increase in Km and Vmax signalling a possible return, albeit delayed,
to the acute values. These results suggest that both ascending and
descending neurons may function in the enzymatic control of GABA
formation. Ascending fibers are known to impinge on interneurons,
which inhibit, presynaptically, afferent fibers in the dorsal spino-
cerebellar tract in Clarke's column (Eccles et al., 1961). These
interneurons may contain GABA. Twelve weeks after transection of the
spinal cord, when presynaptic inhibition is reduced in degree and
duration, the Km and Vmax levels below transection are similar to that
found in acute preparations. This finding would suggest that the
function of the GABAergic inhibitory system at twelve weeks after spinal
lesion should be similar to that in the acute preparations. Smith et al.
(1975), however, found that the GABA concentration at this time is
markedly enhanced. Therefore, a reduction in the release of the
inhibitory transmitter would possibly explain the biochemical and physiological data.

Paradoxically, spinal transection had no effect on the DRP. These
dorsal root antidromic potentials resulting from primary afferent
depolarization are usually associated, physiologically and pharmacologically,
with presynaptic inhibition. There is, however, data which suggest
that transmission through GABAergic interneurons that are involved
with presynaptic inhibition includes events that are, in part, independent
of DRP. For example, Vyklicky et al. (1976) demonstrated that DRP's
evoked in frog spinal cord are not always completely blocked in the
presence of high concentration of Mg^{2+}. This observation suggests that
primary afferent depolarization is not completely dependent on transmitter-
mediated events. Polc et al. (1974) reported an augmentation of
prolonged spinal inhibition without an accompanying enhancement of the
DRP in cats that were treated with aminooxyacetic acid (AOAA). Further,
Belfl and Anderson (1974) found that AOAA doubled cord GABA levels
but had no effect on dorsal root reflex or DRP. In mammalian brain,
AOAA inhibits neuronal GABA-transaminase *in vivo* and probably
augments GABA levels (Baxter and Roberts, 1961). Further work is
necessary to elucidate the reason(s) for the attenuation of presynaptic
inhibition that is seen in chronic spinal cats without a concomitant
reduction of the DRP's.

Verrier et al. (1975) reported that diazepam failed to potentiate
presynaptic inhibition in patients with long-standing (five years)
complete spinal lesions. This is in contrast to the enhancement of
presynaptic inhibition that was observed in the acute spinal cats
(Schmidt, 1967; Schlosser, 1971; Stratten and Barnes, 1971). Our
data in chronic spinal cats (6 to 12 weeks) shows that diazepam
response, indeed appears to be dependent on the normal functioning
of the inhibitory mechanisms; the gradual loss of inhibition after
spinal cord transection is accompanied by a decrease in diazepam's
effectiveness.

Effect of Chronic Spinal Cord Transection on Descending Monoaminergic
Pathways and Flexor Reflex Afferents (FRA)

Dahlstrom and Fuxe (1965), using the histochemical fluorescence
technique, demonstrated in the rat that soon after lesion of the spinal
cord, norepinephrine and 5-hydroxytryptamine accumulate above the
level of transection and disappear caudal to the lesion. Further, they
showed that the monoaminergic terminals belong to bulbospinal pathways,

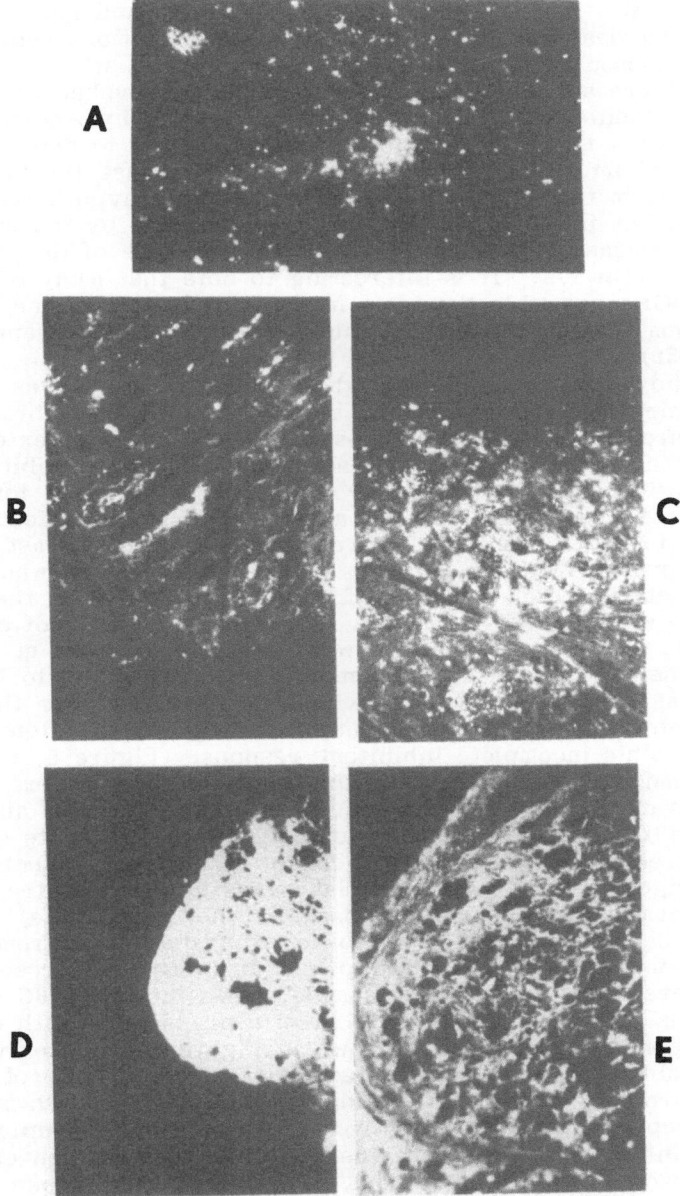

Fig. 6. Catecholamine histofluorescence (formaldehyde induced fluorescence) from cat spinal cord following chronic transection.   A. A cross section of a control speciment showing ventral horn thoracic region (T 12), mag. 160X.   B. Section showing ventral horn region immediately rostral to the lesion taken from specimens four days post-transection, mag. 160X.   C. Ventral horn region from the same preparation as in B showing a section immediately caudal to the lesion, mag. 160X.   D. Ventral horn, five weeks post-transection.   Note intense yellow fluorescence rostral to the lesion, ag. 80X.   E. Five weeks post-transection caudal to transection showing lack of fluorescence, ventral horn, mag. 160X.

with the cell bodies located in the medulla oblongata and lower pons.

The physiological importance of these descending monoaminergic pathways was demonstrated by Carlsson et al. (1963), who observed that L-DOPA increased the flexor reflex, which was evoked by pinching the skin in the acute spinal cat. Later investigation by Anden et al. (1966a,b) revealed that the major effect of L-DOPA is to depress transmission in the short latency paths from FRA and release the long latency paths from the FRA. The following working hypothesis was proposed: L-DOPA inhibits transmission from the FRA by increasing synthesis and release of transmitter from the terminals of descending noradrenergic pathways. It is interesting to note that many of the effects of L-DOPA resemble the tonic inhibition of transmission through the FRA system seen in the decerebrate preparation (Eccles and Lundberg, 1959).

In our study, transmission through the FRA pathways was examined by the inhibitory effect produced via a conditioning volley through cutaneous afferents (sural) on a monosynaptic discharge of extensor motoneurons (GS). In the acute spinal animal, complete inhibition of the monosynaptic reflex from extensor motoneurons was seen for at least a period of 5 msec, followed by a rapid return of the test potential approximately to control values (Figure 5, acute). In contrast, preparations examined one to 12 weeks after transection showed an inhibitory effect, in which duration of complete inhibition of the monosynaptic spike was markedly reduced, followed by a period of enhanced reflex activity. Similar observations were made by Hancock et al. (1973). In addition, there was a phase of transition, occurring two to five days following spinal cord transection, at which time a volley from the FRA did not completely inhibit the monosynaptic reflexes from extensor motoneurons. This incomplete inhibitory response (Figure 5; two to five days), mimics that seen in decerebrate preparations where tonic inhibition of transmission from the FRA was reported (Eccles and Lundberg, 1959), and is also similar to that seen in the acute spinal preparations treated with L-DOPA (Anden et al., 1966a). Therefore, these data suggest a dumping of catecholamines during this transitional phase and interaction of the neurotransmitter (norepinephrine) with interneurons that are involved in inhibition of transmission from FRA to extensor motoneurons. The buildup and dumping of fluorescent material that are seen in the tissue sample shown in Figure 6C support this hypothesis. Figure 6C was taken from a preparation with an inhibitory response similar to that shown in Figure 5 (two to five days).

Most probably, spinal spasticity results from dysfunction of a number of neurotransmitters. Descending monoaminergic pathways containing norepinephrine and 5-hydroxytryptamine are disrupted, removing the inhibitory function of these transmitters (Anden et al., 1966a,b; Carlsson, 1973; Naftchi et al., 1974). Ascending neuronal pathways containing substance P are blocked, with a resultant buildup of this putative neurotransmitter (modulator) below the level of transection (Naftchi et al., 1978). A predominance of excitatory effects have been reported after iontophoretic application of substance P on brain and spinal cord neurons (Henry, 1976; Krnjevic and Morris, 1974; Otsuka and Konishi, 1976). Although inhibitory effects of substance P were rarely observed, when they occurred they consistently blocked the excitatory action of acetylcholine on Renshaw cells, thus preventing the inhibitory action of these interneurons (Belcher and Ryall, 1977; Krnjevic and Lekic, 1977).

Glycine and aspartate concentrations rapidly decline after transection in the canine spinal cord. Within eight weeks following transection, levels of these inhibitory and excitatory transmitters are 50% below control values (Hall et al., 1976). The decrease in glycine correlates with the decrement in postsynaptic and recurrent inhibition observed by Herman et al. (1973) and Veale et al. (1973) in patients with various neurological lesions. Therefore, in addition to changes that were observed in GABAergic transmission, spinal cord lesion also affects other interneuronal neurotransmitters.

REFERENCES

Anden, N.E., Jukes, M.G.M., Lundberg, A., and Vyklicky, L.   The effect of DOPA on the spinal cord.   1. Influence on transmission from primary afferents. *Acta. Physiol. Scand.* 67:373-386 (1966a).

Anden, N.E., Jukes, M.G.M., and Lundberg, A.   The effect of DOPA on the spinal cord.   2. A pharamcological analysis. *Acta. Physiol. Scand.* 67:387-397 (1966b).

Barber, R.P., Vaughn, J.E., Saito, K., McLaughlin, B., and Roberts, E.   GABAergic terminals are presynaptic to primary afferents terminals in the substantia gelatinosa of the rat spinal cord. *Brain Res.* 141:35-55.

Baxter, C.F., and Roberts, E.   Elevation of γ-aminobutyric α-ketoglutaric acid transaminase. *J. Biol. Chem.* 236:3287-3294 (1961).

Belcher, G., and Ryall, R.W.   Substance P and Renshaw cells: A new concept of inhibitory synaptic interactions. *J. Physiol. (Lond.)* 272:105-119 (1977).

Bell, J.A., and Anderson, E.G.   Dissociation between amino-oxyacetic acid-induced depression of spinal reflexes and the rise in cord GABA levels. *Neuropharmacology* 13:885-894.

Bird, E.D., and Iversen, L.I.   Huntington's chorea post-mortem measurements of glutamic acid decarboxylase, choline acetyltransferase and dopamine in basal ganglia. *Brain* 97:457-472 (1974).

Burke, D., and Ashby, P.   Are spinal "presynaptic" inhibitory mechanisms suppressed in spasticity? *J. Neurol. Sci.* 15:321-326 (1972).

Carlsson, A., Falck, B., Fuxe, K., and Hillarp, N.A.   Cellular localization of monoamines in the spinal cord. *Acta. Physiol. Scand.* 60:112-119 (1964).

Carlsson, A., Magnusson, T., and Rosengren, E.   5-Hydroxytryptamine of the spinal cord normally and after transection. *Experientia (Basel)* 19:359-360 (1963).

Cleland, W.W.   The statistical analysis of enzyme kinetic data. *Advances in Enzymology* 29:1-32.

Corrodi, H., and Jonsson, G.   The formaldehyde fluorescence method for the histochemical demonstration of biogenic monoamine.   A review of the methodology. *J. Histochem. Cytochem.* 15:65-78 (1967).

Curtis, D.R., Duggan, A.W., Felix, D., and Johnston, G.A.R.   Bicuculline, an antagonist of GABA and synaptic inhibition in the spinal cord of the cat. *Brain Res.* 32:69-96 (1971).

Dahlstrom, A., and Fuxe, K.   Evidence for the existence of monoamine neurons in the central nervous system.   II.   Experimentally induced changes in the intraneuronal amine levels of bulbopsinal neuron systems. *Acta. Physiol. Scand.* 64 (Suppl.):247 (1965).

Delwaide, P.J.   Human monosynaptic reflexes and presynaptic inhibition. New Developments in Electromyography and Clinical Neurophysiology. *Vol.* 3:508-522, J.E. Desmedt, ed., Karger, Basel (1973).

Eccles, J.C.   Presynaptic inhibition in the spinal cord. Progress in

130 SCHLOSSER et al.

Brain Res., *Vol. 12*: 65-91. J.C. Eccles, and J.P. Shade, ed. Elsevier, Amsterdam.

Eccles, J.C., Oscarsson, O., and Willis, W.D. Synaptic action of Group I and II afferent fibres of muscle on the cells of the dorsal spino-cerebellar tract. *J. Physiol. (Lond.) 158*: 517-543 (1961).

Eccles, R.M., and Lundberg, A. Supraspinal control of interneurones mediating spinal reflexes. *J. Physiol. 147*: 565-584 (1959).

Engberg, I., and Ryall, R.W. The inhibitory action of noradrenaline and other monoamines on spinal neurones. *J. Physiol. (Lond.) 185*: 298-322 (1966).

Falck, B., and Owman, C. A detailed methodological description of the fluorescence method for the cellular demonstration of biogenic monoamines. *Acta. Univ. Lund. II 7*: 3-23 (1965).

Gillies, J.D., Lance, J.W., Neilson, P.D., and Tassinari, C.A. Presynaptic inhibition of the monosynaptic reflex by vibration. *J. Physiol. 205*: 329-339 (1969).

Granit, R. Receptors and sensory perception. Yale University Press, New Haven, pp. X1-366 (1955).

Granit, R. The case for presynaptic inhibition of synapses on the terminals of motoneurons. Structure and function of inhibitory neuronal mechanisms, Vol. 10, pp. 183-195. C. von Euler, S., S. Koglund, and U. Soderberg, eds., Pergamon Press, Oxford (1968).

Granit, R., and Kaada, B.R. Influence of stimulation of central nervous structures on muscle spindles in cat. *Acta. Physiol. Scand. 27*: 130-160 (1952).

Green, D.G., and Kellerth, J.O. Postsynaptic versus presynaptic inhibition in antagonistic stretch reflexes. *Sci. 152*: 1097-1099 (1966).

Hall, P.V., Smith, J.E., Campbell, R.L., Felten, D.L., and Aprison, M.H. Neurochemical correlates of spasticity. *Life Sci. 18*: 1467-1472 (1976).

Hancock, J., Knowles, L., and Gillies, J.D. Segmental reflex changes in acute and chronic spinal cat. *Proc. Australian Assoc. Neurologist 10*: 139-143 (1973).

Henry, J.L. Effects of substance P on functionally identified units in cat spinal cord. *Brain Res. 114*: 439-452 (1976).

Herman, R., Freedman, W., and Meeks, S. Physiological aspects of hemeplegic paraplegic spasticity. New Developments in Electromyography and Clinical Neurophysiology, Vol. 3: 579-588. S. Karger, Basel (1973).

Krnjevic, K., and Lekic, D. Substance P selectively blocks excitation of Renshaw cell by acetylcholine. *Canad. J. Physiol. Pharmacol. 55*: 958-961 (1977).

Krnjevic, K., and Morris, M.E. Extracellular K^+ activity and slow potential changes in spinal cord and medulla. *Canad. J. Physiol. Pharmacol. 53*: 923-934 (1972).

Krnjevic, K., and Morris, M.E. An excitatory action of substance P on cuneate neurones. *Canad. J. Physiol. Pharmacol. 52*: 736-744 (1974).

Lowry, O.H., Rosebrough, N.J., Farr, A.L., and Randall, R.J. Protein measurement with the folin phenol reagent. *J. Biol. Chem. 193*: 265-275.

Magoun, H.W. Caudal and cephalic influences of the brain stem reticular formation. *Physiol. Rev. 30*: 459-474 (1950).

Magoun, H.W., and Rhines, R. An inhibitory mechanism in the bulbar resticular formation. *J. Neurophysiol. 9*: 165-171 (1946).

McCouch, G.P., Austin, G.M., Liu, C.M., and Liu, C.Y.   Sprouting as a cause of spasticity.   *J. Neurophysiol. 21:*205-216 (1958).

McLaughlin, B.J., Barber, R.P., Saito, K., Roberts, E., and Wu, J.-Y.   Immunocytochemical localization of glutamate decarboxylase in rat spinal cord.   *J. Comp. Neurol. 164:*305-322 (1975).

Naftchi, N.E., Abrahams, S.J., St. Paul, N.H., Lowman, E.W., and Schlosser, W.   Localization and changes of substance P in spinal cord of paraplegic cats.   *Brain Res. 153:*507-513 (1978).

Naftchi, N.E., Wooten, G.F., Lowman, E.W., and Axelrod, J.   Relationship between serum dopamine-β-hydroxylase activity, catecholamine metabolism, and hemodynamic changes during paroxysmal hypertension in quadriplegia.   *Circulation Res. 35:*850-861 (1974).

Otsuka, M., and Konishi, S.   Substance P and excitatory transmitter of primary sensory neurons.   *Col Spring Harbour Symp. Quant. Biol. 40:*135-143 (1976).

Ottaway, J.H.   Normalization in the fitting of data by iterative methods. Application to tracer kinetics and enzyme kinetics.   *Biochem. J. 134:*729-736 (1973).

Polc, P., Mohler, H., and Haefely, W.   The effect of diazepam on spinal cord activities: possible sites and mechanisms of action. *Naunyn-Schiedeberg's Arch. Pharmacol. 284:*319-337 (1974).

Schlosser, W.   Action of diazepam on the spinal cord.   *Arch. Int. Pharmacodyn. Therap. 194:*93-102.

Schmidt, R.F., Vogel, M.E., and Zimmermann, M.   Die Wirkung von diazepam auf Die Prasynaptische Hemmung und andere Ruckenmarksreflexe.   *Naunyn-Schmiedeberg's Arch. Pharm. Exptl. Pathol. 258:*69-82 (1967).

Smith, J.E., Hall, P.V., Campbell, R.L., Jones, A.R., and Asprison, M.H.   Levels of γ-aminobutyric acid in the dorsal grey lumbar spinal cord during the development of experimental spinal spasticity. *Life Sci. 19:*1525-1530 (1976).

Stratten, W.P., and Barnes, C.D.   Diazepam and presynaptic inhibition. *Neuropharmacology 10:*685-696 (1971).

Teasdall, R.D., and Stavraky, G.   Responses of deafferented spinal neurons to cortical spinal impulses.   *J. Neurophysiol. 16:*367-375 (1953).

Veale, J.L., Rees, S., and Mark, R.F.   Renshaw cell activity in normal and spastic man.   New Developments in Electromyography and Clinical Neurophysiology, Vol. 3:523-537.   S. Karger, Basel (1973).

Verrier, M., MacLeod, S., and Ashby, P.   The effect of diazepam on presynaptic inhibition in patients with complete and incomplete spinal cord lesions.   *Canad. J. Neurol. Sci. 2:*179-184 (1975).

Vyklicky, L., Sykova, E., and Mellerova, B.   Depolarization of primary afferents in the frog spinal cord under high Mg^{2+} concentrations. *Brain Res. 117:*153-156 (1976).

10

Clinical Trial of an Alpha Adrenergic Receptor Stimulating Drug (Clonidine) For Treatment of Spasticity in Spinal Cord Injured Patients

J. TUCKMAN, D.S. CHU, C.R. PETRILLO, and N.E. NAFTCHI

Spasticity is a clinical symptom that commonly interferes with the development of maximal functional achievement in spinal cord injured subjects during rehabilitation. Several medical and surgical procedures have been tried previously for treatment of spasticity with variable results. This communication presents a report on the effect of clonidine, Catapres[R], on two spinal cord injured patients who were severely spastic and suffered from rhythmic contractions of the lower extremities and trunk. Although alpha adrenergic drugs have been used in spinal cord injured animals to influence their motor activity, these data are the first to be reported on the use of clonidine in humans.

PATIENT I

An 18-year-old male, weighing 50 kg., was admitted on September 1, 1979, two weeks post-onset of acute traumatic quadriplegia, due to the fracture and dislocation of C-5,6 vertebrae with a C-5 complete lesion. One month following trauma, the patient gradually developed increasing spasticity of both lower extremities and trunk extensors and assumed an opisthotonic-like posture of the spine. At this time, he also had continuous rhythmic contractions of the trunk and hip extensors at approximately 30 contractions per minute. The lumbar tap was negative. Diazepam, baclofen, and phenytoin were administered to the patient on different occasions without significant clinical improvement. Five months post-onset, the extensor spasticity remained severe, and the rhythmic contractions persisted, interfering with the rehabilitation program (Figure 1A). The patient was unable to sit in bed or in a wheelchair. Clonidine treatment was started with an initial dose of 0.1 mg., p.o., q 6 hours, and was increased gradually to 0.2 mg., p.o., q 4 hours during a period of two weeks.

Results

Within 36 hours of the beginning of treatment, an obvious decrease in extensor spasticity and rhythmic contractions was noted. After two weeks, the patient could remain in a wheelchair for two hours, and the rhythmic contractions had completely disappeared (Figure 1B-D).
Minimal side effects of clonidine treatment were dryness of the mouth and slight reductions of the blood pressure, which had no clinical significance.

133

PATIENT I

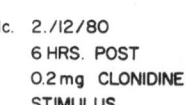

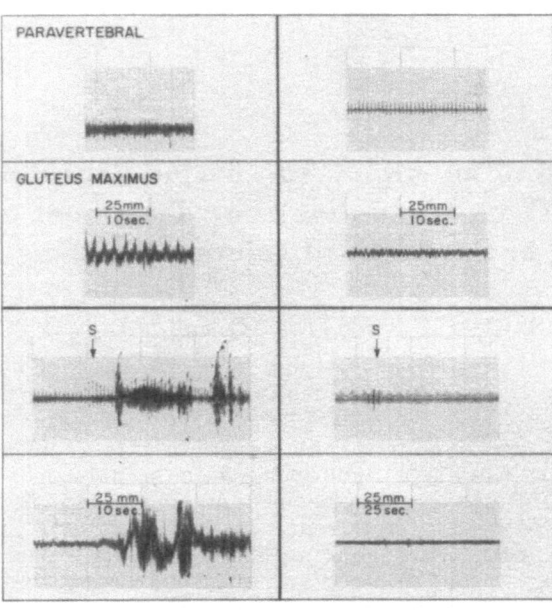

Ia. 1./9/80
PRE-TREATMET
NO STIMULUS

Ib. 2./12/80
CHRONIC TREATMENT
6 HRS. POST 0.2 mg CLONIDINE
NO STIMULUS

Ic. 2./12/80
6 HRS. POST
0.2 mg CLONIDINE
STIMULUS

Id. 2./12/80
2 HRS. POST
0.2 mg CLONIDINE
STIMULUS

Fig. 1. The effects of oral clonidine on spasticity. Patient I: Five
months post-traumatic quadriplegia with a C-5 complete lesion. EMG
activity was recorded with transcutaneous surface electrodes in the
mid-lower thoracic paravertebral and gluteus maximus regions. The
1A recordings were obtained before clonidine was started, and 1B-D
were obtained after 27 days of treatment. The stimulus was moderate
compression of a calf during several seconds. It is apparent (1B)
that chronic treatment diminished spontaneous EMG activity. Further,
near the peak of the drug's concentration in the blood, evoked spastic
activity was inhibited (1D). This was not so at lower blood concentrations (1C). The activity on the paravertebral recordings in
1B and D is the ECG.

PATIENT II

A 32-year-old male, weighing 62 kg., was readmitted on November
26, 1979, approximately three and one-half years post-traumatic
quadriplegia, due to fracture and dislocation of C-5,6 vertebrae with a
C-5 incomplete lesion.
The patient's severe chronic spasticity of both upper and lower
extremities and trunk interfered with most of the activities of daily
living and transfers. Therefore, several modes of treatment had been
attempted, including the administration of diazepam and dantrolene
sodium with no significant clinical improvement. In addition, bilateral
adductor tenotomies with obturator neurectomy were performed one and
one-half years post-onset to alleviate the severe spasticity of the lower
extremities, but this produced only temporary relief.
Nine months prior to the present readmission, the patient started
to experience involuntary rhythmic contractions of the trunk and hip
extensors, at approximately 40 contractions per minute, which continued
throughout the day and night and during sleep (Figure 2, 1A). Clonidine
was administered, starting with an initial dose of 0.05 mg., p.o., q 6
hours, which was increased gradually to 0.1 mg., q 6 hours, during

PATIENT   II

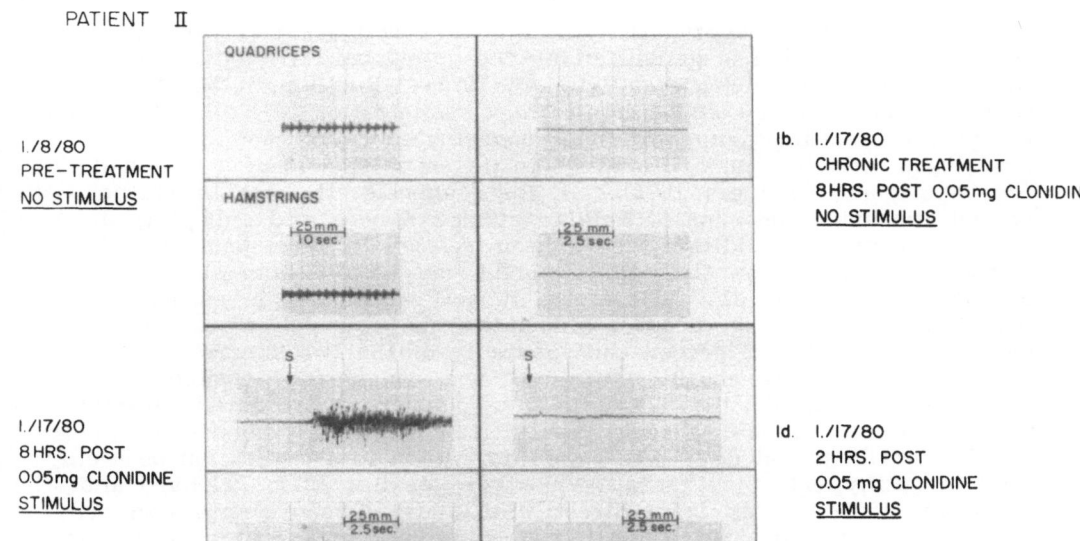

a. 1./8/80
PRE–TREATMENT
NO STIMULUS

Ib. 1./17/80
CHRONIC TREATMENT
8HRS. POST 0.05mg CLONIDINE
NO STIMULUS

c. 1./17/80
8HRS. POST
0.05mg CLONIDINE
STIMULUS

Id. 1./17/80
2 HRS. POST
0.05 mg CLONIDINE
STIMULUS

Fig. 2. The effects of oral clonidine on spasticity.   Patient II: Three and one-half years post-traumatic quadriplegia with a C-5 incomplete lesion.   EMG activity was recorded with transcutaneous surface electrodes in the quadriceps and hamstrings of regions of the same leg.   The 1A recordings were obtained before clonidine was started, and 1B-D were obtained after eight days of treatment.   The stimulus was voluntary waving of the arms during several seconds.   It is apparent (1B) that chronic treatment diminished spontaneous EMG activity.   Further, near the peak of the drug's concentration in the blood, evoked spastic activity was inhibited (ID).   This was not so at lower blood concentrations (IC).

a period of two weeks.   Concimmitantly, an intensive program of therapeutic exercise was maintained.

Results

After the first dose of clonidine, the patient's rhythmic contractions diminished significantly.   During the entire course of treatment, spasticity decreased considerably.   The most marked effect appeared to be on the rhythmic contractions of the trunk and hip extensors (Figure 2, B-D).

While receiving clonidine, the patient had clinically insignificant moderate reductions in his blood pressure.

DISCUSSION AND CONCLUSION

Spasticity in spinal cord injured subjects frequently inhibits the rehabilitation process that is directed toward the normalization of daily activity.   This report presents observations accumulated from the preliminary utilization of a new form of treatment; data was collected from two patients with spinal cord injuries, in whom extreme spasticity prevented significant rehabilitative progress.

It is generally accepted that the alternate activation of various muscles in locomotion is generated by the spinal cord (Brown, 1911; Grillner, 1976; Forssberg and Grillner, 1973). Further, it has been demonstrated that in spinal animals the administration of alpha adrenergic receptor stimulating drugs produces coordinated reflex motions of the hind limbs, which adjust themselves to different speeds of a treadmill (Forssberg and Grillner, 1973). In these animals, the agents caused normal appearing patterns of walking at slow speeds and galloping at higher speeds. In addition, the animals seemed to develop sufficient muscular force to allow them to support themselves without assistance during those movements. Therefore, it was relevant to investigate the effects of an alpha receptor stimulating drug, which crosses the blood-spinal cord barrier, on the spasticity of the two severely incapacitated patients in this study. It was considered possible that the medication might relieve spasticity by allowing coordinated muscular balance without inducing flaccid paralysis of the involved muscles.

The administered drug was clonidine, which is a medication commonly used in antihypertensive therapy (Goldberg et al., 1977; Prichard and Tuckman, 1977). This agent directly stimulates alpha receptors in the spinal cord, and thus its action is not dependent on the alpha receptor stimulation of medullary cell bodies of the bulbo-spinal tracts, or the transport of metabolically active products from those cells to the spinal cord (Forssberg and Grillner, 1973; Goldberg et al., 1977; Prichard and Tuckman, 1977). If the drug did not have such direct alpha receptor action in the spinal cord, it would presumably be useless in patients with complete transections, and its effects would be greatly diminished in those with extensive incomplete high thoracic or cervical lesions.

The results indicate that oral administration of clonidine reduced spasticity in both patients. In acute and chronic oral administration, the onset, enhancement, and duration of the effects approximated the drug's plasma concentration (Goldberg et al., 1977; Rehbinder, 1973). In acute laboratory procedures, a single dose of clonidine eliminated both clinically observed spasticity and EMG evidence of continuous and evoked activity (Figures 1, 2); it did not cause clinically obvious flaccid paralysis. When the drug was given "chronically" in divided doses, which varied between q 4-6 hours, it also decreased spasticity in both subjects, as estimated by clinical and EMG observations (Figures 1,2), and permitted the patients to participate more actively in their rehabilitation programs.

The primary aim of this investigation was to test the hypothesis that alpha receptor stimulating drugs could reduce spasticity in patients with spinal cord lesions, without simultaneously causing flaccid paralysis. The observations that are noted above answered that question affirmatively. However, this short study was not directed toward the more general problem of whether continued administration of alpha receptor stimulating drugs would offer practical long-term treatment of spasticity in these patients and hasten their rehabilitation. Nonetheless, the results are encouraging and indicate that a formal investigation should be undertaken in this regard, not only in spinal cord injured subjects but also in patients with other neurological conditions in which spasticity causes significant clinical complications.

REFERENCES

Brown, T.G. The intrinsic factors in the act of progression in the
    mammal. *Proc. Roy. Soc. B* 84:308-319 (1911).

Forssberg, H., and Grillner, S.   The locomotion of the acute spinal
    cat injected with clonidine *in vitro*.   *Brain Research 50:* 184-186
    (1973).
Goldberg, L.I., Rick, J.H., and Oparil, S.   Management and treatment
    of hypertension.   In *Hypertension* J. Genest, E. Koiw, and O.
    Kuchel, eds., pp. 990-1024, McGraw-Hill Book Co., New York,
    1977.
Grillner, S.   Some aspects on the descending control of the spinal
    circuits generating locomotion.   In *Advances in Behavioral Biology,*
    Volume 18, pp. 351-375, Plenum Press, New York, 1976.
Prichard, B.N.C., and Tuckman, J.   Management and mechanisms of
    drug treatment of hypertension.   In *Hypertension* J. Genest,
    E. Koiw, and O. Kuchel, eds., pp. 1085-1117, McGraw-Hill Book
    Co., New York, 1977.
Rehbinder, D.   Biochemistry of clonidine, in New Aspects for the
    Treatment of Arterial Hypertension.   Round Table Discussion.
    Institute of Cardiovascular Research, University of Milan, Nov.
    1973, Boehringer-Ingelheim, Florence, 1973.

SECTION THREE

Hemodynamic Changes During Autonomic Dysreflexia

11

Relationship Between Serum Dopamine-β-Hydroxylase Activity, Catecholamine Metabolism, and Hemodynamic Changes During Paroxysmal Hypertension in Quadriplegia

N.E. NAFTCHI, G.F. WOOTEN, E.W. LOWMAN, and J. AXELROD

ABSTRACT

During the chronic phase of spinal cord injury, serum dopamine-β-hydroxylase activity, arterial blood pressure, and blood flow in the fourth finger, the ballux, and the calf were measured in nine quadriplegic subjects before, during, and after expansion of the urinary bladder. In addition, in five chronic quadriplegic subjects, serum dopamine-β-hydroxylase activity, urinary catecholamine metabolites, and arterial blood pressure were measured before and during spontaneous hypertensive episodes. There was a significant correlation between the different stages of hypertension, the serum dopamine-β-hydroxylase activity, and the concentration of urinary catecholamine metabolites. The highest levels were found at the height of intracystic pressure when the arterial blood pressure was at its maximum but the pulse rate had dropped to its lowest level. At the same time the blood flow in the upper and lower extremities and the calf musculature was below detection limits, and peripheral vascular resistance was markedly enhanced. Serum dopamine-β-hydroxylase and arterial blood pressure levels correlated directly with urinary concentrations of normetanephrine but not with those of metanephrine. The data provide evidence for an in vivo simultaneous, proportional release of dopamine-β-hydroxylase and norepinephrine, suggesting release by exocytosis. The data further show that dopamine can also be released together with norepinephrine and dopamine-β-hydroxylase as evidenced by increased urinary concentrations of its major catabolite, homovanillic acid, during hypertensive stress. The hypertensive response in quadriplegic subjects during routine test of bladder function renders these subjects ideal models for self-controlled studies of neurogenic hypertension and its biochemical parameters. The results indicate that hypertension in quadriplegia, whether spontaneous or induced, is caused by increased release of norepinephrine and that the half-life of dopamine-β-hydroxylase released during stress is shorter than that previously reported.

INTRODUCTION

Autonomic hyperreflexia, characterized by paroxysmal hypertension, has been well documented ever since Head and Riddoch (1917) first described the symptoms in quadriplegia. Patients with high level spinal cord injury, above the sympathetic outflow at the level of thoracic six dermatome (T6), very often develop spontaneous hypertensive crises due to any one of several noxious stimuli (Guttman and Whitteridge, 1947). These stimuli usually arise from the urinary bladder because

This paper is reprinted by permission of the American Heart Association from Circulation Research 35: 850-861, Dec. 1974.

of cystitis or kidney stone formation or from the rectum because of
rectal impaction. Since the quadriplegic patients are usually hypotensive,
the high pressures that develop represent pressure changes of a magnitude that can cause cerebrovascular accident and death of the subject.
    Considerable evidence (Gitlow et al., 1964; De Champlain et al.,
1969; Spector et al., 1972; Engleman et al., 1970; Schamberg et al.,
1974) has implicated norepinephrine-containing nerves in certain forms
of hypertension and suggested that elevated levels of plasma and urinary
catecholamines and serum dopamine-β-hydroxylase activity reflect
increased activity of the sympathetic nervous system. Further more,
it has been inferred (Schamberg et al., 1974) that measurement of serum
dopamine-β-hydroxylase activity may be of diagnostic value in differentiating various types of hypertension.
    Synthesis of norepinephrine is catalyzed by the enzyme dopamine-β-
hydroxylase (E.C.1.14.2.1) from the precursor 3,4-dihydroxyphenylethyl-
amine (dopamine) (Kaufman and Friedman, 1965). Dopamine-β-hydroxylase
has been found in the catecholamine-containing granules in the heart
(Potter and Axedrod, 1963) and in the synaptosomes of the brain (Coyle
and Axelrod, 1972) and the splenic nerves (Stjarne and Lishaiko, 1967).
It is also present in cell bodies and nerve terminals (Molinoff et al.,
1970) and localized in chromaffin granules of the adrenal medulla
(Kirshner, 1957). The enzyme is found in the serum of a variety of
mammalian species (Weinshilboum and Axelrod, 1971). Analysis of
dopamine-β-hydroxylase has provided evidence for the simultaneous
release of the neurotransmitter norepinephrine and dopamine-β-hydroxylase
from sympathetic nerve endings by the process of exocytosis (Weinshilboum
et al., 1971; Viveros et al., 1968; Gewirtz and Kopin, 1970; Geffen
et al., 1969). Kvetnansky and Mikulaj (1979) have shown that
immobilization stress produces an increased release of catecholamines
in the rat. Weinshilboum et al. (1971) have also demonstrated an
enhancement of serum dopamine-β-hydroxylase activity under the
same stress conditions. Wooten and Cardon (1973) have found an
elevation in serum dopamine-β-hydroxylase activity during cold pressor
test and exercise in man.
    We have previously reported a rise in the excretion of catecholamine
metabolites in chronic quadriplegic subjects (Naftchi et al., 1969;
Naftchi et al., 1972). These levels are further enhanced during spontaneous hypertensive episodes (Naftchi et al., 1971; Sell et al., 1972).
Tyrosine hydroxylase activity is also elevated in the rat brain, brainstem,
and adrenal glands after transection of the spinal cord (Naftchi et al.,
1972). Therefore, as an index of sympathetic activity, we decided to
examine changes in serum dopamine-β-hydroxylase activity in quadriplegic subjects with cervical spinal cord injury. The present paper
describes an enhancement in serum dopamine-β-hydroxylase activity and
in excretion of catecholamine metabolites in quadriplegic humans that
correlates directly with arterial blood pressure during spontaneous
hypertensive episodes or during hypertension resulting from distention
of the urinary bladder.

METHODS

    Excretory cystometry is a procedure performed routinely on quadri-
plegic subjects to measure the vesicular pressure produced by a given
volume of urine and thereby to determine whether a urinary bladder is
hypertonic, normotonic, or hypotonic and whether the distention of the
urinary bladder produces reflex contractions.
    A group of nine quadriplegic subjects were self-compared during

routine excretory cystometry before and after expansion of the urinary bladder by water intake. (Informed consent was obtained from all subjects with approval from the Human Studies Committee.) All of the subjects had complete physiological transections at the cervical fifth to seventh dermatomes (C5-7) during the chronic phase (at least 6 months after onset of injury). Subjects that showed signs and symptoms of renal or cardiovascular involvement were eliminated from the study.

Intracystic pressure was measured using a cystometric apparatus attached to an intraurethralcatheter or an intraurethral catheter attached to a mercury-in-rubber Whitney gauge and a Honeywell recorder. Digital blood flow in the fourth finger and the great toe were measured calorimetrically (Naftchi et al., 1972). In four C5-7 subjects, blood flow in the thumb, the hallux, and the calf was simultaneously monitored before, during, and after hypertensive episodes by venous occlusion plethysmography with a Whitney mercury-in-rubber strain gauge attached to a Honeywell recorder. Brachial blood pressure was determined by the auscultatory technique, and digital blood pressure was determined with a Gartner capsule using the flush-throb method (Naftchi et al., 1972). Mean arterial and digital blood pressures were measured by adding one-third of the pulse pressure to the diastolic pressure, i.e., 1/3(systolic − diastolic) + diastolic. Effective mean digital blood pressure was derived by subtracting a calculated venous pressure correction from the mean digital blood pressure (Naftchi et al., 1972). Digital vascular resistance was calculated from the ratio of the effective mean digital pressure and the digital blood flow.

Control blood samples were drawn after the subject had been recumbent for 30 minutes and his bladder had been emptied and was free from all autonomic symptoms. The test samples during routine cystometric studies were not obtained at constant time intervals, since the time required for the rise in intracystic pressure varies in different individuals and depends on the type of bladder. The time relationship between dopamine-β-hydroxylase data reported in the figures is clear. A comparison between Figures 1-4 shows the variations in time and in the nature of the response between different subjects. The "moderate" samples were taken as soon as a 30-40 mm Hg increase in systolic blood pressure was noted. The last or "peak" samples were withdrawn from the catheter when the subject felt discomfort, and the test was terminated (Table I).

Serum dopamine-β-hydroxylase activity was analyzed before and during spontaneous hypertensive crises and when the subject's blood pressure was at resting control levels, i.e., when the urinary bladder was empty and no adverse autonomic signs were present. Serum dopamine-β-hydroxylase activity was determined by a modification (Weinshilboum and Axelrod, 1971) of the sensitive isotopic method of Molinoff et al (1973). This technique utilizes the conversion of phenylethanolamine. The latter is converted to ^{14}C-labeled N-methyl-phenylethanolamine by purified bovine adrenal phenylethanolamine-N-methyltransferase in the presence of the active methyl donor s-adenosylmethionine methyl-^{14}C. Serum dopamine-β-hydroxylase units are given in nmoles phenylethanolamine/ml serum hour-^{1}. The standard error of the mean for a repetitive analysis of dopamine-β-hydroxylase activity in a given blood sample was 1.8 nmoles/ml hour-^{1} (ten assays).

Control urine specimens were withdrawn directly from the urinary bag attached to a urethral catheter. The urinary bag was immediately emptied, and the urine that had collected in the bag during hypertensive episodes was used as the crisis sample. Urine specimens were only obtained from the subjects who underwent spontaneous crises; thus, the

TABLE I

Changes in Dopamine-β-Hydroxylase Activity and Arterial Blood Pressure in Nine C5-7 Quadriplegic Subjects During Bladder Distention by Water Intake

Subjects	Brachial blood pressure (mm Hg)			Serum dopamine-β-hydroxylase activity (nmoles phenylethanolamine/ml serum hour⁻¹)		
	Control	Moderate	Peak	Control	Moderate	Peak
1	110/70	140/90		341	362	
2	96/60	146/94		619	719	
3	134/98	194/126	210/130	428	540	560
4	100/60	160/100	184/120	218	302	425
5	98/70	154/96	174/104		891	910
6	106/74	144/102	210/126	307	367	
7	116/80	160/100	188/116	629	663	
8	94/62	178/110	188/116	410		1069
9	110/70	138/100	156/110	759	851	938
MEAN ± SD	107 ± 13/72 ± 12	157 ± 19/102 ± 11	187 ± 21/118 ± 10	464 ± 186	587 ± 229	780 ± 274
P		<0.001	<0.001		<0.001	<0.01

P = probability that the difference is not due to chance. P values are paired samples and compare moderate and peak levels with control levels.

control values could have been somewhat higher than they should have been, since a spontaneous crisis cannot be predicted before its occurrence. This possibility was also reflected in higher than usual control values of arterial blood pressure. The specimens were acidified with a few drops of concentrated HCl and the creatinine concentration was determined by the method of Jaffe (Jaffe, 1886). Urinary metabolites of catecholamines, 4-hydroxy-3-methoxymandelic acid (vanilmandelic acid) and 4-hydroxy-3-methoxyphenylacetic acid (homovanillic acid) were analyzed by bidimensional paper chromatography (Armstrong et al., 1956). Urinary 4-hydroxy-3-methoxyphenylethylene glycol was analyzed by gas-liquid chromatography (Wilk et al., 1968). The urine samples were incubated overnight with 0.1-0.2 ml of glusulase, a mixture of aryl sulfatase and β-glucuronidase, derived from the digestive juices of *Helix pomatia* (Endo Corporation) at pH 5.2 and 37°C to hydrolyze conjugated 4-hydroxy-3-methoxyphenylethylene glycol. The free 4-hydroxy-3-methoxyphenylethylene glycol was then extracted with ethyl acetate at pH 6. By a modification of the latter method, a derivative of the extracted 4-hydroxy-3-methoxyphenylethylene glycol was made by reacting 4-hydroxy-3-methoxyphenylethylene glycol with trifluoroacetic anhydride. After drying with nitrogen gas, the 4-hydroxy-3-methoxyphenylethylene glycol-trifluoroacetate derivative was brought into solution by the addition of redistilled ethyl acetate and chromatographed on a 3% OV-17 coiled steel column (6 ft × 4 mm, o.d.) at 125°C. Nitrogen was used as the carrier gas; the flow rate of the nitrogen was regulated at 60 ml/min. and an electron capture detector was used for the detection of the 4-hydroxy-3-methoxyphenylethylene glycol-trifluoroacetate derivative in a model 1400 varian gas-liquid chromatograph.

Urinary free metanephrine (3-O-methylepinephrine) and normetanephrine (3-O-methylnorepinephrine) were also analyzed, a urine sample was subjected to acid hydrolysis for 20 minutes in a boiling water bath, adsorbed on Amberlite CG-50 at pH 6.0-6.5, and eluted with ammonium hydroxide. Separation of metanephrine and noremetanephrine was achieved by the modification (Wilk and Bertani, 1968) of the Taniguchi and Armstrong technique (Taniguchi et al., 1964).

RESULTS

Self-compared brachial blood pressure changes and changes in serum dopamine-β-hydroxylase activity in nine quadriplegic subjects before and during hypertension precipitated by excretory cystometry are shown in Table I. After bladder distention, the brachial blood pressure and dopamine-β-hydroxylase activity were higher in all nine subjects examined. During spontaneous hypertensive crises, autonomic hyperreflexia, serum dopamine-β-hydroxylase activity, and excretion of metabolites of dopamine, norepinephrine, and epinephrine were elevated in five C5-7 quadriplegic subjects (Table II). For one C5-6 quadriplegic subject who developed hypertensive episodes on five separate occasions, serum dopamine-β-hydroxylase activity and catecholamine metabolite excretion are listed in Table III in the order of severity of the crises and are compared with the control values. There was an increase in catecholamine excretion and in all but one serum dopamine-β-hydroxylase; the increases in both serum dopamine-β-hydroxylase and urinary catecholamines were proportional to the severity of the crisis. The increase in dopamine-β-hydroxylase activity during spontaneous or induced hypertension correlated directly with elevated levels of normetanephrine, a metabolite of norepinephrine, but not with those of metanephrine, a metabolite of epinephrine (Table IV). The ratio of normetanephrine to

TABLE II

Serum Dopamine-β-Hydroxylase Activity and Urinary Catecholamine Metabolites
Before and During Hypertensive Crises in Spinal Man

Subject	Brachial blood pressure (mm Hg)		VMA (μg/mg creatinine)		HVA (μg/mg creatinine)		HMPG (μ/mg creatinine)		DβH (nmoles phenylethanolamine/ml serum hour^{-1})	
	Before	During	Before	During	Before	During	Before	During	Before	During
1	108/68	230/130	1.5	5	2	10	2	6	718	1652
2	144/102	210/126	3	7	6	16	4	8	1155	1916
3	128/80	176/122	3	5	4	7	2	3	594	646
4	136/98	172/110	2.5	5	6	12	3	5.5	1394	1617
5	112/78	150/90	2	2.5	2	5	2	4	307	484
MEAN ± SD	126 ± 15/85 ± 14	188 ± 32/116 ± 16	2.2 ± 0.91	4.9 ± 1.6	4.0 ± 2.0	10 ± 4.3	2.6 ± 0.89	5.3 ± 1.9	833 ± 437	1263 ± 650
P		<0.001		<0.001		<0.001				<0.05

VMA = vanilmandelic acid, HVA = homovanillic acid, HMPG = 4-hydroxy-3-methoxyphenylethylene glycol, DβH = dopamine-β-hydroxylase, and P = probability that the difference is not due to chance.

metanephrine increased from 4.49 to 11.1 during hypertension.

Figure 1 illustrates the effect of gradual bladder filling and thereby stretching of the vesicular wall in one C7 quadriplegic subject; the filling was accompanied by a progressive rise in brachial blood pressure and serum dopamine-β-hydroxylase activity. These changes were inversely proportional to pulse rate and blood flow in the fourth finger; blood flow dropped to immeasurable amounts at the height of intracystic pressure. Similar results were obtained in one C6-7 quadriplegic subject (Figure 2); the blood flow in the great toe significantly decreased

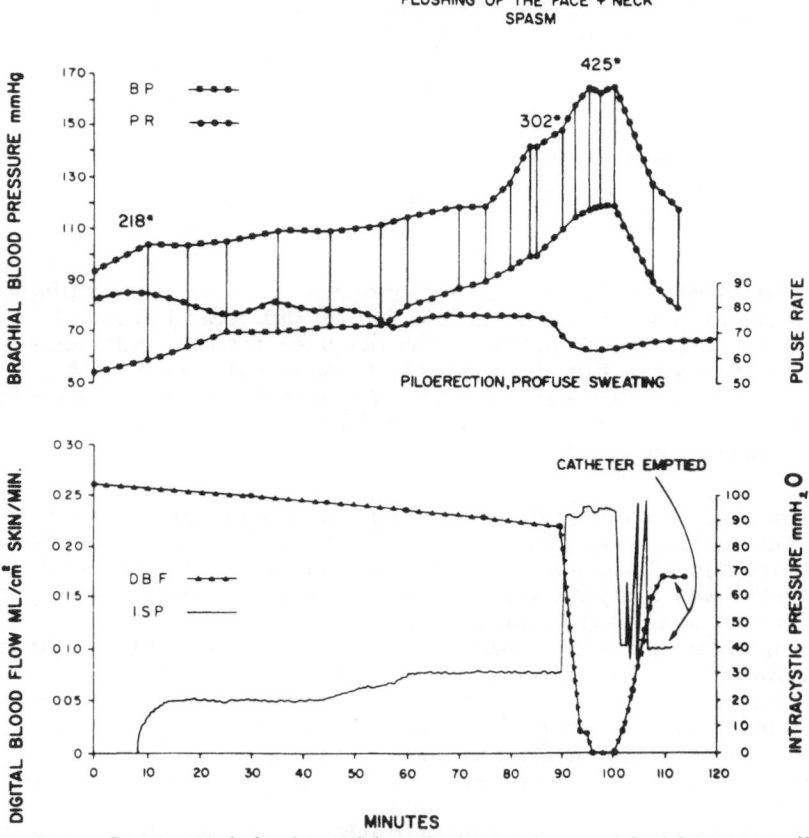

Fig. 1. In a C7 quadriplegic subject, the urinary bladder was distended by water intake during excretory cystometry. The brachial blood pressure was measured by the auscultatory technique and the blood flow in the fourth finger was determined calorimetrically. A cystometric apparatus attached to an indwelling catheter was used for measurement of intracystic pressure. B.P. = blood pressure, P.R. = pulse rate, D.B.F. = digital blood flow, and I.S.P. = intracystic pressure. An asterisk indicates the numbers that represent units of dopamine-β-hydroxylase activity (nmoles phenylethanolamine formed/ml serum hour^{-1}).

from a control value of approximately 0.10 ml/cm^{2}min^{-1} to 0.02 ml/cm^2 min^{-1} at the height of intracystic and brachial blood pressures. The high level of dopamine-β-hydroxylase activity dropped to the control level or below the control level after the urinary bladder was emptied. In another C7 subject (Figure 3), the base-line level of serum dopamine-

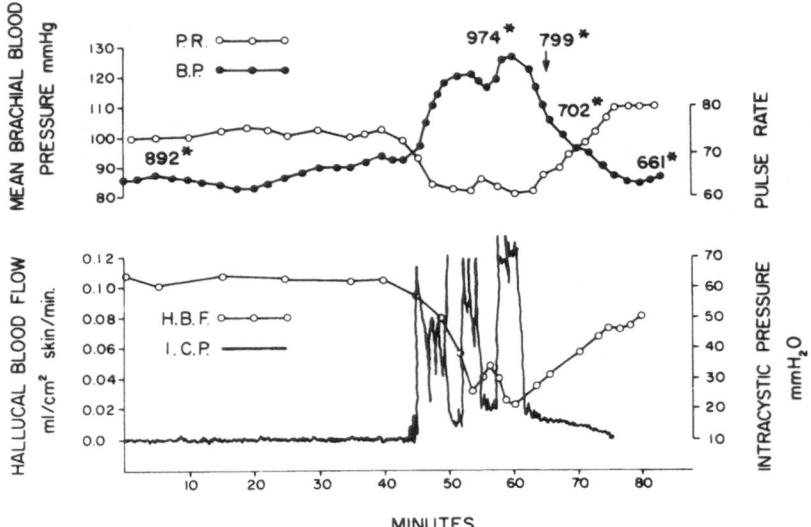

Fig. 2. At the height of autonomic dysfunction in a C6-7 quadriplegic subject, the blood flow in the great toe fell as did fourth finger blood flow in Figure 1.   Serum dopamine-β-hydroxylase activity enhanced 9% during the hypertension but dropped 18% (5 minutes) and 28% (8 minutes) after the bladder was emptied.   Abbreviations and measurement of hemodynamics are the same as those in Figure 1, except that I.C.P. = intraceptic pressure and H.B.F. = hallux blood flow.

β-hydroxylase was low and did not change appreciably at the height of dysreflexia or bladder emptying.   By contrast, in the C5-7 quadriplegic subject (Figure 2), whose base-line level of serum dopamine-β-hydroxylase was high, there was a significant rise in dopamine-β-hydroxylase activity at the height of the hypertension and autonomic dysfunction.   After the urinary bladder had been emptied, serum dopamine-β-hydroxylase activity dropped below the base-line level.   In another C5-6 subject whose base-line serum dopamine-β-hydroxylase activity was 718 nmoles phenylethanolamine/ml serum hour^{-1}, serum dopamine-β-hydroxylase activity increased to 1652 nmoles/ml hour^{-1} during 25 minutes of sustained spontaneous hypertension.   The arterial blood pressure had risen to 230/130 mm Hg at the height of the crisis.   This 15-year-old subject experienced extreme headache, profuse flushing, and diaphoresis of the face and upper extremeities.   He was in a state of complete exhuastion, and, approximately 5 minutes after the remission of the crisis following the removal of a rectal impaction, his serum dopamine-β-hydroxylase activity and brachial blood pressure had dropped to 137 nmoles/ml hour^{-1} and 86/54 mm Hg, respectively.

Similar to findings in other subjects, in a C5-6 quadriplegic subject (Figure 4), the gradual increase in intracystic pressure was accompanied by a proportional rise in arterial blood pressure and serum dopamine-β-hydroxylase activity.   There was a concomitant decrease in the pulse rate and the blood flow of the calf, the thumb, and the great toe.   In three other C5-6 quadriplegic subjects, the distention of the urinary bladder by water intake was accompanied by the same autonomic and hemodynamic changes (Figure 4).   In all subjects the finger was more sensitive in response than were the hallux and the calf.

The changes in digital blood flow, digital blood pressure, and digital

blood pressure, and digital vascular resistance consequent to the
expansion of the vesicular wall in a C5-6 quadriplegic subject are
illustrated in Figure 5.   In this subject the digital vascular resistance
increased markedly at pressures greater than 105 mm Hg; when the
effective mean digital blood pressure reached 115 mm Hg, the digital
vascular resistance rose sharply and became almost asymptotic.

The increase in serum dopamine-β-hydroxylase activity during hypertension in some subjects exceeded 150% of control values (Tables I, II,
and IV).

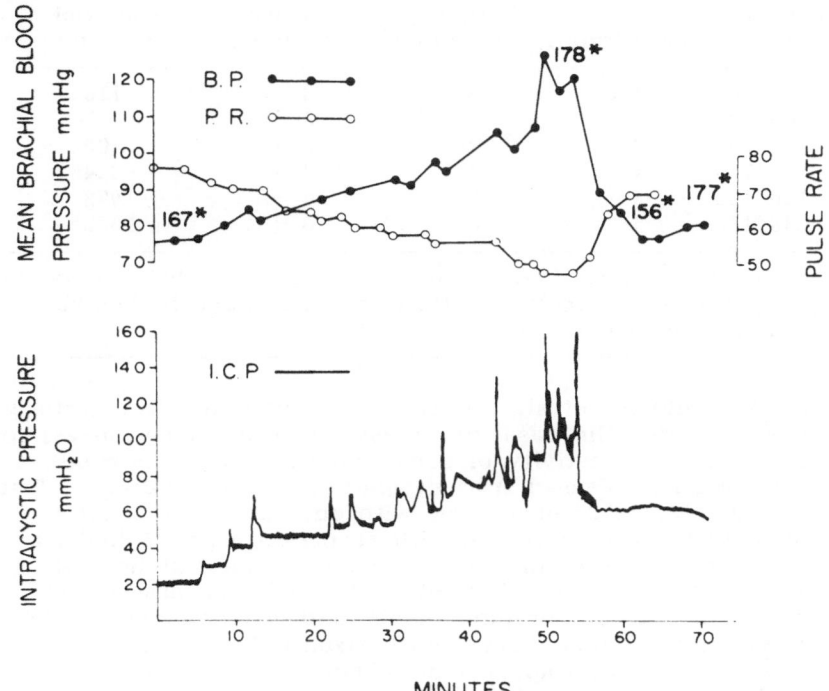

MINUTES

Fig. 3. In this C7 quadriplegic subject there was a significant rise in
arterial blood pressure and a compensatory fall in the pulse rate.   The
low base-line activity of serum dopamine-β-hydroxylase did not change
significantly either at the height of bladder distention or after the
bladder was emptied.   This subject was spastic and received diazepam
therapy (80 mg/day).   Abbreviations are the same as those in Figure 2.

DISCUSSION

During the past decade a greal deal of evidence has accumulated
to implicate dysfunction in norepinephrine storage, release, and
metabolism in certain forms of hypertension (Gitlow et al., 1964; De
Champlain et al., 1969; Spector et al., 1972).   Recently, Engelman et
al. (Engelman et al., 1970), DeQuattro and Chan (1972), and Louis
et al. (1973) have shown an increase in the concentrations of plasma
catecholamines in essential hypertension.   The recent work of Geffen
et al. (1973) has shown that, although circulating catecholamines are
greatly increased in subjects with phaeochromocytoma, plasma dopamine-
β-hydroxylase is not significantly elevated.   By contrast, they found
a correlation between dopamine-β-hydroxylase and plasma catecholamines
in essential hypertension (Geffen et al., 1973).   These findings agree

TABLE III

Serum Dopamine-β-Hydroxylase Activity and Urinary Catecholamine
Metabolites During Hypertensive Crises in One C5-6
Quadriplegic Subject

Crisis*	Brachial blood pressure (mm Hg)	VMA (μg/mg creatinine)	HVA (μg/mg creatinine)	HMPG (μg/mg creatinine)	DβH (nmoles phenylethanol-amine/ml serum hour-[1])
Control	108/68	1.5	3	2	718
1	160/120	4	8	3	
2	168/108	3	4	2.5	705
3	164/110	4	4.5	2.5	944
4	190/126	5	7	4	1072
5	230/130	5	10	6	1652

VMS = vanilmandelic acid, HVA = homovanillic acid, HMPG = 4-hydroxy-3-methoxyphenylethylene glycol, and DβH = dopamine-β-hydroxylase.
*Crisis are listed in order of severity.

with those of Weinshilboum et al. (1971) who found that adrenalectomy
in the rat does not alter the base-line levels of serum dopamine-β-hydroxylase and, therefore, the activity of serum dopamine-β-hydroxylase
represents the amounts released from sympathetic nerve endings. These
results (Geffen et al., 1973) also agree with our finding of a direct
correlation of arterial blood pressure with serum dopamine-β-hydroxylase
activity and concentrations of urinary normetanephrine but not with
levels of urinary metanephrine. Normetanephrine is the immediate
3-O-methylated catabolite of norepinephrine, and metanephrine is the
comparable metabolite of epinephrine synthesized only in the adrenal
medulla. Since there was no appreciable change in metanephrine during
hypertension (Table IV), the release of epinephrine from adrenal
glands did not contribute to the hyptertension in quadriplegia and, in
the subjects examined in the present study, the hypertensive stress
was not sympathoadrenal but rather it was purely sympathetic and due
to norepinephrine release. A physiological corollary of these findings
is the occurrence of bradycardia at the height of hypertension, an
effect generally seen after norepinephrine infusion; the administration
of epinephrine causes tachycardia.

During autonomic dysreflexia induced by infusion of saline into the
urinary bladder, Garnier and Girtsch (1964) have reported increased
excretion of urinary norepinephrine in some quadriplegic subjects they
have studied. They did not, however, find an appreciable change in
the urinary concentration of epinephrine and vanilmandelic acid.
Sizemore and Winternitz (1970) found no change in catecholamine and
vanilmandelic acid concentrations in 24-hour urine specimens from two
quadriplegic subjects, although they succeeded in suppressing all
adverse autonomic symptoms by treatment with the α-receptor blocker,
phenoxybenzamine.

Our studies in quadriplegia clearly demonstrate that during spontaneous
or induced hypertension there is a definite, direct correlation between
serum dopamine-β-hydroxylase activity, concentration of urinary normetanephrine, and levels of arterial blood pressure. These findings are

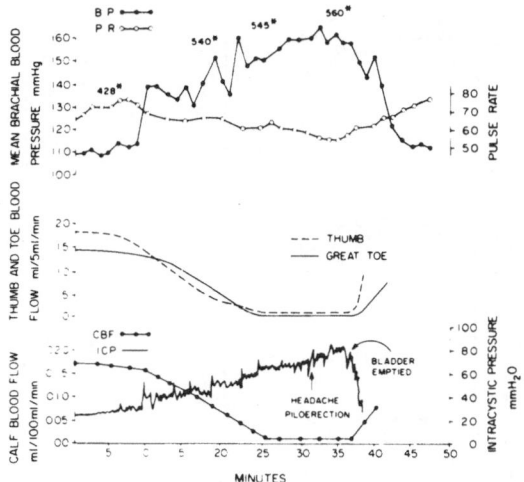

Fig. 4. In this C5-6 quadriplegic subject, the blood flow in the thumb, the great toe, and the calf and the intracystic pressure were simultaneously monitored by a Whitney mercury-in-rubber strain gauge attached to a Honeywell recorder. The arterial blood pressure response followed the sudden spikes of intracystic pressures by 3-6 seconds. As the intravesicular pressure rose there was a simultaneous increase in arterial blood pressure and serum dopamine-β-hydroxylase activity. First there was an increase and then a compensatory fall in the pulse rate as the peak pressures were sustained. At this time a concomitant and severe vasoconstriction in the upper and lower extremities and the calf musculature occurred. This state of marked autonomic dysfunction was accompanied by flushing, profuse diaphoresis, piloerection, severe headache, and chest pain, which were relieved soon after the bladder was emptied. Abbreviations are the same as those in Figure 2, except that CBF = calf blood flow.

These findings are consistent with the concept that there is a proportional release of the neurotransmitter norepinephrine together with dopamine-β-hydroxylase from the sympathetic nervous system of man, possibly by the process of exocytosis. The process of exocytosis involves a fusion of the norepinephrine storage vesicle with the neuronal membrane. Nerve depolarization is followed by an opening of the cell membrane whereupon norepinephrine and all the soluble vesicular contents are extruded into the postjunctional cleft; one such vesicle-specific soluble protein is dopamine-β-hydroxylase. This process has already been demonstrated in other mammalian species (15-18). Since the concentration of urinary homovanillic acid, the major catabolite of dopamine, is sharply elevated during hypertensive episodes, the results suggest that dopamine, which serves as a substrate for the biosynthesis of norepinephrine, is also released concomitantly with norepinephrine and dopamine-β-hydroxylase during sympathetic nerve stimulation. The rapid fall in serum dopamine-β-hydroxylase activity after hypertensive episodes (Figures 2 and 3) suggests that the half-life for circulating dopamine-β-hydroxylase released during stress is shorter than that previously reported (Ruch and Feffen, 1972; Roffman et al., 1973).

In quadriplegia there were large individual variations in serum dopamine-β-hydroxylase activity as previously described by Weinshilboum and Axelrod (1971) and Freedman et al. (1972) for normal subjects.

TABLE IV

Relationship Between Serum Dopamine-β-Hydroxylase Activity and Excretion of and Normetanephrine in Five C5-7 Quadriplegic Subjects

Subject	Metanephrine (μg/100 mg creatinine)		Normetanephrine (μg/100 mg creatinine)		Ratio of normetanephrine to metanephrine		Dopamine-β-hydroxylase (nmoles phenylethanolamine/ml serum hour^{-1})	
	Before	During	Before	During	Before	During	Before	During
1	12.2	16.4	42.0	175	3.44	10.7	718	1652
2	13.0	12.1	24.7	110	1.90	9.1	307	484
3	9.1	14.0	75.1	230	8.25	16.4	1394	1617
4	13.7	12.3	43.5	91	3.18	7.4	410	1069
5	15.3	18.2	87.0	220	5.69	12.1	1155	1916
MEAN ± SD	12.7 ± 2.3	14.6 ± 2.7	54.5 ± 27.7	165.2 ± 62.9	4.49 ± 2.51	11.1 ± 3.43	796.8 ± 469.2	1347.6 ± 572.7
P		<0.15		<0.0001		<0.001		<0.001

The ease with which a hypertensive response is brought about in these subjects during routine test of their bladder function makes a self-controlled study of hypertension very facile and provides the unique advantage of studying the changes in sympathetic activity and biochemical parameters under conditions that are not readily available in other models of hypertension.

An intense vasoconstriction in the upper and lower extremities of all nine subjects accompanied by a simultaneous decrease in the blood flow of the calf musculature was observed during the expansion of the urinary bladder. This generalized vasoconstriction below the level of the lesion correlated with elevated levels of arterial blood pressure, enhanced serum dopamine-β-hydroxylase levels, and increased excretion of catecholamine metabolites, notably normetanephrine. Roussan et al. (1966) showed that blood flow in the calf of one quadriplegic subject was decreased during autonomic hyperreflexia. They speculated that consequent to the expansion of the urinary bladder there was a gradual facilitation of the spinal cord which served as a primary cause for the reduced circulation in the calf musculature. They also suggested that the cause of or the increase in hypertension was the result of sudden shifts of large blood volumes from skeletal muscle circulation to the capacitance vessels. Our findings of marked vasoconstriction in the upper and lower extremities and the calf musculature indicate that the blood shift into the capacitance vessels at the height of hypertension must be of enormous magnitude; it may act as positive feedback causing compensatory vasodilation, profuse flushing, and diaphoresis in the head and neck and, ultimately, chest pain and headache. Due to the lack of data on venous blood volume and compliance of these vessels, however, this line of reasoning remains speculative.

Dahlstrom and Fuxe (1965), using the histochemical fluorescence technique, have demonstrated in the rat that soon after a transection of the spinal cord, norepinephrine and 5-hydroxytryptamine accumulate above the level of the lesion, not only in the descending fibers but also in certain norepinephrine and 5-hydroxytryptamine terminals of the sympathetic lateral column and the ventral horn. Furthermore, the increase in fluorescence intensity is accompanied by swollen varicosities. It has been shown (Naftchi et al., 1972; Dahlstrom and Fuxe, 1965; Anden et al., 1964; Magnusson and Rosengren, 1963) that norepinephrine and 5-hydroxytryptamine disappear from the cord below the level of transection and accumulate rostrally. Their disappearance suggests that one of these biogenic amines may be an inhibitory neurotransmitter within the spinal cord, since both norepinephrine and 5-hydroxytryptamine depress anterior horn cells and Renshaw cells(Phillis et al., 1968; Weight and Salmoiraghi, 1966). The loss of the inhibitory neurotransmitter(s) after spinal cord injury may cause permanent facilitation of the cord below the level of the lesion. In subjects with injuries to the cervical spinal cord, this absence or curtailment of inhibition within the greater segment of the cord (thoracolumbar and sacral) coupled with the lack of control from higher centers could be the primary reason why noxious stimuli easily produce extreme autonomic responses. For example, stimuli arising from the mucosa and the muscle coats of the stretched vesicular wall reach the spinal cord via presacral and pelvic nerves. Unimpeded by suprasegmental inhibitory influences or by an inhibitory neurotransmitter within the cord, these impulses travel rostrally by way of lateral spinothalamic tracts to the level of transection and reflexly stimulate the intact sympathetic chain. This process results in arteriolar vasoconstriction in the skin vessels and the splanchnic bed in direct proportion to the amount of norepinephrine released. The

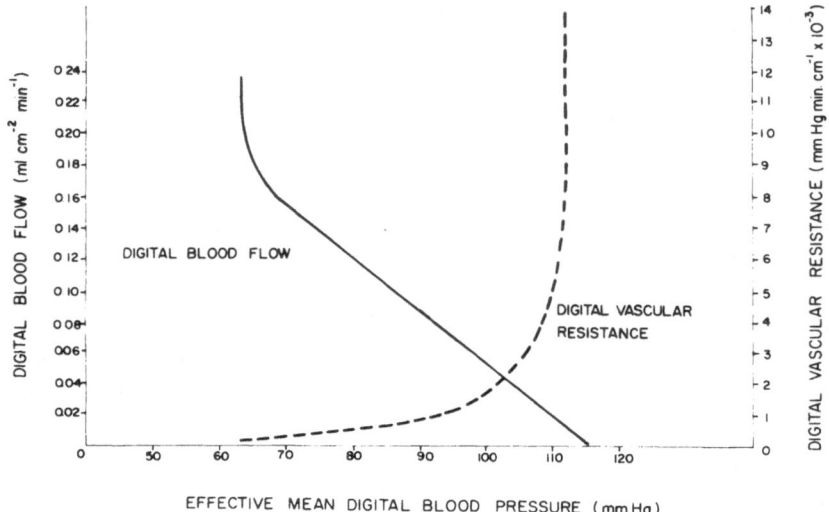

EFFECTIVE MEAN DIGITAL BLOOD PRESSURE (mm Hg)

Fig. 5. Digital blood flow–blood pressure relationships for a C5-6 quadriplegic subject. The urinary bladder was distended by water intake. The increase in intravesicular pressure was accompanied by elevations in arterial and digital blood pressures and was commensurate with a precipitous fall in digital blood flow during hypertension. At digital pressures greater than 105 mm Hg, the digital vascular resistance increased rapidly and because asymptotic above 110 mm Hg.

peak of the vasoconstriction below the level of the lesion coincides with the peak of intracystic pressure at which time the increased release of norepinephrine has caused the highest rise in arterial blood pressure and maximal peripheral resistance (Figure 5). The hypertension sensed by the receptors in the carotid sinus, the aortic arch, and the sinoatrial node is transferred via the ninth and tenth cranial nerves to the vasomotor center in the medulla; efferent impulses via the vagus then cause bradycardia. The afferent discharges from the baroreceptors to the vasomotor center cause vasodilation in the face and the neck, pulsating temporal arteries, a histaminelike flush, profuse diaphoresis, and headache in contrast to the pallor, chest pain, extreme vasoconstriction, and piloerection below the level of transection. However without the removal of the stimulus or the administration of ganglioplegic or sympatholytic drugs, these remaining regulatory mechanisms cannot appreciably lower the blood pressure.

ACKNOWLEDGMENTS

    This study was supported in part by The Edmond A. Guggenheim Clinical Research Endowment and by the Social and Rehabilitation Service, Department of Health, Education, and Welfare.

REFERENCES

Anden, N.E., Haggendal, E., Magnusson, T., and Rosengren, E. Time course of the disappearance of noradrenaline and 5-hydroxytryptamine in spinal cord after transection. *Acta. Physiol. Scand.* *62:* 115-118 (1964).

Armstrong, M.D., Shaw, K.N.F., and Wall, P.E.   The phenolic acids.
   J. Biol. Chem. *218:*293-303 (1956).
Coyle, J. T., and Axelrod, J.   Dopamine-β-hydroxylase in the rat
   brain: Developmental characteristics. *J. Neurochem.* *19:*449-459
   (1972).
Dahlstrom, A., and Fuxe, K.   Evidence for the existence of monoamine
   neurons in the central nervous system: II. Experimentally induced
   changes in the intraneuronal amine levels of bulbospinal neuron
   systems. *Acta. Physiol. Scan. (Suppl.)* *64:*1-85 (1965).
De Champlain, J., Karkoff, L., and Axelrod, J.   Interrelationships of
   sodium intake, hypertension, and norepinephrine storage in the
   rat. *Circ. Res.* *24: (suppl I):*75-92 (1969).
DeQuattro, V., and Chan, S.   Raised plasma catecholamines in some
   patients with primary hypertension. *Lancet 1:*806-809 (1972).
Engelman, K., Portnoy, B., and Sjoerdsma, A.   Plasma catecholamine
   concentrations in patients with hypertension. *Circ. Res. 27 (suppl
   I):*141-146 (1970).
Freedman, L.S., Ohuchi, T., Goldstein, M., Axelrod, F., Fish, I.,
   and Dancis, J.   Changes in human serum dopamine-β-hydroxylase
   activity with age. *Nature (Lond.)* *236:*310-311 (1972).
Garnier, V.B., and Gertsch, R.   Autonome Hyperreflexie und
   Katecholaminausscheidung beim Paraplegiker. *Schweiz Med. Wochenschr
   94:*124-130 (1964).
Geffen, L.B., Livett, B.G., and Rush, R.A.   Immunohistochemical
   localization of protein components of catecholamine storage vesicles.
   J. Physiol. (Lond.) *204:*593-605 (1969).
Geffen, L.B., Rush, R.A., Louis, W.J., and Doyle A.E.   Plasma
   catecholamines and dopamine-β-hydroxylase amounts in phaeo-
   chromocytoma. *Clin. Sci.* *44:*421-424 (1973).
Gewirtz, G.P., and Kopin, I.J.   Release of dopamine-β-hydroxylase
   with norepinephrine during cat splenic nerve stimulation. *Nature
   (Lond.)* *227:*406-407 (1970).
Gitlow, S.E., Mendlowitz, M., Wilk, E.K., Wilk, S., Wolf, R.L., and
   Naftchi, N.E.   Plasma clearance of D,L-β-H^3-norepinephrine in
   normal human subjects and patients with essential hypertension.
   J. Clin. Invest. *43:*2009-2015 (1864).
Guttmann, L., and Whitteridge, D.   Effects of bladder distension on
   autonomic mechanisms after spinal cord injuries. *Brain 70:*361-405
   (1947).
Head, H., and Riddoch, J.   Autonomic bladder, excessive sweating,
   and some other reflex conditions in gross injuries of the spinal
   cord. *Brain 40:*188-263 (1917).
Jaffe, M.   Uber den Niederschlag, welchen Pilerinsaure in normalen
   Harnerzeugt und uber eine neue Reaction des Kreatinis. *Z. Physiol.
   Chem. 10:*391-400 (1886).
Kaufman, S., and Friedman, S.   Dopamine-β-hydroxylase. *Pharmacol.
   Rev. 17:*71-100 (1965).
Kirshner, N.   Pathway of noradrenaline formation from dopa. *J. Biol.
   Chem. 226:*821-825 (1957).
Kvetnansky, R., and Mikulaj. L.   Adrenal and urinary catecholamines in
   rats during adaptation to repeated immobilization stress. *Endocrinology
   87:*738-743 (1970).
Louis, W.J., Doyle, A.E., and Anavekar, S.   Plasma norepinephrine
   levels in essential hypertension. *N. Engl. J. Med. 288:*599-601
   (1973).
Magnusson, T., and Rosengren, E.   Catecholamines of the spinal cord
   normally and after transection. *Experimentia 19:*229-230 (1963).

Molinoff, P.B., Brimijoin, W.S., Weinshilboum, R.M., and Axelrod, J.
Neurally mediated increase in dopamine-β-hydroxylase activity.
*Proc. Natl. Acad. Sci. USA 66:*453-458 (1970).

Naftchi, N.E., Demeny, M., Kertesz, A., and Lowman, E.W.   CNS
and adrenal tyrosine hydroxylase activity and norepinephrine,
serotonin and histamine in the spinal cord after transection (abstr.)
*Fed. Proc. 31:*3483 (1972).

Naftchi, N.E., Lowman, E.W., Rusk, H., and Reich, T.   Urinary
catecholamine metabolites in spinal cord injured human (abstr.)
*Fed. Proc. 28:*544 (1969).

Naftchi, N.E., Lowman, E.W., Sell, H., and Rusk, H.   Hypertensive
crisis associated with increased urinary catecholamine catabolites
in spinal man (abstr.) *Fed. Proc. 30:*678 (1971).

Naftchi, N.E., Lowman, E.W., Sell, G.H., and Rusk, H.A.   Peripheral
circulation and catecholamine metabolism in paraplegia and quadriplegia.
*Arch Phys. Med. Rehabil. 53:*357-362 (1972).

Phillis, J.W., Tebecis, A.K., and York, D.H.   Depression of spinal
motoneurones by noradrenaline, 5-hydroxytryptamine and histamine.
*Eur. J. Pharmacol. 4:*471-475 (1968).

Potter, J.T., and Axelrod, J.   Properties of norepinephrine storage
particles in the rat heart. *J. Pharmacol. Exp. Ther. 142:*299-305
(1963).

Roffman, M., Freedman, L.S., and Goldstein, M.   Effect of acute and
chronic swim stress on dopamine-β-hydroxylase activity. *Life Sci.
12:*369-376 (1973).

Roussan, M.S., Abramson, A.S., Lippmann, H.I., and DiOronzio, G.
Somatic and autonomic responses to bladder filling in patients with
complete transverse myelopathy. *Arch. Phys. Med. 47:*450-456
(1966).

Rush, R.A., Geffen, L.B.   Radioimmunoassay and clearance of circulating
dopamine-β-hydroxylase. *Circ. Res. 31:*444-452 (1972).

Schanberg, S., Stone, R., Kirshner, N., Gunnels, J., and Robinson,
R.   Plasma dopamine-β-hydroxylase: A possible aid in the study
and evaluation of hypertension. *Science 183:*523-525 (1974).

Sell, G.H., Naftchi, N.E., Lowman, E.W., and Rusk, H.   Autonomic
hyperreflexia and catecholamine metabolites in spinal cord injury.
*Arch. Phys. Med. Rehabil. 53:*415-418 (1972).

Sizemore, G.W., and Winternitz, W.W.   Autonomic hyperreflexia:
Suppression with alpha-adrenergic blocking agents. *N. Engl. J.
Med. 282:*795 (1970).

Spector, S., Tarver, J., and Berkowitz, B.   Catecholamine biosynthesis
and metabolism in vasculature of normotensive and hypertensive rats.
In *Spontaneous Hypertension: Its Pathogenesis and Complications,*
edited by K. Okamoto. Tokyo, Igaku Shoin, Ltd., 1972, pp. 41-45.

Stjarne, L., and Lishajko, F.   Localization of different steps in
noradrenaline synthesis to different fractions of a bovine splenic
nerve homogenate. *Biochem. Pharmacol. 16:*1719-1798 (1967).

Taniguchi, K., Kakimoto, Y., and Armstrong, M.   Quantitative determination of metanephrine and normetanephrine in urine. *J. Lab.
Clin. Med. 64:*469-484 (1964).

Viveros, O.H., Arqueros, L., and Kirshner, N.   Release of catecholamine
and dopamine-β-oxidase from adrenal medulla. *Life Sci. 7:*609-618
(1968).

Weight, F.F., and Salmoiraghi, G.C.   Adrenergic responses of Renshaw
cells. *J. Pharmacol. Exp. Ther. 154:*391-396 (1966).

Weinshilboum, R.M., and Axelrod, J.   Serum dopamine-β-hydroxylase
activity. *Circ. Res. 28:*307-315 (1971).

Weinshilboum, R.M., and Axelrod, J. Reduced plasma dopamine-β-hydroxylase activity in familial dysautonomia. *N. Engl. J. Med.* *285:* 938-942 (1971).

Weinshilboum, R.M., Kvetnansky, R., Axelrod, J., and Kopin, I.J. Elevation of serum dopamine-β-hydroxylase activity with forced immobilization. *Nature (New Biol.) 230:* 287-288 (1971).

Weinshilboum, R.M., Thoa, N.B., Johnson, D.G., Kopin, I.J., and Axelrod, J. Proportional release of norepinephrine and dopamine-β- hydroxylase from sympathetic nerves. *Science 174:* 1349-1351 (1971).

Wilk, E., Gitlow, S.E., Clarke, D.D., and Paley, D.H. Determination of urinary 3-methoxy-4-hydroxyphenylethyleneglycol by gas-liquid chromatography and electron capture detections. *Clin. Chim. Acta. 16:* 403-408 (1967).

Wilk, E., Gitlow, S., and Bertani, L. Modification of the Taniguchi method for the determination of noremetanephrine and metanephrine. *Clin. Chim. Acta. 20:* 147-148 (1968).

Wooten, G.F., and Cardon, P. Plasma DβH activity: Elevation in man during cold pressor test and exercise. *Arch. Neurol. 28:* 103-106 (1973).

12

Autonomic Hyperreflexia: Hemodynamics, Blood Volume, Serum Dopamine-β-Hydroxylase Activity, and Arterial Prostaglandin PGE_2

N.E. NAFTCHI, M. DEMENY, M. BERARD,
D. MANNING, and J. TUCKMAN

ABSTRACT

The syndrome of autonomic dysreflexia often occurs in quadriplegic subjects and is characterized by paroxysmal hypertension, headache, vasoconstriction below and flushing of the skin above the level of transection, and bradycardia. These attacks may cause hypertensive encephalopathy, cerebral vascular accidents, and death. In five patients during crises, the mean arterial pressure changed from 95 to 154 mmHg, heart rate 72 to 45 beats/min., cardiac output 4.76 to 4.70 litres/min., and peripheral resistance 1650 to 2660 dynes·sec·cm^{-5}. In eight subjects, the control plasma, red cell, and total blood volumes were 19.1, 10.5, and 29.6 ml/cm body height, respectively, and, when hypertensive, the plasma protein concentration increased by 9.9% and the hematocrit by 9.5%. It was estimated that plasma volume was reduced 10-15%. At that time, arterial dopamine-β-hydroxylase (DβH) activity increased 65% and prostaglandin E_2 concentration by 68%. Thus, the augmented DβH activity primarily represented elevated sympathetic tone rather than hemoconcentration of that protein. It is also suggested that the rise in prostaglandin may be a contributing cause of the severe headaches during hypertensive episodes.

INTRODUCTION

Most patients with high transverse lesions of the spinal cord above the origins of the thoracolumbar preganglionic sympathetic neurones eventually develop symptoms of autonomic hyperreflexia or dysreflexia (Bors, 1956). That is, the stimulation of dermatomes and muscles that are supplied by nerves from below the injury, and, especially, manipulation of the perineum, genitalia and distension of the bladder or rectum evokes a syndrome that includes hypertension, profuse sweating, flushing, piloerection (cutis anserina), and headache (Head and Riddoch, 1917; Guttman and Whitteridge, 1947). The increase in arterial pressure is often severe and prolonged, and it may cause cerebral vascular accidents and death (Bors, 1956; Johnson et al. 1975). This syndrome has been mistakenly diagnosed as pheochromocytoma and, during delivery, as toxemia of pregnancy (Oppenheimer, 1971). Also, it becomes a major complication during surgical procedures when it is induced by traction of the viscera (Desmond, 1970).

The hypertensive crises, during episodes of autonomic dysreflexia, are unusual since an increase in sympathetic activity occurs simultaneously with elevated, rather than lowered, parasympathetic tone. The adrenergic activity originates below the level of transection, and the cholinergic activity is due to stimulation of the supra-spinally mediated carotid sinus and aortic arch baroreceptor reflexes, which produce a dramatic brady-cardia. The prinicple aim of the present investigation was to measure the effect of this anomalous parallel increase in autonomic activity on cardiac output. Another objective was to determine if blood volume decreased during autonomic hyperreflexia, as happens when arterial blood pressure is raised by intravenous infusion of noradrenalin in normotensive subjects (Finnerty et al., 1958; Cohn, 1966). If during the hypertensive episodes in quadriplegic patients, a reduction in plasma volume occurred, it would cause hemoconcentration of high molecular weight plasma proteins, including dopamine-β-hydroxylase (DβH), and alter interpretation of the latter's significance as an index of sympathetic activity (Weinshilboum et al., 1971; Wooten and Cardon, 1973; Naftchi et al., 1974; Viveros et al., 1968; Gerwirtz and Kopin, 1970). In addition, the existence of such a hypovolemia could be of direct clinical significance, since even a small diminution in blood volume might produce severe *hypotension* when the hypertensive stimulus, e.g. bladder distension, was abruptly removed (Freis et al., 1951; Freis and Rose, 1957).

Severe headache is a characteristic symptom of autonomic hyper-reflexia and some experimental data are consistent with the hypothesis that it results from passive dilatation of cerebral vessels to the high systemic arterial pressure (Schumacher and Guthrie, 1951). However, elevated sympathetic and parasympathetic activity both release prosta-glandins (Bennet et al., 1967) and infusions of PGE$_1$ and PGE$_2$ in man cause headache (Carlson et al., 1968; Hillier and Embrey, 1972; Karim and Filshie, 1972). Therefore, the arterial concentration of PGE$_2$ was measured to determine if the magnitude of its increase during the hypertensive episodes could provide a contributory explanation for the headache.

MATERIALS AND METHODS

The protocol of this investigation was approved by the Human Studies Committee of the New York University Medical Center. Eleven male quadriplegic subjects participated in the study after they gave their informed consent. The procedures were done before and during the episodes of autonomic hyperreflexia that were associated with routine tests of urinary bladder function which was carried out in these patients by cystometry.

The patients, 18 to 25 years of age, all had physiologic transverse lesions of the spinal cord at the level of the fifth to eighth cervical segments. The injuries had occurred at least six months prior to the test, and the patients were in an unremarkable chronic stable condition. None had evidence of cardiovascular disease or decreased renal function. Drugs affecting the cardiovascular system were discontinued before the procedures began, and the subjects were studied after they had been fasting 10 to 12 hours.

Blood volume determinations were done in eight of the eleven subjects. Cardiac output studies, without blood volume determinations, were also performed in three of these eight patients on another occasion and in two other subjects. Arterial samples for measurements of serum dopamine-β-hydroxylase (DβH) activity and plasma prostaglandin

PGE_2 concentration were obtained from the five patients at the time of the cardiac output procedures and from one subject in whom neither cardiac output nor blood volume determinations were done.

The procedures took place in the morning, approximately one hour after the insertion of a Foley catheter coated with lidocaine gel. The control period began after the subjects had been supine for at least 30 minutes and 15 minutes after all needles and other catheters were in place. Urine flowed freely in this period, and there were no signs of autonomic hyperreflexia (hypertension, diaphoresis, piloerection, and headache). Autonomic dysreflexia was produced by gradually filling the bladder with isotonic saline during cystometry. The type of bladder reaction (hypo-, normo-, or hypertonic) determined the magnitude of the rise in arterial blood pressure as well as duration of autonomic dysreflexia, before the episode was ended by again permitting the free flow of urine. Brachial arterial pressure was measured by auscultation at least every two minutes, and the fourth Korotkoff sound was used to determine diastolic pressure. Mean arterial pressure was calculated by adding one-third of the pulse pressure to the diastolic pressure.

Direct red cell and plasma volumes were measured simultaneously with chromate labelled red blood cells (^{51}Cr-RBC) and iodinated human serum albumin (^{125}I-HSA) (Sterling and Gray, 1950; Tuckman et al., 1959; Tuckman and Blumberg, 1976). One hour before the procedure, ten drops of Lugol's solution were given in small amounts of drinking water, to block the uptake of ^{125}I by the thyroid glands. Two blank venous samples were obtained without stasis immediately before the injectate was given. Twenty minutes later, four 5 ml samples were taken, also without stasis, at four-minute intervals from a contralateral antecubital vein. Plasma volume was calculated by extrapolating the ^{125}I-HSA disappearance slope to the time of injection. Red cell volume was determined from the average ^{51}Cr-RBC radioactivity in the four post-injection samples. Hematocrits of each sample were also determined using microhematocrit capillary tubes spun in an Adams Micro-Centrifuge (Clay Adams, Inc., New York) at 15,000g. No correction was made for trapped plasma (Dacie and Lewis, 1975). The total body/large vessel, hematocrits ratios were calculated from the relationship of the direct blood volume measurements and the microhematocrits:

$$\frac{\frac{red\ cell\ volume}{red\ cell\ volume + plasma\ volume}}{microhematocrit}$$

Plasma protein concentrations of the samples were measured by the method of Lowry et al. (1951).

Following the control period, several additional venous samples were obtained during each of the hypertensive episodes to estimate the changes in plasma volume. This was done by comparing the changes in plasma protein concentrations and hematocrits with the respective control measurements.

Supine cardiac output was measured before and during autonomic hyperreflexia in five patients by the indicator-dilution method. Indocyanine green (cardio-green; Hyson, Westcote & Dunning, Inc., Baltimore, Md.) was injected through a small PE50 (Clay Adams, Inc., New York) catheter that had been "floated" into an intrathoracic vein, and brachial or femoral arterial blood was withdrawn through a Waters' densitometer by a pump at a rate of 40ml/minute. The blood was collected in a sterile manner and returned to the subjects after each cardiac output determination. The area under the curves was calculated by numerical summation at one second intervals until the

exponential downslope began and from there, by integration, to infinity
(Lillienfield and Kovach, 1956). Calibration was done by drawing two
different concentrations of the dye in the patient's blood through the
arterial tube-densitometer system at the same rate that was used in
recording of the indicator-dilution curves. In each subject, two or
three cardiac outputs were determined during the control period, and
two or three others were determined, within several minutes, at the
height of the hypertension. Peripheral resistance was calculated from
the ratio of mean arterial pressure and cardiac output and was expressed
in dynes $\cdot$ sec $\cdot$ cm^{-5}.

The arterial samples for analysis of serum DβH activity and plasma
PGE$_2$ concentration were obtained during the control periods and at the
times of greatest elevation of blood pressure. Serum DβH activity
was determined by a modification (Weinshilboum and Axelrod, 1971)
of the sensitive isotopic method of Molinoff et al. This technique
utilizes conversion of phenylethylamine by DβH to phenylethanolamine.
The latter is converted to ^{14}C-labelled N-methyl-phenylethanolamine by
purified bovine adrenal phenylethanolamine-N-methyltransferase in the
presence of the active methyl donor s-adenosyl-methionine methyl-^{14}C.
Serum DβH activity is expressed in n moles of phenylethanolamine/ml
serum/hour. The concentration of PGE$_2$ in plasma was determined by
the sensitive radio-immunoassay of Levine et al. (1971). This method
involves incubation of the deproteinized sample with (^{3}H)-labelled rabbit
antibody to PGE$_2$ and goat antirabbit globulin. The precipitate
containing the antibody-bound ^{3}H-PGE$_2$ is separated by centrifugation,
and it is then dissolved in NaOH and assayed by liquid scintillation
spectrometry.

The statistical analysis of the results was by the paired "t" test.

RESULTS

The means for the control supine red cell, plasma, and total blood
volumes are presented in Table I. The volumes are expressed as ml/cm
body height. Blood volumes are relatively independent of body height
and have been found to be a better reference index for expressing
results than weight or surface area in most groups of subjects (Chien
et al., 1966; Tarazi et al., 1968; Tuckman et al., 1973). The one
abnormal finding was that the red cell volume of 10.5 ml/cm (range
9.3-11.7) was somewhat decreased. The average total body/large
vessel hematocrits ratio was 0.87 and was less than unity in all of the
patients (0.81-0.91). This indicated that the hematocrit in the larger
vessels was greater than that in the smaller vessels, as is the case in
normal subjects and in patients with different types of disease
(Tuckman et al., 1959; Gibson et al., 1946; Verel, 1954; Gregersen and
Rawson, 1959).

A primary aim of this study was to determine if the hypertension
of autonomic hyperreflexia caused a reduction in plasma volume. In
the eight blood volume procedures, the blood pressure was considerably
elevated during periods of nine, nine, 13, 16, 21, 22, 26, and 33
minutes. The average increase of 73% in mean arterial pressure
(Table I) was calculated from several measurement that were obtained
in each patient at the end and height of the hypertensive episodes.
The average elevations of plasma protein concentration and hematocrit at
those times were 9.9% and 9.5%, respectively.

The results from the five hemodynamic investigations are presented
in Table II and Figure 1. Blood pressure was significantly elevated in
all the procedures during periods of 21, 22, 40, and 55 minutes. The

TABLE I[1]

Eight Male Quadriplegic Subjects: Control Blood Volumes and
Changes in Hematocrit and Plasma Protein Concentration in Autonomic Hyperreflexia

	N	CONTROL MEAN ± S.E.M.	A.H.+ MEAN ± S.E.M.	P	PERCENT CHANGE
MAP++ mmHg	8	77 ± 6.5	133 ± 9.8	<0.001	+73%
Heart Rate Beats/Min.	7	79 ± 5.8	55 ± 2.0	<0.01	-24 beats/min.
Plasma Protein g/100ml	7	7.1 ± 0.32	7.8 ± 0.36	<0.01	+9.9%
Hematocrit %	8	40.9 ± 1.03	44.8 ± 1.15	<0.001	+9.5%
Red Cell Volume ml/cm*	8	10.5 ± 0.29			
Plasma Volume ml/cm	8	19.1 ± 0.55			
Total Blood Volume ml/cm	8	29.6 ± 0.76			
TB/LVH**	8	0.87 ± 0.01			

+A.H. :   autonomic hyperreflexia; measurements obtained at the height of the hypertensive period.
++MAP :   supine mean arterial pressure (diastolic + 1/3 pulse pressure).
*ml/cm :   supine volumes with reference to centimeter of body height.
**TB/LVH :   total body/large vessel hematocrits ratio.

data in Table II and Figure 1, during autonomic hyperreflexia, represent the means of two or three measurements that were obtained within several minutes at the end and height of the hypertension. The average increase in blood pressure was 62%, which was accompanied by a substantial bradycardia in all patients that averaged -27 beats/minute. A similar bradycardia occurred during the blood volume studies (Table I).

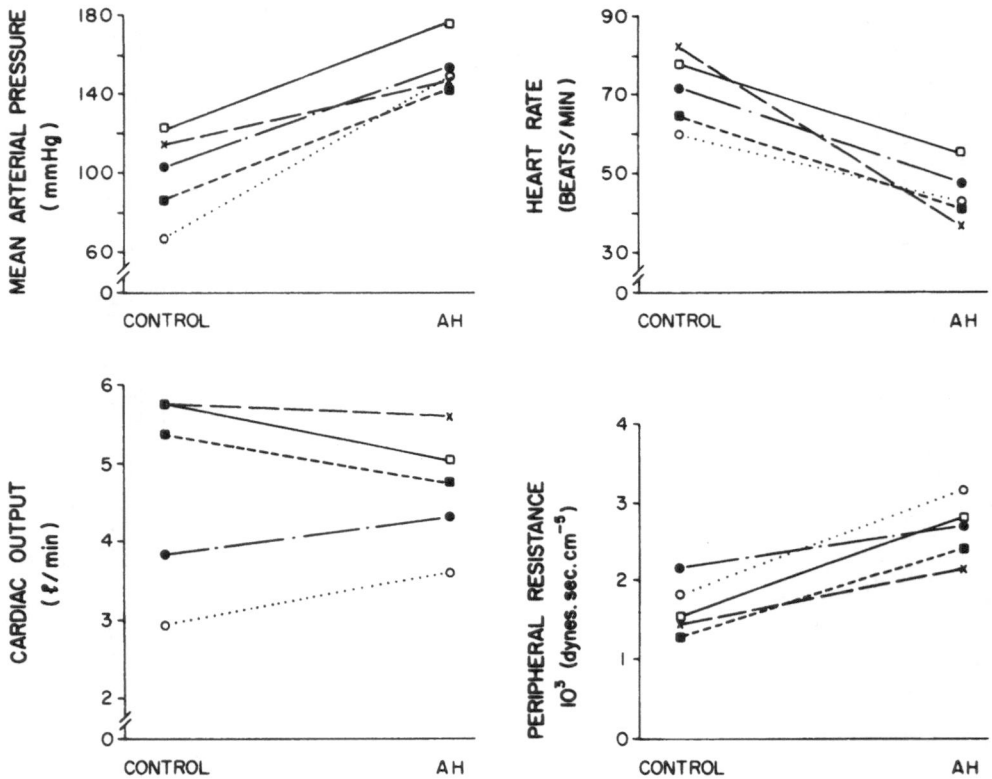

Fig. 1. Hemodynamic changes during autonomic hyperreflexia in five quadriplegic subjects. Bladder distension evoked a large increase in mean arterial pressure (+62%), which, in turn, produced a striking reflex bradycardia (-27 beats/min.). The hypertensive episode was also accompanied by a significant rise in peripheral resistance (+61%) and no change in cardiac output.

The control mean cardiac output of 4.76 litres/minute remained essentially unchanged during the hypertensive episodes when it was 4.70 litres/minute. The individual changes were modest and included reductions of 0.18, 0.57 and 0.79, and elevations of 0.50 and 0.73 litres/minute. These were also small changes when expressed as percentages in four of the subjects and varied between -3 and +13%. In the fifth patient (subject 4), there was a 25% increase in cardiac output, but this larger relative rise was due to a low control measurement (2.95 litres/minute) rather than a large absolute change (+0.73 litres/minute). In all subjects, mean peripheral resistance rose

TABLE II[1]

Cardiac Output, Cardiac and Stroke Work, and Peripheral Resistance During Autonomic Hyperreflexia in Five Quadriplegic Subjects

Subject	MAP++ mmHg		Heart Rate Beats/Min.		Cardiac Output ℓ/Min.		"Minute Cardiac Work"* ℓ·mmHg		"Stroke Work"* ℓ·mmHg		Peripheral Resistance dynes·Sec.·cm−5	
	C.+	A.H.+	C.	A.H.	C.	A.H.	C.	A.H.	C.	A.H.	C.	A.H.
1	108	147	84	38	5.82	5.64	629	829	7.48	21.82	1483	2083
2	112	179	79	56	5.84	5.05	654	904	8.28	16.14	1533	2833
3	102	152	72	48	3.88	4.38	396	666	5.50	13.87	2101	2773
4	67	147	60	43	2.95	3.68	198	541	3.29	12.58	1815	3192
5	88	144	64	43	5.33	4.76	469	685	7.33	16.32	1320	2418
Mean	95	154	72	45	4.76	4.70	469	725	6.38	16.15	1650	2660
SEM	8.2	6.4	4.5	3.1	0.58	0.33	83.3	64.0	0.90	1.58	138.0	189.4
P	<0.001		<0.01		N.S.		<0.001		<0.01		<0.01	
	+62%		-27 b/min.		-1%		+55%		+153%		+61%	

+C.: control
+A.H.: autonomic hyperreflexia: measurements obtained at height of hypertensive period
+MAP: supine mean arterial pressure (diastolic + 1/3 pulse pressure)
*minute cardiac work: MAP (mmHg) x cardiac output (ℓ/minute)
stroke work: MAP (mmHg) x stroke volume (ℓ)

considerably (61%) between 32% to 85%.

Serum DβH activity and plasma PGE$_2$ concentration in arterial blood samples increased in all patients during autonomic hyperreflexia, and the average changes were +65% and +68%, respectively (Table III).

Hyperhidrosis, piloerection and flushing were present in various degrees over the face, neck, and upper trunk during all the episodes of autonomic hyperreflexia. Half of the patients also experienced heacaches. No attempt was made, however, to correlate the severity of this symptom with the rises in arterial plasma PGE$_2$ concentration.

DISCUSSION

High spinal cord injuries before World War II were usually fatal within a short period of time after the onset of the injury. This is no longer true, since improved emergency treatment after the accident is now more readily available. Furthermore, chronic complications (infections, amyloidosis, pulmonary, and renal impairment) are avoided by adequate physical rehabilitation and the use of antibiotics (Tribe, 1963; Freed et al., 1966; Burke et al., 1960). As a result, there are an increasing number of quadriplegic subjects in the community who lead a productive life and have an apparently normal life expectancy.

During subacute (three to six months after the onset) and chronic (six months or longer after onset) phases of the injury, the subjects become sensitive to stimulation below the level of transection. Thus, they may suffer from somatic hyperreflexia and spasticity because afferent stimuli, free from supra-spinal control, spread widely through the distal spinal stump producing excessive and uncoordinated activation of the anterior horn cells. Similarly, the afferent stimuli can produce widespread activation of preganglionic sympathetic neurones in the intermediolateral cell columns and autonomic hyperreflexia (dysreflexia).

The main symptoms of autonomic hyperreflexia are systemic hypertension, bradycardia, headache, and in the dermatomes that are innervated from above the spinal cord lesion, piloerection, hyperhidrosis, and vasodilatation. Stimulation of the dermatones and muscles innervated by nerves from *below* the injury will bring about the syndrome, but it is most severe and consistently evoked after excitation of the genitoanal region, distension of the bladder (blocked passage of urine) or rectum (enema, rectal impaction). Attacks of autonomic dysreflexia occur in subjects with transections at and above the T6 segment (Bors, 1956; Guttman and Whitteridge, 1947; Johnson et al., 1975; Schumacher and Guthrie, 1951). As indicated above, the excessive sympathetic activity in the distal spinal stump is due to lack of control by the hypothalamus, medulla, and other supra-spinal "vasomotor centres." In addition, preganglionic sympathetic neurones may also be supersensitive to stimulation since the content of noradrenalin and other neurotransmitters within the spinal cord below the lesion have been depleted (Naftchi et al., 1969; Anden et al., 1964; Magnusson and Rosengren, 1963; Hall et al., 1976).

A generalized increase in sympathetic tone could, therefore, alter hemodynamics and raise arterial pressure by: (1) reducing the distensibility of postarteriolar capacity vessels (augmented cardiac filling pressures); (2) directly increasing myocardial contractility; and (3) elevating arteriolar resistance. However, analysis of the hypertension in autonomic hyperreflexia is more complex since it also involves a parallel increase in parasympathetic tone. The latter causes a striking bradycardia that depends presumably on excessive stimulation of the carotid sinus and aortic-arch baroreceptor reflexes, i.e., elevated

TABLE III[1]

Changes in Arterial Prostaglandin and Dopamine-β-Hydroxylase Levels
During Hypertension in Quadriplegia

Patient	ng PGE_2/ml Plasma		Arterial Serum DβH*	
	Before	During	Before	During
1	0.43	0.56	695	1580
2	0.31	0.40	1145	1418
3	0.40	0.64	702	1106
4	0.10	0.36	905	1456
5	0.37	0.69	794	1235
6	0.44	0.75	640	1270
MEAN	0.34	0.57	814	1344
±SEM	0.05	0.06	76	70
P	<0.001		<0.001	

*units = nmoles phenylethanolamine/ml serum/hour

afferent IX and X and efferent X cranial nerve activity.

In fact, there have been relatively few hemodynamic investigations
of autonomic dysreflexia. The blood flow has been measured in fingers
and toes by calorimetry (Naftchi et al., 1974), in the calf by venous
occlusion plethysmography (Naftchi et al., 1974; Cunningham et al.,
1953; Roussan et al., 1966). In plantar, thigh, chest, forearm, and
palmar surfaces, the cutaneous blood flow has been "assessed" by
photoelectric plethysmography (Wurster and Randall, 1975). In all of
these studies, the blood flow was found to be diminished, and, since
it occurred simultaneously with considerable elevations in arterial
pressures, this indicated that there were large increases in arteriolar
vascular resistance in those regions. Other investigations of blood
flow in the forearm and kidney have been too few to permit adequate
analysis of the data (Cunningham et al., 1953; Hodgson and Wood, 1958).
Further, results of venous tone determinations have not been sufficient
(Cunningham et al., 1953; Roussan et al., 1966) to indicate whether
venous tone was changed during autonomic hyperreflexia.

Several groups of workers have measured cardiac output and
total peripheral resistance. Agrest and Roncoroni (1960), used the
direct Fick and indicator-dilution methods in two patients in whom the
syndrome was evoked by bladder distension. They found that the
cardiac output varied between -21% and +7% and peripheral resistance
varied between +9% and +58%. It is difficult to draw conclusions from
so few results. In addition, the patients did not become hypertensive
during the episodes of dysreflexia; the highest pressures were only
116/88 and 112/78 mmHg. Other investigators have used methods of
doubtful validity to measure cardiac output (Cunningham et al., 1953)
or did not publish adequate details of their methods or results (Mertens
et al., 1960; Debarge et al., 1974).

In the present hemodynamic studies, bladder distension induced
considerable increases in mean arterial pressure in all five subjects

(from +36 to +119%). Heart rate also decreased in all the procedures
(from -17 to -46 beats/minute, Table II, Figure 1). These large
changes in mean arterial pressure and heart rate were associated with
an insignificant, and very small fall in cardiac output of 0.06 litres/
minute. Nonetheless, "minute cardiac work" (cardiac output x mean
arterial pressure) rose in all subjects from 32% to 174% (average 55%)
and because of the bradycardia, the elevation in "stroke work" (stroke
volume x mean arterial pressure) was even greater and averaged +153%.

The total peripheral resistance increased in all of the subjects from
+32 to +85%, and the average change was +61% (Table II). Hypertensive
episodes of autonomic hyperreflexia are, therefore, accompanied by a
significant degree of "overall" arteriolar vasoconstriction. This
conclusion could not be drawn from previous studies that measured
cardiac output (Cunningham et al., 1953; Agrest and Roncoroni, 1960;
Mertens et al., 1960; Debarge et al., 1974) or from the relatively few
hemodynamic investigations of local circulations.

The average control cardiac index in the five quadriplegic subjects
was 2.61 litres/minute/M^2 (range 1.74-3.36) and was approximately
15-20% less than that usually reported for normal males of similar age
range, between 18 to 25 years (Griedberg, 1966; Guyton et al.).
However, until cardiac output measurements are obtained from normal
subjects in this laboratory, it would seem unwise to speculate on this
apparent difference.

Another objective of this study was to determine if the increased
sympathetic activity and circulating noradrenalin levels during
dysreflexia reduced plasma volume, which occurs during intravenous
infusions of noradrenalin in man. Finnerty et al. (1958) and Cohn
(1966) reported that infusions that raised mean arterial pressures by
56% and 36% decreased plasma volumes by 15% and 9.6%, respectively.
These losses were most likely caused by the drug-induced elevation of
capillary hydrostatic pressure (Cohn, 1966), and, not unexpectedly,
they were associated with increases in plasma protein concentrations
and large vessel hematocrits. Only Finnerty et al. (1958) measured
the plasma protein concentration, by a relatively crude method, and it
rose by 6%. However, both studies followed the changes in hematocrit,
which increased by 8% in one (Finnerty et al., 1958) and 2.7% in the
other (Cohn, 1966). Partly, this difference could have reflected
dissimilar potencies of the infusions, but, even when an adjustment
that is simply based on the discrepancy between the decreases in plasma
volumes is made, the rise of hematocrit in Cohn's study would be
altered to only slightly above 4%. Although it would be surprising if
the changes in plasma protein concentrations and hematocrits exactly
corresponded to these reductions in plasma volumes for several reasons,
among which are increased diffusion of the proteins from the capillaries
(Finnerty et al., 1958; Pappenheimer, 1953) and shifts of blood volumes
between vascular beds with different hematocrits (Verel, 1954;
Gregersen and Rawson, 1959), there can be little doubt that noradenalin
infusions in man cause hemoconcentration and significant elevations of
those two measurements.

In the eight procedures done here (Table I), there were considerable elevations of mean arterial pressures for periods of nine to 33
minutes, and, during the final five to ten minutes the average increases
in blood pressure, plasma protein concentration and hematocrit were
73%, 9.9%, and 9.5%, respectively. When these data are compared with
those observed by Finnerty et al. (1958) and Cohn (1966), and
consideration is taken of their plasma volume measurements, it does
not seem unreasonable to conclude that plasma volume decreased during
autonomic hyperreflexia and to estimate that the reduction was between
10 to 15%.

Serum DβH activity rose by 65% (Table 3) during autonomic hyper-reflexia in the present study. This confirmed previous findings from this laboratory (Naftchi et al., 1974). However, since the protein has a molecular weight of 290,000 daltons (Friedman and Kaufman, 1965), it seemed logical to consider how the blood volume changes might influence interpretation of its elevated activity as true release with noradrenalin by exocytosis and how much reflected hemoconcentration. The "maximal" possible decrease of plasma volume that was estimated in this investigation strongly suggests that the hemoconcentration could only have accounted for, at most, one-quarter of the 65% rise in serum DβH activity.

A 5% to 9% reduction in total blood volume, which corresponds to a 10-15% decrease in plasma volume in subjects with hematocrits of 41% (Table I) would not significantly reduced arterial blood pressure in those who had normal control volumes and intact compensatory sympathetic cardiovascular reflexes (Freis et al., 1951; Freis and Rose, 1957). Since quadriplegic patients, in general, have a diminished muscle mass, it was considered necessary for this study to determine if they were hypovolemic. The results in Table I show that the total blood volume was normal in these male patients. However, in nonquad-riplegic subjects who received drugs that reduce resting vascular tone and reflex sympathetic activity (Freis et al., 1951), this small degree of blood loss can cause severe hypotension and syncope, even when supine. This did not occur here when the hypertensive episodes were quickly ended by allowing the bladder to empty, despite the inability of the carotid sinus and aortic arch baroreceptors, and receptors in the low-pressure vascular compartment to mediate a compensatory excitation of the preganglionic sympathetic neurones below the spinal cord transection. This indicated that the quadriplegic patients had essentially normal levels of adrenergic cardiovascular tone when not in a state of autonomic hyperreflexia or that they had the ability to compensate for minor blood volume disturbances or both. The compen-satory mechanisms could include cardio-cardiac and cardio-arteriolar excitatory spinal sympathetic reflexes, which have been demonstrated in animals (Brown and Malliani, 1971; Malliani et al., 1972), and the supra-spinally regulated reduction of efferent vagal tone.

In any event, it would seem unwise to place these subjects in a seated or head-up "tilt" position immediately after a dysreflexic attack, because of the peripheral venous pooling of blood. Furthermore, it would seem possible that conditions that reduce resting blood volume, arteriolar and venous tone, or depress the myocardium, may lead to extreme hypotension during the hypovolemic period after autonomic hyperreflexia. Such conditions would exist in excessively hot environ-ments, if the subjects had infections and fever, or if they received drugs that affected the cardiovascular system. Such considerations will assume greater clinical relevance as quadriplegic subjects continue to live longer and enter older age ranges. They should then have an increasing incidence of coronary heart disease and hypertension and will be candidates for drug regimes that importantly affect the heart and blood vessels.

During autonomic hyperreflexia, the systemic hypertension is adequately explained by the high degree of arteriolar vasoconstriction and increased cardiac work, and the bradycardia by supra-spinal reflexes. However, it is not obvious why the hyperhidrosis, piloerection, and flushing are limited to the upper dermatomes that are innervated by somatic nerves from above the spinal cord lesion, and cutaneous vasoconstriction occurs in the more caudal regions. This is because all regions are supplied by the sympathetic nerves, and, in the subjects with cervical cord injuries, presumably nearly all of the preganglionic fibers originate below the transection.

In any case, the diaphoresis and piloerection in the more cephalad dematomes, above the level of transection, would seem logical consequences of increased sympathetic cholinergic (and probably adrenergic) nervous system activity (Robertshaw, 1975). It can be speculated that the vasodilatation is secondary to stimulation of the sweat glands by the cholinergic sympathetic fibers and the secretion of bradykinin (Fox and Hilton, 1958). This could be the basis for observations (Head and Riddoch, 1917; Guttman and Whitteridge, 1947) that as an attack of autonomic hyperreflexia continues a gradual caudad spread of both the diaphoresis and vasodilatation occur, which might result from the diffusion of acetycholine and bradykinin.

It is also possible to consider that the blood vessels in the upper dermatomes react differently to many stimuli than those elsewhere and to consider other mechanisms which might cause the vasodilatation. Psychological stimuli frequently cause blushing that is limited to these areas. Also infusions of adrenalin (Allen and Roddie, 1972) and attacks in patients with pheochromocytoma (Prout and Wardell, 1969) cause vasodilatation that is sometimes limited to these regions. In addition, it is possible that the arterial prostaglandins of the E series, which increased (E_2) by 68% in this study, contributed to the flushing. Infusions of these substances in man cause vasodilatation of similar distribution (Carlson et al., 1968). Also, they can increase acetylcholine output from some nerves (Weeks, 1972), and there are relationships between the prostaglandins and bradykinin. On the one hand, bradykinin can release prostaglandins (Vane and McGift, 1975, and, on the other hand, prostaglandins enhance the vascular actions and other inflammatory effects of bradykinin (Ikeda et al., 1975; Goldyne, 1975).

It is noted that some workers have concluded that the flushing during autonomic hyperreflexia is the result of passive vasodilataion, but they offered no reason why the vascular bed in cephalad dermatomes was so weak. Still others have suggested that the redness is due to active compensatory vascular mechanisms and that the relevant vessels have a dual sympathetic and parasympathetic autonomic innervation (Kurnick, 1956; Braddon and Johnson, 1969). Present descriptions of the autonomic control of cutaneous blood vessels, however, are based primarily on simple sympathetic innervation and on the premise that vasodilatation is brought about by the diminution of sympathetic activity alone.

Headache is a characteristic symptom of autonomic hyperreflexia and can be so severe that is has been described as excruciating (Schumacher and Guthrie, 1951). Although headache is a frequent complaint, it does not always occur during the episodes of dysreflexia, and its presence, absence, or degree of severity, has not been correlated with the level of hypertension (Hutch, 1955; Ariefe et al., 1962). One-half of the subjects in the present study volunteered that they had the symptom during the hypertensive episode. Many investigators have hypothesized that it results from passive vasodilatation of cerebral vessels during the systemic hypertension. They have used the presence of cutaneous vasodilatation in the cephalad dermatomes, as well as the less frequent symptom of nasal congestion, to support this reasoning. As discussed previously, there is no clear evidence to indicate that the cutaneous vasodilatation is passive. It would seem equally inadequate to use nasal congestion as evidence. It is not a sign which usually occurs during other types of paroxysmal hypertension. Theoretically, nasal congestion might take place during autonomic hypererflexia because of increased parasympathetic activity (Koelle, 1975), but then the attendant elevated blood flow to the mocous glands would be associated with copious nasal secretion. This is not a feature of the syndrome.

However, the cerebral vessels are primarily controlled by nonneural, myogenic auto-regulation (Lassen, 1973) and, therefore, are presumably independent of the increased sympathetic vasoconstricting effect, which acts on the cutaneous vascular beds during autonomic hyperreflexia. Also, there is some evidence that supports the conclusion that passive vasodilatation of cerebral vessels could occur during systemic hypertension. For example, intravenous infusion of angiotensin II (in man) sometimes produces elevations of blood pressure that break through the cerebral auto-regulatory mechanism and increase blood flow to the brain (Lassen, 1973; Strandgaard et al., 1973). It is noted, in this regard, that angiotensin II has no direct vasoconstricting effect on the cerebral arterioles (Oleson, 1972). Also, initial analysis of results reported by Schumacher and Guthrie (1951) provide strong support for this hypothesis of the cause of the headache. In six subjects, during attacks of autonomic hyperreflexia, the investigators increased the lumbar subarachnoidal spinal fluid pressure by forced saline infusions. This procedure eliminated headache in the four patients who had an open communication between the lumbar and cranial subarachnoidal spaces, despite continued systemic hypertension but not in the other two subjects in whom the spinal canal was blocked. Moreover, in two of the patients, the internal carotid arterial pulsations were repeatedly obliterated by bilateral manual compression during 10 to 20 second periods, and these maneuvers, in the majority of attempts, temporarily stopped or diminished the headaches.

Further consideration of the above data, however, suggests that they may not provide a convincing basis for the hypothesis. In most subjects, if the initial rate of intravenous infusions of angiotensin or noradrenalin is gradually increased over several minutes, attendant quite high arterial blood pressure can be maintained during prolonged periods without causing headache (Finnerty et al., 1958; Tuckman and Finnerty, 1959). Noradrenalin as well as angiotensin does not have a direct vasoconstricting effect on cerebral arterioles (Oleson, 1972). Furthermore, the levels of spinal pressure that successfully ended headache during autonomic dysreflexia were not higher than 50 cm H_2O and were at least as low as 30 cm H_2O (Schumacher and Guthrie, 1951). Increasing cerebrospinal fluid pressure within this range, and even to 100mmHg, did not reduce cerebral blood flow in dogs, probably because the decrease in the cerebral artery–venous pressure gradient was compensated for by the normal autoregulatory mechanism and consequent arteriolar vasodilatation (Haggendal et al., 1970). Thus, it is concluded that at present, there is no single direct explanation for the mechanism of the headache that is associated with hyperreflexia. In this study, the arterial concentration pf PGE_2 rose by 68% (from 0.34 to 0.57 ng/ml plasma, Table III). It is also known that infusions of PGE_1 or PGE_2 (in man) at sufficiently high rates, typically produce flushing in the face, neck and upper trunk, and headache (Carlson et al., 1968; Horton, 1972; Robinson et al., 1973), but data are conflicting as to whether they decrease the tone of cerebral vessels (Denton et al., 1972; Pelofsky et al., 1972; Yamamoto et al., 1972; Nakano et al., 1973; Handa et al., 1975). Nonetheless, intravenous infusions of PGE_2 at rates of 5-20 µg/min. would cause headache (Karim and Filshie, 1972; Hillier and Embrey, 1972) and, assuming 90% destruction during each pulmonary transit (Ferreira and Vane, 1967), produce arterial concentrations of the prostaglandins similar to those measured here at the time of autonomic hyperreflexia. The symptom could be the result of a direct biochemical effect or of the possible relexation of vascular smooth muscles, which would reduce the autoregulatory control of cerebral blood flow (Lassen, 1973). In the latter circumstance, the headache might then, indeed, be due to the passive vasodilatation of cerebral vessels during the hypertensive episodes.

The presence of high arterial concentrations of prostaglandins during autonomic hyperreflexia may have a much greater significance since they may be part of a compensatory mechanism that abates adrenergic activity. Previous studies indicated that the release of prostaglandins is modulated by sumpathetic tone and that they are also liberated by stimulation of parasympathetic nerves (Bennet et al., 1967). The parallel elevation of the activities of both branches of the autonomic nervous system is a prominent feature in autonomic dysreflexia. The high arterial concentrations of PGE_2, therefore, may reflect heightened activity of the two systems. A mechanism through which the high concentration of prostaglandins diminish sympathetic activity is indicated by *in vitro* results, which have shown that they may inhibit the calcium dependent release of noradrenalin and $D\beta H$ by the process of exocytosis (Johnson et al., 1971). Finally, previous data from this laboratory (Naftchi et al., 1974) documented a rapid decline in serum $D\beta H$ activity coincident with the reduction of autonomic symptoms when the bladder was allowed to empty. Since high concentrations of the large molecular weight of $D\beta H$ would still be present at this time, it is possible that the sharp decline in serum $D\beta H$ activity may be the result of inhibition of the process of exocytosis by the prostaglandins or the sudden release of large amounts of endogenous inhibitor(s) (Harralson and Brown, 1975) after cessation of autonomic dysreflexia, or both.

REFERENCES

Agrest, A., and Roncoroni, A.J.   Effect of bladder distension on pulmonary vascular bed. *Circ. Res. 8:*501-505 (1960).

Allen, A.J., and Roddie, I.C.   The role of circulating catecholamines in sweat production in man. *J. Physiol. 227:*801-814 (1972).

Anden, N.E., Haggendal, E., Magnusson, T., and Rosengren, E.   Time course of the disapperance of noradrenaline and 5-hydroxy-tryptamine in spinal cord after transection. *Acta Physiol. Scand. 62:* 115-118 (1964).

Ariefe, A.J., Tigay, E.L., and Pyzik, S.W.   Acute hypertension induced by urinary bladder distension. *Arch. Neurol. 2:*248-256 (1962).

Bennet, A., Friedman, C.A., and Vane, J.R.   Release of prostaglandin E from the rat stomach. *Nature (Lond) 216:*873 (1967).

Bevegard, S., and Oro, L.   Effect of prostaglandin E_1 on forearm blood flow. *Scand. J. Clin. Invest. 23:*347-353 (1969).

Bors, E.   The challenge of quadriplegia. *Bull. Los. Angeles Neurol. Soc. 21:*105-123 (1956).

Brown, A.M., and Malliani, A.   Spinal sympathetic relexes initiated by coronrary reflexes. *J. Physiol. 212:*685-705 (1971).

Braddon, R.L., Johnson, E.W.   Mecamylamine in control of hyperreflexia. *Arch. Phys. Med. Rehab. 50:*448-453 (1969).

Burke, M.H., Hicks, A.F., Robins, M., and Kessler, H.   Survival of patients with injuries of the spinal cord. *JAMA 172:*121-124 (1960).

Carlson, L.A., Ekelund, L.G., and Oro, L.   Clinical and metabolic effects of different doses of prostaglandin E_1 in man. *Acta Med.*

*Scand. 183:*423-430 (1968).

Carlson, L.A., Ekelund, L.G., and Oro, L.   Circulatory and respiratory effects of different doses of prostaglandin E_1 in man.   *Acta Physiol. Scand. 75:*161-169 (1969).

Chien, S., Usami, S., Simmons, R.L., McAllister, F.F., and Gregersen, M.I.   Blood volume and age: repeated measurements on normal men after 17 years.   *J. Appl. Physiol. 21:*583-588 (1966).

Cohn, J.N.   Relationship of plasma volume changes to resistance and capacitance vessel effects of sympathomimetic amines and angiotensin in man.   *Clin. Science 30:*267-278 (1966).

Cunningham, D.J.C., Guttman, L., Whitterridge, D., and Wyndham, C.H.   Cardiovascular responses to bladder distension in paraplegic patients.   *J. Physiol. 121:*581-592 (1953).

Dacie, J.V., and Lewis, S.M.   *Practical Hematology.*   Fifth Edition.   Churchill Livingstone, Edinburgh, London, and New York, 1975, pp. 39-41.

Debarge, O., Christensen, N.J., Corbett, J.L., Eidelman, B.H., Frankel, H.L., and Mathias, C.J.   Plasma catecholamines in tetraplegics.   *Paraplegia 12:*44-49 (1974).

Denton, I.C., White, R.P., and Robertson, J.T.   The effects of prostaglandins E_1, A_1 and F_2 α on the cerebral circulation of dogs and monkeys.   *J. Neurosurgery 36:*34-42 (1972).

Desmond, J.   Paraplegia: problems confronting the anaesthesiologist.   *The Canadian Anaesthesiologists' Soc. Jrl. 17:*435-451 (1970).

Ferreira, S.H., and Vane, J.R.   Prostaglandins: Their disappearance from and release into the circulation.   *Nature 216:*868-873 (1967).

Finnerty, F.A., Jr., Buchholz, J.H., and Giullaudeau, R.L.   The blood volumes and plasma protein during levarteronol.   *J. Clin. Invest. 37:*425-429 (1958).

Fox, R.H., and Hilton, S.M.   Bradykinin formation in human skin as a factor in heat vasodilatation.   *J. Physiol. 142:*219-232 (1958).

Freed, M.M., Bakst, H.J., and Barrie, D.L.   Life expectancy, survival rate and causes of death in civilian patients with spinal cord trauma.   *Arch. Phys. Med. 47:*457-463 (1966).

Freis, E.D., Standon, J.R., Finnerty, F.A., Jr., Schnaper, H.W., Johnson, R.L., Roth, C.E., and Wilkens, R.W.   The collapse produced by venous congestion of the extremities and by venesection following hypotensive agents.   *J. Clin. Invest. 30:*435-444 (1951).

Freis, E.D., and Rose, J.C.   The sympathetic nervous system, the vascular volume and the venous return in relation to cardiovascular integration.   *Am. J. Med. 22:*175-178 (1957).

Friedberg, C.K.   Diseases of the heart.   Third Edition.   W.B. Saunders Company, Philadelphia 1966, p. 313.

Friedman, S., and Kaufman, S.   3,4-Dihydroxyphenylethylamine β-hydroxylase.   Physical properties, copper content, and role of copper in the catalytic activity.   *J. Biol. Chem. 240:*4763-4773 (1965).

Gewirtz, G.P., and Kopin, I.J.   Release of dopamine-β-hydroxylase with norepinephrine during cat splenic nerve stimulation.   *Nature (London) 227:*406-407 (1970).

Gibson, J., Peacock, W., Seligmann, A., and Sack, T.   Circulating red cell volume measured simultaneously by the radioactive iron and dye methods.   *J. Clin. Invest. 25:*838-847 (1946).

Goldyne, M.E.   Prostaglandins and cutaneous inflammation.   *J. Invest. Derm. 64:*377-385 (1975).

Gregersen, M.I., and Rawson, R.A.   Blood volume.   *Physiol. Rev. 39:*307-342 (1959).

Guttman, L., and Whitterridge, D.   Effects of bladder distension on

autonomic mechanisms after spinal cord injuries. *Brain 70:*361-405
(1947).

Guyton, A.C., Jones, C.E., and Coleman, T.G.   Circulatory Physiology:
Cardiac output and its regulation. Second Edition. W.B. Saunders
Company, Philadelphia, pp. 8-9.

Haggendal, E., Lofgren, J., Nilsson, N.J., and Zwetnow, N.N. Effects
of varied cerebrospinal fluid pressure on cerebral blood flow in
dogs. *Acta. Physiol. Scand. 79:*262-271 (1970).

Hall, P.V., Smith, J.E., Campbell, R.L., Felten, D.L., and Aprison,
M.H. Neurochemical correlates of spasticity. *Life Sci. 18:*1467-
1472 (1976).

Harralson, J.D., and Brown, F.C. Inhibitors of dopamine-β-hydroxylase
human plasma. *Proc. Soc. Exp. Bio. and Med. 149:*643-645 (1975).

Handa, J., Yoneda, S., Matsuda, M., and Handa, H. Effects of
prostaglandins A_1, E_1, E_2 and F_2 α on canine carotid arterial blood
flow, cerebrospinal fluid pressure and intraocular pressure. *J.
Neurosurgery 38:*32-39 (1973).

Horton, E.W. In *Prostanglandins.* Springer-Verlag, Berlin, New York,
1972, p. 150.

Head, H., and Riddoch, J. Autonomic bladder, excessive seating, and
some other reflex conditions in gross injuries of the spinal cord.
*Brain 40:*188-263 (1917).

Hodgson, N.B., and Wood, J.A. Studies of the nature of paroxysmal
hypertension in paraplegics. *J. Urology 79:*719-721 (1958).

Hutch, J.A. A study of the hyperactive autonomic reflex initiated by
bladder distension in patients with lesions in the cervical and high
thoracic cord. *J. Urology 73:*1019-1025 (1955).

Ikeda, K., Tanaka, K., and Katori, M. Potentiation of bradykinin-
induced vascular permeability increase by prostaglandin E_2 and
arachidonic acid in rabbit skin. *Prostaglandins 10:*747-758 (1975).

Johnson, B., Pallares, V., Thomason, R., and Sadove, M.S.
Autonomic hyperreflexia: a review. *Military Medicine 140:*345-349
(1975).

Johnson, D., Thoa, N., Weinshilboum, R.M., Axelrod, J., Kopin, I.J.
Enhanced release of dopamine-β-hydroxylase from sympathetic
nerves by calcium and phenoxybenzamine and its reversal by
prostaglandins. *Proc. Nat. Acad. Sci. 68:*2227 (1971).

Karim, Sm.m., and Filshie, G.M. The use of prostaglandin E_2 for
therapeutic abortion. *J. Obst. Gynec. Brit. Commonwealth 79:*
1-13 (1972).

Koelle, G.B. Neurohumoral transmission and the autonomic nervous
system. In *The Pharmacological Basis of Therapeutics,* Fifth
Edition, L.S. Goodman and A. Gilman, MacMillan Publishing Company,
Inc., New York, Chapter 21, p. 407.

Kurnick, N.B. Autonomic hyperreflexia and its control in patients
with spinal cord lesions. *Annals. of Internal Med. 44:*678-685
(1956).

Lassen, N.A. Control of cerebral circulation in health and disease.
*Circ. Res. 34:*749-760 (1973).

Levine, L., Gutierrez-Cernosek, R.M., and Van Vunakis, H.
Specificities of prostaglandins B_1, F_1 α antigen-antibody reactions.
*J. Biol. Chem. 246:*6782 (1971).

Lillienfield, L., Kovach, R. Simplified method for calculating flow,
mean circulating time and downslope from indicator dilution curves.
*Proc. Soc. Exper. Biol. and Med. 91:*595-598 (1956).

Lowry, O.H., Rosebrough, N.J., Farr, A.L., and Randall, R.J.
Protein measurement with the Folin pehnol reagent. *J. Biol. Chem.*

*193:*265 (1951).

Magnusson, T., and Rosengren, E. Catecholamines of the spinal cord normally and after transection. *Experimentia 19:*229-230 (1963).

Malliani, A., Peterson, D.F., Bishop, V.S., and Brown, A.M. Spinal sympathetic cardiocardiac reflexes. *Circ. Res. 30:*158-166 (1972).

Mertens, H.G., Harms, S., Harms, H., and Jungmann, H. The regulation of the circulation in patient swith cervical cord transection. *Ger. Med. Monthly 5:*189-193 (1960).

Naftchi, N.E., Lowman, E.W., Rusk, H., and Reich, T. Urinary catecholamine metabolites in spinal cord injured human (abstr.) *Fed. Proc. 28:*544 (1969).

Naftchi, N.E., Wooten, G.F., Lowman, E.W., and Axelrod, J. Relationship between serum dopamine-β-hydroxylase activity, catecholamine metabolism and hemodynamic changes during paroxysmal hypertension in quadriplegia. *Circ. Res. 35:*850-861 (1974).

Nakano, J., Chang, A.C.K., and Fisher, R.G. Effects of prostaglandins E_1, E_2, A_1, A_2 and F_2 α on canine carotid arterial blood flow, cerebrospinal fluid pressure and intraocular pressure. *J. Neurosurgery 38:*32-39 (1973).

Oleson, J. The effect of intracarotid epinephrine, norepinephrine and angiotensin on the regional cerebral flow in man. *Neurology 22:*978-987 (1972).

Oppenheimer, W.A. Pregnancy in paraplegic patients. *Am. J. Obst. Gynec. 110:*784-786 (1971).

Pappenheimer, J.R. Paggage of molecules through capillary walls. *Phys. Rev. 33:*387-423 (1953).

Robertshaw, D. Catecholamines and control of sweat glands in Endocrinology. Vol. VI *Handbook of Physiology,* pp. 591-603, Washington, D.C., 1975.

Prout, B.J., and Wardell, W.M. Sweating and peripheral blood flow in patients with phaeochromocytoma. *Clin. Sci. 36:*109-117 (1969).

Robinson, B.F., Collier, J.G., Karim. S.M.M., and Somers, K. Effect of prostaglandins A_1, A_2, E_1, E_2 and F_2 α on the forearm bed and superficial hand veins in man. *Clin. Sci. 44:*367-376 (1973).

Pelofsky, S., Jacobson, E.D., and Fisher, R.G. Effects of prostaglandins E_1 on experimental cerebral vasospasm. *J. Neurosurgery 36:*635-639 (1972).

Roussan, M.S., Abramson, A.S., Lippman, H.I., and D'Oronzio, G. Somatic and autonomic responses to bladder filling in patients with complete tranverse myelopathy. *Arch. Phys. Med. Rehab. 47:*450-456 (1966).

Schumacher, G.A., and Guthrie, T.C. Studies on headache: mechanisms of headache and observations on other effects induced by distension of bladder and rectum in subjects with spinal cord injuries. *AMA Arch. Neurol. Psych. 65:*568-580 (1951).

Sterling, K., and Gray, S.J. Determination of the circulating red cell volume in man by radioactive chromium. *J. Clin. Invest. 29:*1614-1619 (1950).

Strandgaard, S., Oleson, J., Skinhoj, E., and Lassen, N.A. Autoregulation of brain circulation in severe arterial hypertension. *Brit. Med. J. 1:*507-510 (1973).

Tarazi, R.C., Frohlich, E.D., and Dustan, H.P. Plasma volume in men with essential hypertension. *N. Eng. J. Med. 278:*762-765 (1968).

Tribe, C.R. Causes of death in the early and late stages of paraplegia. *Paraplegia 1:*19-47 (1963).

Tuckman, J., Finnerty, F.A., Jr., and Buchholz, J.H. Discrepancy between body and venous hematocrits. Dilution curves of simultaneously administered I^{131}-HSA and Cr^{51}-labeled erythrocytes. *J. Appl. Physiol. 14:* 585 (1959).

Tuckman, J., and Blumberg, A. Serial measurements of total blood volume in patients on maintenance hemodialysis. *Klin. Wochenschr 54:* 735-738 (1976).

Tuckman, J., Benninger, J.L., and Reubi, F. Haemodynamic and blood volume studies in long-term haemodialysis patients, and in patients with successfully transplanted kidneys. *Clin. Sci. Mol. Med. 45:* 155s-157s (1973).

Tuckman, J., and Finnerty, F.A., Jr. The cardiac index (indicator dilution method) during intravenous levarteronol infusion. *Circ. Res. 7:* 988-991 (1959).

Vane, J.R., and McGiff, J.C. Possible contributions of endogenous prostaglandins to the control of blood pressure. *Circ. Res. 36:* Suppl. 1, 68-75 (1975).

Verel, J. Observations on the distribution of plasma and red cells in disease. *Clin. Sci. 13:* 51-59 (1954).

Viveros, O.H., Arqueros, L., and Kirshner, N. Release of catecholamine and dopamine-β-hydroxylase from and adrenal medulla. *Life Sci. 7:* 609-618 (1968).

Weeks, J.R. Prostaglandins. *Annl. Rev. Pharm. 12:* 317-336 (1972).

Weinshilboum, R.M., Kvetnansky, R., Axelrod, J., and Kopin, I.J. Elevation of serum dopamine-β-hydroxylase activity with forced immobilization. *Nature (New Biology) 230:* 287-288 (1971).

Weinshilboum, R.M., and Axelrod, J. Reduced plasma dopamine-β-hydroxylase activity in familial dysautonomia. *N. Eng. J. Med. 285:* 938-942 (1971).

Weinshilboum, R.M., Thoa, N.B., Johnson, D.G., Kopin, I.J., and Axelrod, J. Proportional release of norepinephrine and dopamine-β-hydroxylase from sympathetic nerves. *Science 174:* 1349-1351 (1971).

Wooten, G.F., and Cardon, P. Plasma DβH activity: Elevation in man during cold pressor tests and exercise. *Arch. Neurol. 28:* 103-106 (1973).

Wurster, R.D., and Randall, W.C. Cardiovascular responses to bladder distension in patients with spinal transection. *J. Appl. Physiol. 228:* 1288-1292 (1975).

Yamamoto, Y.L., Feindel, W., Wolfe, L.S., Katoh, H., and Hodge, C.P. Experimental vasoconstriction of cerebral arteries by prostaglandins. *J. Neurosurgery 37:* 385-397 (1972).

Hillier, K., and Embrey, M.P. High dose intravenous administration of prostaglandin E_2 and F_2 α for the termination of mid-trimester pregnancies. *J. Obst. Gynec. Birt. Commonwealth 79:* 14-22 (1972).

[1]Reprinted by permission of the American Heart Association from Naftchi, NE, Demeny, M, Lowman, EW, and Tuckman, J. Hypertensive Crises in Quadriplegic Patients. Circulation 57: 336-341, February 1978.

SECTION FOUR

Bone Mineral and Matrix
Changes Following Spinal
Cord Injury: Possible Modes
of Treatment

13

Disodium Etidronate in the Prevention of Postoperative Recurrence of Heterotopic Ossification in Spinal Cord Injured Patients

S.L. STOVER, K.M.W. NIEMANN, and J.M. MILLER, III

ABSTRACT

Disodium etidronate (EHDP) was used in clinical trials to study its effectiveness in preventing the recurrence of mineralization after surgical removal of heterotopic ossification in spinal cord injury patients. Four patients with hip ankylosis had seven surgical wedge resections on a controlled, or double-blind, study. Wedge resections without EHDP treatment prevented recurrence as long as the drug was administered, up to 39 weeks. After discontinuation of EHDP therapy, recurrence was variable but was less than expected. EHDP is the first therapeutic agent that may delay and partially prevent postoperative heterotopic ossification recurrence.

Heterotopic ossification can be classified in three forms: (1) Neurogenic heterotopic ossification, which occurs with severe neurological conditions; (2) traumatic myositis ossificans, which occurs after direct muscle trauma or other types of tissue injury; and (3) myositis ossificans progressiva, a congenital form of unknown etiology.

Following spinal cord injury, neurogenic heterotopic ossification is reported to occur with an incidence ranging between 16% and 53% (Venier and Ditunno, 1971). Prospective roentgenogram surveys have shown that the hip joints are most frequently involved, followed by knees, shoulders, elbows, and spine (Stover et al., 1975). It appears most frequently one to four months after injury but has been detected as early as 19 days or, rarely, several years after injury (Hardy and Dickson, 1963).

Ossification may be minimal, identified only as coincidental roentgenographic findings, and may have no clinical effect in a majority of patients. With more extensive ossification, severe limitation of motion and ankylosis occurs in about 3% of all spinal cord injury patients (Wharton and Morgan, 1970). Therefore, in spinal cord injury patients who develop any degree of heterotopic ossification, ankylosis may develop in 8-20% secondary to the size of the mass or its relationship to a major joint (Hardy and Dickson, 1963; Wharton and Morgan, 1970). Restricted joint motion, or deformity, may cause further functional impairment and skin breakdown, limiting rehabilitation goals; therefore, the patient may benefit from operative intervention.

The early clinical appearance of larger masses of heterotopic ossification are characteristic of any soft tissue inflammatory reaction. The extremity, within a short period of time, becomes warm and swollen, and fever may occur. Within several days, a more localized, firmer mass is palpable within the area of edema with a gradual decrease in passive range of motion. An elevated serum alkaline phosphatase may be of value in differentiating early heterotopic ossification from other clinical entities (Nicholas, 1973). Early calcification often is not seen on routine roentgenograms for seven to ten days after clinical signs have appeared. Radioisotope bone scanning may be the only definitive method of early diagnosis (Rossier, 1975).

The etiology and pathogenesis are still unknown. An inflammatory-type reaction causes connective tissue edema and cell metaplasia with immature-appearing connective tissue, chondrogenesis, and osteogenesis (Rossier et al., 1973). Mineralization of the tissue involves an amorphous calcium phosphate phase, which is gradually replaced by enlarging hydroxyapatite crystals. This leads to the formation of lamellar cortico-spongiosal bone. The process usually arises at the periphery of muscle, gradually becoming distinct from the main muscle mass, but occasionally has atrophic muscle fibers incorporated within the bony mass. The joint space and capsule are preserved as bone forms in periarticular areas adjacent or more distal to the joint in predisposed areas.

MATERIAL AND METHODS

Disodium Etidronate

The diphosphonates are simple chemical compounds that are characterized by phosphorus-carbon-phosphorus bonds. They possess properties similar to the naturally occurring inorganic pyrophosphate, which is hypothesized to be a regulator of biological calcification, but disodium etidronate has the advantage of being absorbed intact from the gut. Unlike inorganic pyrophosphate, the diphosphonates are almost totally stable to chemical and enzymatic degradation.

One of the diphosphonates, disodium etidronate, disodium ethane-1-hydroxy-1,1-diphosphonate* (EHDP) is known to have profound effects on crystal behavior *in vitro* and in experimentally induced soft tissue calcification. *In vitro*, EHDP blocks the transformation of amorphous calcium phosphate into crystalline hydroxyapatite without inhibiting the formation of the initial or nucleation phase (Francis et al., 1969). In addition, EHDP also inhibits the dissolution of calcium phosphate crystals. *In vivo*, EHDP inhibits aortic and renal calcification in rats that have been given large doses of vitamin D_3 (Fleisch and Russell, 1969), calcium deposition in skin induced by dihydrotachysterol (Casen et al., 1972), and prevents periarticular calcification and articular changes that are associated with adjuvant arthritis in rats (Francis et al., 1964). In clinical studies, EHDP has been shown to partially prevent mineralization of heterotopic bone in myositis ossificans progressiva (Geho and Whiteside, 1973) and decreases bone turnover rate in disorders of increased bone resorption such as Pagets' disease (Altman et al., 1973; Khairi et al., 1974; Russell et al., 1974). EHDP may actually have important direct or indirect effects on bone cells (Russell et al., 1974). The only tissue where it accumulates to any appreciable extent is bone (Michael et al., 1972; Wellman et al., 1973). EHDP is not metabolized and is excreted in the urine unchanged.

Although the exact mechanism of action of EHDP is still unknown (Francis et al., 1973), the *in vitro* and experimental animal model data

---

*Investigational drug, Proctor and Gamble Company.

suggested that diphosphonates might be effective in preventing the recurrence of heterotopic ossification after surgical excision. Therefore, EHDP was selected for the clinical study.

Methods of Study

The first two patients served as their *own control* (history of previous surgical removal). Without drug treatment, wedge resections had been followed by postoperative recurrent (Table I). Repeat surgery was deferred until the alkaline phosphatase had returned to normal, ranging in time from 15 to 22 months. The patients were then started on EHDP, approximately 20 mg/kg/day for two weeks preoperatively and continued on the same dosage postoperatively for six, 30, and 39 weeks, respectively. Medication was administered orally one hour before breakfast with a glass of fruit juice.

Encouraging results from the above protocol led to the development of a double-blind study, which was used for the last two patients and is a continuing study. Patients entering the study were assigned randomly to a treatment group (placebo or EHDP). Medication was administered as above in a approximate dosage of 20 mg/kg/day, starting four weeks preoperatively and continuing twelve weeks postoperatively.

Surgery

Wedge resections of the central part of the heterotopic bone mass were performed allowing hip flexion to at least 90°, as recommended by Hardy and Dickson (1963). Each case had an anterior iliofemoral bar that restricted hip motion. These masses were all approached through a standard anterior iliofemoral incision.

After reflection of the sartorius, the bony mass was generally encountered within the layers of the rectus femoris muscles. An attempt was made to keep the dissection extraperiosteal as far as possible. In several instances, the femoral nerve or its major branches were encountered on the medial aspect of the mass but in no instance was the nerve or major branches of the nerve found to be incorporated or running through the ossified mass. The muscle masses could be rather easily reflected medially and laterally, and the resections were started at the midportion, centered over the inferior aspect of the hip joint, and heterotopic bone was removed with an osteotome, forming a "V". In all cases, the hip joint capsule could be easily identified, and the bony mass could be separated from its external surface. As soon as the hip joint was freed, motion was tested, and resection was continued, both proximally and distally until 90° of hip flexion could be obtained.

In several instances, the hip joint capsule was opened and the articular surfaces were found to be in good condition, although the articular cartilage was somewhat thin. In one instance, a subcapital fracture was produced by the maneuver of flexion of the hip during the removal process. After sufficient bone was removed to achieve the desired range of motion, a hemovac drain was inserted through the lateral thigh into the depths of the wound and laid on the anterior hip joint capsule. The muscle fascia was then reapproximated with absorbable sutures as was the subcutaneous tissue. Closure was by silk sutures. When the masses were large, considerable dead space remained. Routine dressings were applied with the hemovac drains in place. Blood loss at surgery was replaced immediately. All surgery except J.B. - eleven month (Table I), was performed by one of the authors (Kurt Nieman, M.D.) so that the operative technique would be standardized.

Preoperative and Postoperative Care

Careful attention was given preoperatively to the conditions of the skin and urinary tract. Surgery was delayed in patients with open pressure ulcers until healing was complete. Urine cultures and sensitivities were obtained at least one week preoperatively so that specific antibiotic treatment could be given before surgery to sterilize the urinary tract. This antibiotic treatment was continued approximately one week postoperatively. The hemovac drains remained in place until they ceased to function, usually two to four days, but in one patient, as long as eleven days. Following hemovac drain removal, if tension developed along the suture lines in the area of the resected dead space, sterile aspirations of accumulated fluid were performed. These aspirations were performed following five of the seven wedge resections, up to a total of eight times in one patient and generally were not necessary longer than four weeks postoperatively. Half of the skin sutures were removed seven to fourteen days postoperatively, and all sutures were removed 14 to 21 days postoperatively. Mild passive range of motion exercises were started about one week postoperatively with progression during the second week to more aggressive exercises and wheelchair sitting, dependent upon the condition of the incision and the amount of resected dead space fluid accumulation.

RESULTS

Four spinal cord injury patients had a total of seven wedge resections for heterotopic ossification in five hips. Two patients served as their *own control*. Two patients were on the double-blind study, one received EHDP and the other received placebo. The postoperative results, following three wedge resections in three untreated or placebo patients, are compared with those results from patients who were treated with EHDP (Table I).

Roentgenographic evidence of heterotopic ossification recurrence became evident less than three weeks postoperatively in all three non-treated and placebo patients, progressing on to recurrent ankylosis despite efforts to maintain range of motion. Serial roentgenograms are shown to document this progression in one patient (J.B., Figures 1A, 1B, 1C, and 1D). Four wedge resections were performed in three patients who were receiving EHDP therapy. There was no evidence of roentgenogram recurrence during EHDP treatment lasting six to 39 weeks. After withdrawal of EHDP, variable recurrence was again noted. In this patient, recurrence was much less after 30 weeks of EHDP treatment (trace recurrence), compared with six weeks of treatment (moderate recurrence) (Figures 1E, 1F, 1G, 1H, and 1I, 1K, 1L). Patient J.B., at 30 weeks of treatment, sustained a traumatic spiral fracture of the right femur, which led to the withdrawal of EHDP therapy. The fracture was stabilized with an intramedullary rod ten days after injury. Early massive callus formation appeared about the fracture site with only a trace recurrence of heterotopic ossification of the right hip (Fig. 1L). Another patient P.R. had no roentgenogram evidence of recurrence during 39 weeks of treatment, using approximately 20 mg/kg/day for 26 weeks and 10 mg/kg/day for the final 13 weeks. Complete drug withdrawal allowed moderate recurrence, while maintaining adequate functional range of motion. In this patient, EHDP again

Fig. 1A through 1L: A thirty-one year old man with T-6 paraplegia who developed heterotopic ossification, causing bilateral hip ankylosis.

Fig. 1A through 1D: Right hip control study (no drug treatment).

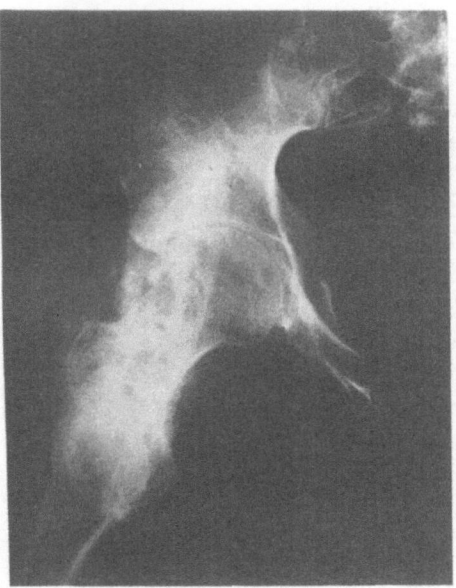

Fig. 1A. Preoperative.

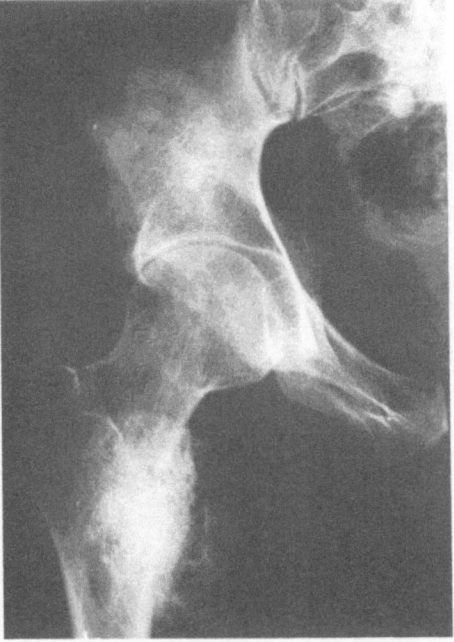

Fig. 1B. Three weeks postoperative with early recurrence of heterotopic ossification already evident.

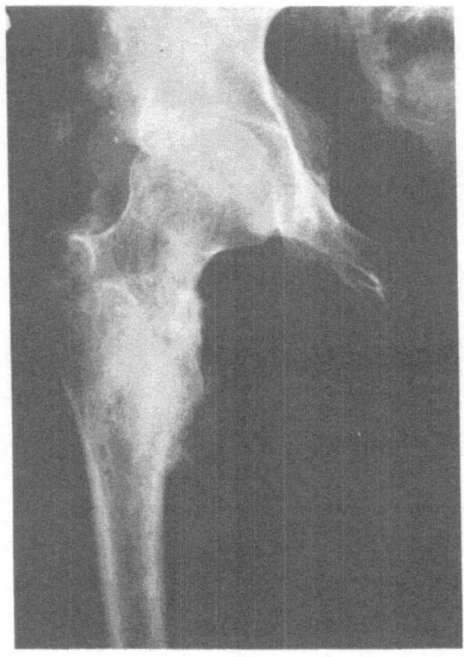

Fig. 1C. Five weeks postoperative showing gradual increase in extent and maturation of recurrent heterotopic ossification.

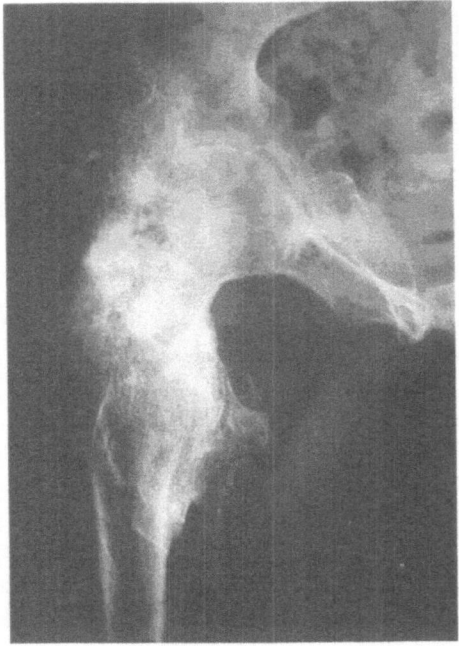

Fig. 1D. Twelve months postoperative with recurring ankylosis.

Fig. 1E through 1H: Left hip with EHDP treatment.

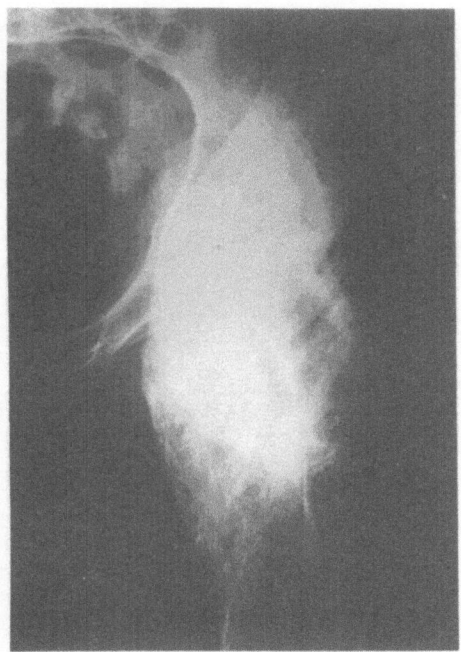

Fig. 1E: Preoperative.

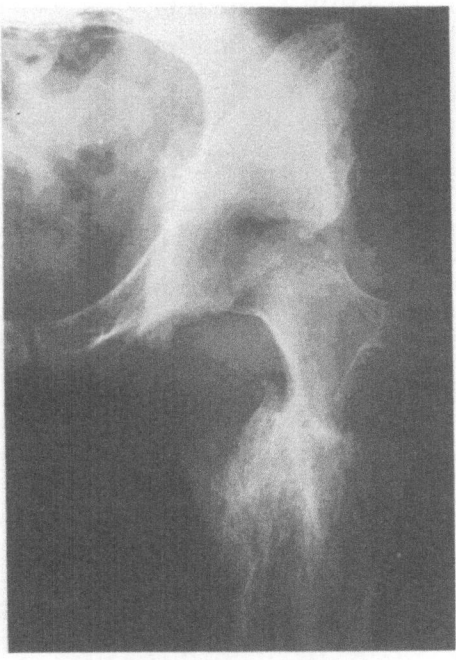

Fig. 1F: One week postoperative baseline study demonstrating extent of surgical wedge resection.

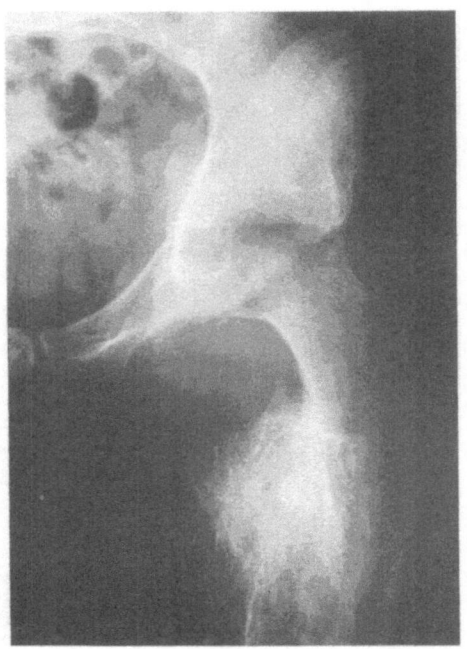

Fig. 1G: Six weeks postoperative with no evidence of recurrence during six weeks of EHDP treatment.

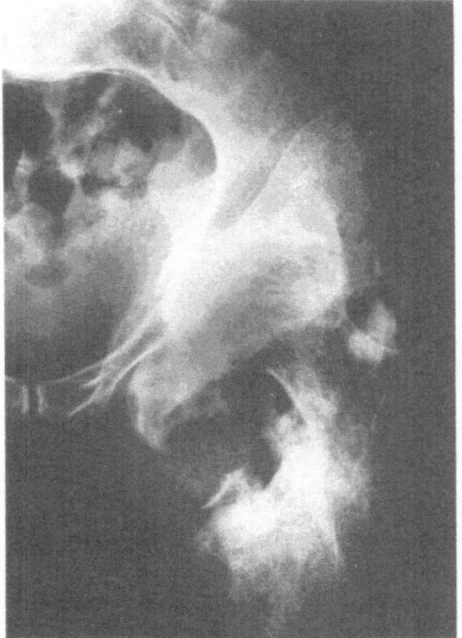

Fig. 1H: Twelve months postoperative with moderate recurrence following withdrawal of EHDP treatment after six weeks.

Fig. 1I through 1L: Right hip with EHDP treatment. Surgery repeated on right hip 36 months after right hip control study (Fig. 1A through 1D).

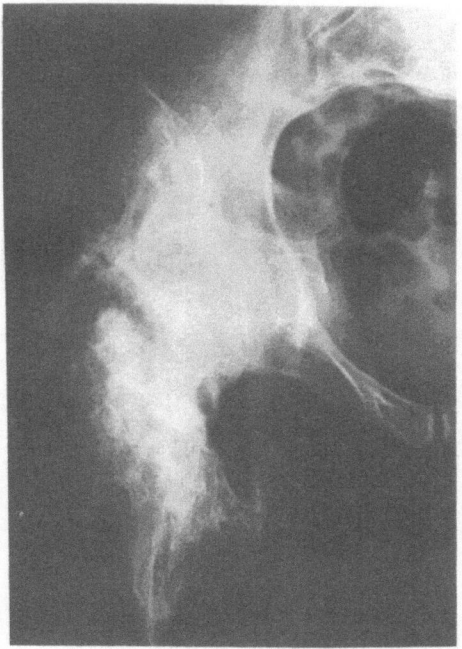

Fig. 1I: Preoperative.

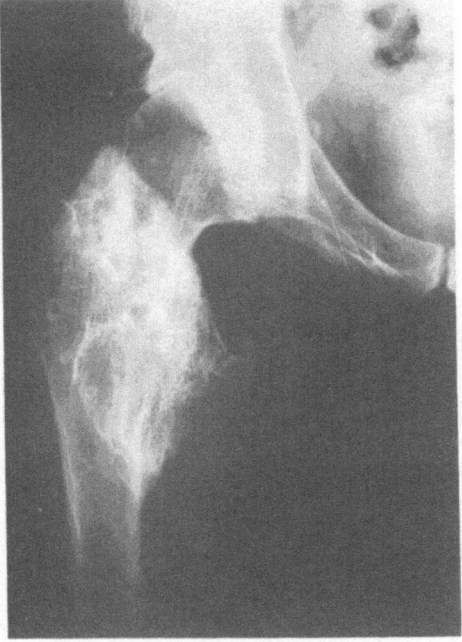

Fig. 1J: Three weeks postoperative baseline study demonstrating extent of surgical wedge resection.

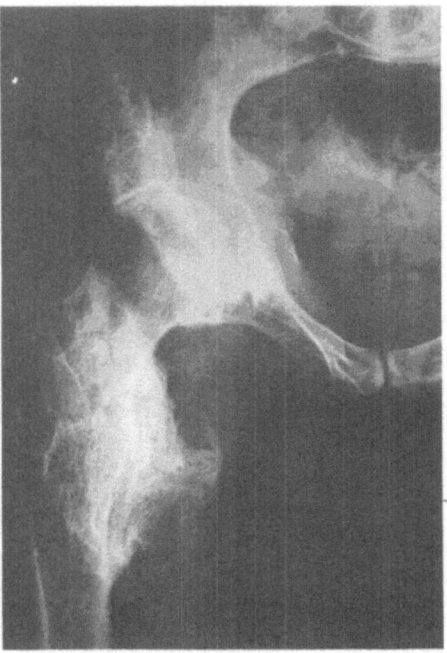

Fig. 1K: 30 weeks postoperative with no evidence of recurrence during thirty weeks of EHDP treatment.

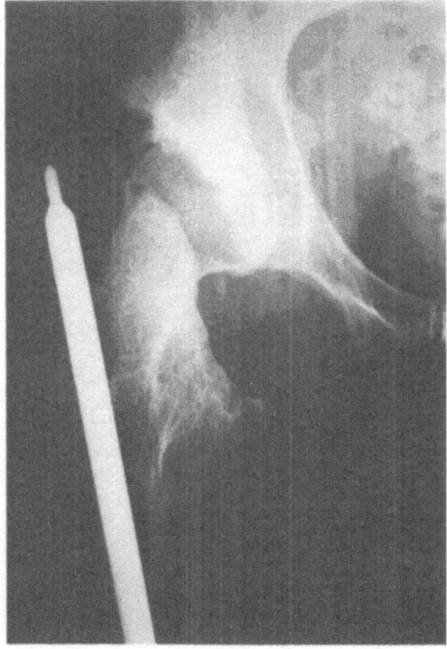

Fig. 1L: 13 months postoperative with traces of recurrence, following withdrawal of EHDP treatment after 30 weeks. A traumatic femoral fracture had no delay in fracture callus formation.

prevented recurrence during twelve weeks of treatment, but complete recurrence and ankylosis followed drug withdrawal. This occurred in spite of the fact that heterotopic ossification was thought to be mature and had been evident radiographically in the hips more than seven years prior to surgical removal.

Surgical complications were limited to: (1) hemorrhage postoperatively from the drain sites requiring blood transfusions in two patients; and (2) anticipated serosanguineous fluid accumulation in the dead space following drain removal.

Side effects of EHDP included only expected elevations of serum phosphate (Recker et al., 1973), which had no known clinical effects, and mild nausea and abdominal discomfort in one patient, which was controlled by giving EHDP in divided doses. Lack of other laboratory or clinical side effects in the parameters studied suggest EHDP's safety for clinical use as further documented in clinical trials with Paget's Disease (Altman et al., 1973; Khairi et al., 1974; Russell et al., 1974).

DISCUSSION

Reluctance toward surgical treatment of heterotopic ossification has been supported by reports of frequent recurrence, hematoma formation, and infections (Street, 1958; Armstrong-Ressy et al., 1959; Damanski, 1961). Limiting resection to a central wedge of bone permitting flexion of the hip to 90° (Hardy and Dickson, 1963) led to satisfactory results if timed properly. In their report on eight patients, recurrence remained a problem, but all patients gained increased functional abilities. Freehafer et al. (1966), stated surgical excision was useful but must be delayed until the bone was mature, well circumscribed, and trabeculated. In a retrospective review of 447 consecutive spinal cord injury patients by Wharton and Morgan (1970), 18 patients were found with ankylosis. Few of those had surgery, while most were obligated to prolonged periods of immobilization. They advocated successive, forceful manipulation causing fractures of the heterotopic bone, which, if followed by manipulation and range of motion exercises, led to fragmentation of the ossification. Ossification recurred but fragmenting allowed a satisfactory range of motion, possibly eliminating the need for surgery. This was not applicable, however, to patients with sensory sparing.

Determination of the maturity of heterotopic ossification remained a problem until parameters of maturation were further clarified by Rossier et al (1973). They suggested that an elevated alkaline phosphatase was a sign of pathological bone growth and, therefore, a contraindication to surgery; however, a normal alkalaine phosphatase was not proof of maturity. Serial bone scans with decreasing isotope uptake gradually approaching normal bone was the most reliable parameter of maturity. They reported surgical experience in seven patients who had eleven affected joints (nine hips and two elbows), with recurrence in two patients (one hip and one elbow). They felt the recurrences were due to operative intervention before they relied on bone scans to determine heterotopic bone maturity.

Bone scans may now assist in determining maturity of heterotopic ossification; however, time required to reach maturity remains variable and often prolonged. During this time, the spinal cord injury patient often remains severely impaired with his limitation of motion and probability of skin complications. Many authors suggest 18 months as a reasonable time to reach maturity while Rossier et al. (1973), state "mineralization after 30 months approaches that of normal, young adult bone." Nonetheless, in two of our patients (P.R. and R.K.), heterotopic ossification was present 59 months and 91 months, respectively, with complete recurrence and ankylosis postoperatively. A bone scan of R.K. continued to show increased uptake more than seven years after onset. EHDP prevented recurrence in R.K. while receiving medication, but recurrence was severe after drug withdrawal.

Our data show that EHDP prevents the appearance of roentgenogram evidence of heterotopic ossification postoperatively in all patients as long as the drug is administered. What occurs in the dead space and matrix during EHDP treatment is still unknown, but mineralization is delayed, and range of motion is maintained without difficulty. The maturity of heterotopic ossification does not seem to influence the affect of EHDP but may influence the extent of recurrence after drug withdrawal. Other factors which may influence the amount of recurrence after drug withdrawal are the length of treatment and the size of the initial mass.

Other early clinical studies with EHDP support these findings. Russell and Smith (1973) reported EHDP retarded mineralization of ectopic bone matrix after surgical removal in myositis ossificans progressiva. EHDP was also used six weeks preoperatively and six to 12 weeks postoperatively as a control study to prevent heterotopic ossification in patients having total hip replacements (1974). They demonstrated a reduction in radiologically visible ossification. Their final prevalence of ossification was not significantly different in 20 of 42 patients receiving EHDP, but the treated group had less pain postoperatively and ultimate function of the hip was better than in untreated patients.

There is now evidence that EHDP also prevents some of the formation of heterotopic ossification following spinal cord injury when administered prophylactically during the first six months after injury (Stover et al.). These findings may be valuable in further studies of the etiology and pathogenesis of heterotopic ossification.

CONCLUSION

Surgical wedge resections of heterotopic ossification were performed in seven ankylosed hips of four spinal cord injury patients. EHDP delayed postoperative recurrence, with maintenance of good range of motion as long as the drug was administered, up to 39 weeks. Surgery without EHDP led to radiological evidence of recurrence within three weeks. Following discontinuation of EHDP therapy, recurrence was variable with some evidence that it was inversely proportional to the size of the initial bone mass and the length of therapy. EHDP is the first therapeutic agent with definite effectiveness in delaying and partially preventing recurrent postoperative heterotopic ossification. Longer treatment periods may further decrease the extent of recurrence, allowing these patients improved joint mobility and the achievement of better functional goals.

ACKNOWLEDGEMENTS

The disodium etidronate (EHDP) used in this investigation was supplied by Procter & Gamble Company, Cincinnati, Ohio, United States of America.

This research project was supported in part by Grant No. 16-P-56807/4-9 from the Department of Health, Education, and Welfare, Rehabilitation Services Administration.

Altman, R.D., Johnston, C.C., Khairi, M.R.A., Wellman, H.N., Serafini, A.N. and Sankey, R.R. Influence of Disodium Etidronate on Clinical and Laboratory Manifestations of Paget's Disease of Bone (Osteitis Deformans). *New Eng. J. Med.* 289:1379-1384 (1973).

Armstrong-Ressy, C.T., Weiss, A.A., and Ebel, A. Results of Surgical Treatment of Extraosseous Ossification in Paraplegia. *N.Y. St. J. Med.* 59:2548-2553 (1959).

Bijvoet, O.L.M., Nollen, A.J.G., Slooff, J.J.H., and Feith, R. Effect of diphosphonate on Para-articular Ossification After Total Hip Replacement. *Acta. Orthop. Scand.* 45:926-934 (1974).

Casey, P.A., Casey, G., Fleisch, H., and Russell, R.G.G. The Effect of Polyphloretin Phosphate, Polyoestradiol Phosphate, a Diphosphonate and a Polyphosphate on Calcification Induced by Dihydrotachysterol in Skin, Aorta and Kidney of Rats. *Experientia* 28:137-138 (1972).

Damanski, M. Heterotopic Ossification in Paraplegia: A Clinical Study. *J. Bone and Joint Surg.* 43-B:286-299 (1961).

Fleisch, H.A., Russell, R.G.G., Bisaz, S., Mulhaubauer, R.C., and Williams, D.A. The Inhibitory Effect of Phosphonates on the Formation of Calcium Phosphate Crystals *In Vitro* and on Aortic and Kidney Calcification *In Vivo*. *Eur. J. Clin. Invest.* 1:12-18 (1970).

Francis, M.D., Russell, R.G.G., and Fleisch, H. Diphosphonates Inhibit Formation of Calcium Phosphate Crystals *In Vitro* and Pathological Calcification *In Vivo*. *Science* 165:1264-1266 (1969).

Francis, M.D. Flora, L., and King, W.R. The Effects of Disodium Ethane-1-Hydroxy-1,1-Diphosphonate on Adjuvant Induced Arthritis in Rats. *Calci. Tissue Res.* 9:109 (1972).

Francis, M.D., Briner, W.W., and Gray, J.A. Chemical Agents in the Control of Calcification Processes in Biological System. In *Hard Tissue Growth, Repair and Remineralization*, p. 57-90, Associated Scientific Publishers, Amsterdam (1973).

Freehafer, A.A., Yurick, R., and Mast, W.A. Para-articular Ossification in Spinal Cord Injury. *Med. Serv. J. Can.* 22:471-477 (1966).

Geho, W.B., and Whiteside, J.A. Experience with Disodium Etidronate in Diseases of Ectopic Calcification. *In Clinical Aspects of Metabolic Bone Disease*, p. 506, Excerpta Medica, Amsterdam (1973).

Hardy, A.G., and Dickson, J.W. Pathological Ossification in Traumatic Paraplegia. *J. Bone and Joint Surg.* 45-B:76-87 (1963).

Khairi, M.R.A., Johnston, Jr., C.C., Altman, R.D., Wellman, H.N., Serafini, A.N., and Sankey, R.R. Treatment of Paget Disease of Bone (Osteitis Deformans). *J. Am. Med. Ass.* 230:562-567 (1974).

Michael, W.R., King, W.R., and Wakim, J.M. Metabolism of Disodium Ethane-1-Hydroxy-1,1-Diphosphonate (Disodium Etidronate) in the Rat, Rabbit, Dog, and Monkey. *Toxic. Appl. Pharmac.* 21:503-515 (1972).

Nicholas, J.J. Ectopic Bone Formation in Patients with Spinal Cord Injury. *Arch. Phys. Med. Rehabil.* 54:354-359 (1973).

Recker, R.R., Hassing, G.S., Lau, J.R. et al. The Hyperphosphatemic Effect of Disodium Ethane-1-Hydroxy-1,1-Diphosphonate (EHDP^{TM}): Renal Handling of Phosphorus and the Renal Response to Parathyroid Hormone. *J. Lab Clin. Med.* 81:258-266 (1973).

Rossier, A.B. *Personal Communication* (1975).

Rossier, A.B., Bussat, P., Infante, F. et al. Current Facts on Para-osteo-arthropathy (POA). *Paraplegia* 11:36-78 (1973).

Russell, R.G., and Smith, R. Diphosphonates: Experimental and Clinical Aspects. *J. Bone and Joint Surg.* 55-B:66-86 (1973).

Russell, R.G.G., and Fleisch, H. Pyrophosphate and Diphosphonates in Skeletal Metabolism, Physiological, Clinical and Therapeutic Aspect. *Clinical Orthopaedics 108:*241-263 (1975).

Russell, R.G.G., Smith, R., Preston, C., Walton, R.J., and Woods, C.G. Diphosphonates in Paget's Disease. *The Lancet 1:*894-898 (1974).

Stover, S.L., Hahn, H.R., and Miller, J.M., III. Disodium Etidronate in the Prevention of Heterotopic Ossification Following Spinal Cord Injury. Accepted for publication in *Paraplegia.*

Stover, S.L., Hataway, C.J., and Zeiger, H.E. Heterotopic Ossification in Spinal Cord Injured Patients. *Arch. Phys. Med. Rehabil. 56:* 199-204 (1975).

Street, D.M. Para-articular Bone Formation. *Proc. A. Clin. Paraplegia Conf. 7:*31 (1958).

Venier, L.H., and Ditunno, J.F., Jr. Heterotopic Ossification in the Paraplegic Patient. *Arch. Phys. Med. Rehabil. 52:*475-479 (1971).

Wellman, H.N., Anger, R.T., Browne, A., Tofe, A., Francis, D., Klairi, R., and Johnson, C. Evaluation of Bone Malignancy with 99mTc-Sn-EHDP Compared with Na18F. *J. Nucl. Med. 14:*464-465 (1973).

Wharton, G.W., and Morgan, T.H. Ankylosis in the Paralyzed Patient. *J. Bone and Joint Surg. 52-A, 1:*105-112 (1970).

14

Reversal by Thyrocalcitonin of Depressed Calcium, Magnesium, and Phosphorus Balances in Paraplegic Rats

N.E. NAFTCHI, A.T. VIAU, and E.W. LOWMAN

INTRODUCTION

Bone is the storehouse of calcium, magnesium, phosphorus, and a number of other ions. This highly vascular tissue is in a dynamic state of continuous renewal. Spinal cord injury results in a disruption of this dynamic bone remodelling; that is, injury to the spinal cord is followed by a dysfunction of homeostatic mechanism, involving the metabolism of bone, cartilage, and mineral ions. The associated complications, such as hypercalciuria, bone resorption, bone pain, and renal calculi, occur early during the acute phase of the injury.

Thyrocalcitonin, a thyroid hormone, usually counteracts the actions of parathormone, both hormones acting to keep plasma calcium concentration at a constant level. It was felt, therefore, that during the acute phase, treatment with thyrocalcitonin might arrest the process of osteoporosis.

In the rat, spinal cord injury results in hypercalciuria and depressed calcium balance (Naftchi et al., 1972). The purpose of the present study was to investigate whether thyrocalcitonin would improve calcium, magnesium, and phosphorus balances in the rat, following spinal cord transection.

MATERIALS AND METHODS

Twenty male Wistar-Lewis rats, weighing 290-300 gm, were made paraplegic by transecting the spinal cord at the level of the thoracic fifth (T5) vertebra. Ten sham-operated rats served as controls. The animals were placed in individual metabolic cages and were fed ad libitum a semipurified 18% casein diet (Allison et al., 1964). Bladders of the paraplegic rats were expressed manually, three to four times daily. Food consumption was recorded, and urine and feces specimens were collected daily in toto.

One group of the paraplegic rats was injected subcutaneously twice a day with two units (Medical Research Council, MRC) of salmon thyrocalcitonin (Armour Pharmaceutical Company) that was dissolved in 16% gelatin vehicle. A second group of paraplegic rats, as well as the sham-operated controls, were injected with the vehicle. Because a dose of 0.1 MRC unit of thyrocalcitonin proved to be ineffective in preventing osteoporosis after spinal cord injury in the rat (Braddon et al., 1973), a dose of 4 MRC units per animal (10 MRC units/kg) was used in this study.   Rats treated with thyrocalcitonin were sacrificed three hours after the last administration of the drug; all the animals were sacrificed on day 12 of the experiment.

Calcium and magnesium concentrations were determined by atomic absorption spectrophotometry in diluted urine and feces specimens, which were first dried, ashed, and dissolved in concentrated nitric acid.   Samples of the diet were also analyzed.   Phosphorus determinations were performed in samples of urine, feces, and diet, using the method of Fiske and Subbarow (1925).   Total serum calcium was determined by atomic absorption spectrophotometry, and serum ionized calcium was measured potentiometrically, using an Orion flow-through electrode. Calcium, magnesium, and phosphorus balances were calculated from the differences between the dietary intake and the sum of fecal and urinary excretion of each compound.   Results are expressed as mean ± standard error.   Significance was determined by using the Student 't' test.

RESULTS

Calcium Balance

Paraplegia in the rat resulted in marked hypercalciuria, which lasted from day five to day 10 after the spinal cord transection.   Administration of 4 MRC units of thyrocalcitonin to spinal rats further increased the urinary excretion of calcium (Figure 1).   Fecal excretion of calcium was significantly greater in paraplegic rats than in sham-operated controls starting five to eight days after the onset of the injury.

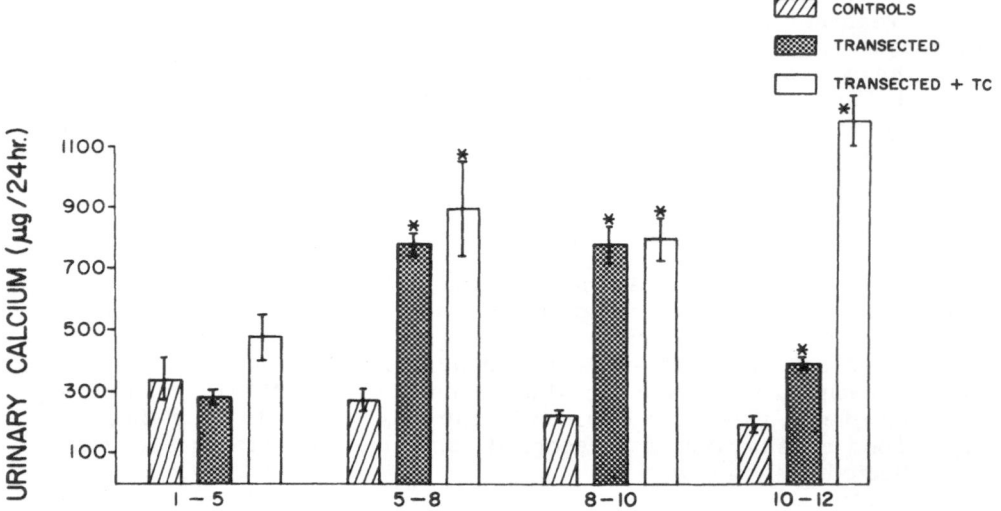

Fig. 1. Urinary excretion of calcium in controls, transected, and thyro-calcitonin-treated transected rats: the animals were made paraplegic by transecting the spinal cord at the T5 level.   Each bar represents mean ± SEM μg of urinary calcium per 24 hours in 10 rats.   TC = salmon thyrocalcitonin, 4 MRC units per rat daily.   Note the hypercalciuria in untreated paraplegic and thyrocalcitonin-treated rats .
($*$ = p<0.01)

Reprinted by permission of Archives of Physical Medicine and Rehabilitation 61:576. 1980

Thyrocalcitonin, however, decreased fecal excretion of calcium to one half of control levels from one to eight days after transection and to control levels thereafter (Figure 2). Although thyrocalcitonin increased the urinary excretion of calcium, it decreased the fecal excretion of this cation to a much greater degree. As a result, calcium balance which was significantly depressed starting five to eight days after spinal cord transection was completely restored in animals treated with thyrocalcitonin (Table I).

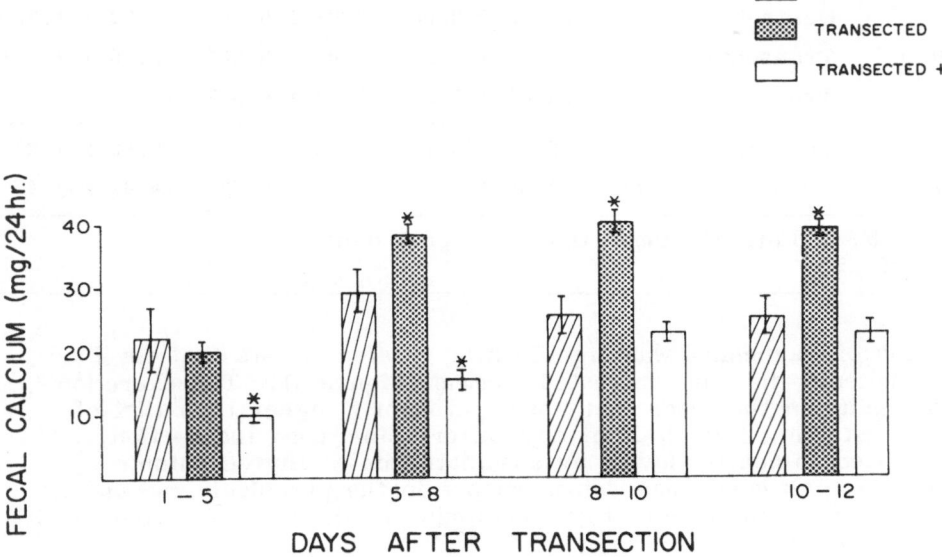

Fig. 2. Fecal excretion of calcium in controls, transected, and thyrocalcitonin-treated transected rats: the animals were made paraplegic by transecting the spinal cord at the T5 level. Each bar represents mean ± SEM μg of fecal calcium per 24 hours in 10 rats. TC = salmon thyrocalcitonin, 4 MRC units per rat daily. Thyrocalcitonin reduced fecal losses of calcium in paraplegic rats.
(* = p<0.01)

Reprinted by permission of Archives of Physical Medicine and Rehabilitation 51: 576. 1980

Magnesium Balance

In paraplegic rats, five to ten days after spinal cord lesion, urinary excretion of magnesium was sharply higher than that of sham-operated controls and was not reduced after administration of thyrocalcitonin. On the contrary, 10 to 12 days after spinal cord transection, urinary

TABLE I

Effect of Thyrocalcitonin on Calcium, Magnesium,
and Phosphorus Balance in The Spinal Rat

Days After Transection	Group	Balance (mg/24 hours)		
		Calcium	Magnesium	Phosphorus
	Control	17.17 ± 1.03	1.12 ± 0.05	-1.80 ± 1.10
1- 5	Transected	17.39 ± 1.72	1.46 ± 0.20	-1.54 ± 1.09
	Transected + TC	19.91 ± 1.23	0.97 ± 0.11	-4.74 ± 1.22*
	Control	14.39 ± 2.05	1.71 ± 0.23	-3.48 ± 1.36
5- 8	Transected	10.35 ± 1.29*	0.43 ± 0.27*	-4.38 ± 1.14
	Transected + TC	25.18 ± 0.66*	1.55 ± 0.15	+3.98 ± 1.53*
	Control	26.45 ± 2.90	3.01 ± 0.29	+6.02 ± 1.69
8-10	Transected	18.03 ± 1.23*	1.01 ± 0.26*	-3.45 ± 1.24*
	Transected + TC	24.00 ± 1.23	1.71 ± 0.54*	+3.01 ± 1.10
	Control	26.71 ± 2.70	3.10 ± 0.33	+6.45 ± 1.81
10-12	Transected + TC	31.34 ± 2.48	2.10 ± 0.27	+4.42 ± 1.46

TC = 4 MRC units of salmon thyrocalcitonin daily
*P   <0.05

excretion of magnesium was significantly greater in rats that received thyrocalcitonin than in nontreated animals (Figure 3). The excretion of magnesium in the feces that was significantly higher than that of controls, starting five to eight days after spinal cord transection, was reduced to control levels by administration of thyrocalcitonin (Figure 4). Although magnesium balance in the paraplegic rat was improved by treatment with thyrocalcitonin, it did not reach control levels (Table I).

Phosphorus Balance

Neither spinal cord transection nor administration of thyrocalcitonin to paraplegic rats altered significantly the urinary excretion of phosphorus (Figure 5). Fecal excretion of phosphorus was significantly lower one to five days after spinal cord lesion and was sharply higher eight to twelve days after, compared with control levels. Thyrocalcitonin administration normalized the fecal phosphorus content (Figure 6). Phosphorus balance was negative in both sham-operated controls and transected animals from one to eight days after the operation, after which it became positive in sham-operated animals but remained negative in spinal cord transected animals. Administration of thyrocalcitonin restored positive phosophorus balance five to eight days after spinal cord lesion (Table I).

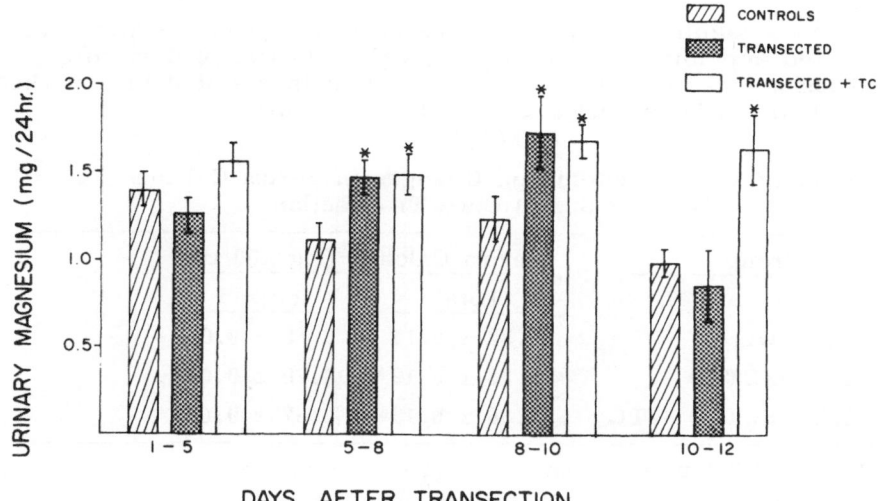

Fig. 3. Urinary excretion of magnesium in controls, transected, and thyrocalcitonin-treated transected rats: the animals were made paraplegic by transecting the spinal cord at the T5 level. Each bar represents mean ± SEM μg of urinary magnesium per 24 hours in 10 rats. TC = salmon thyrocalcitonin, 4 MRC units per rat daily. (* = p<0.01)

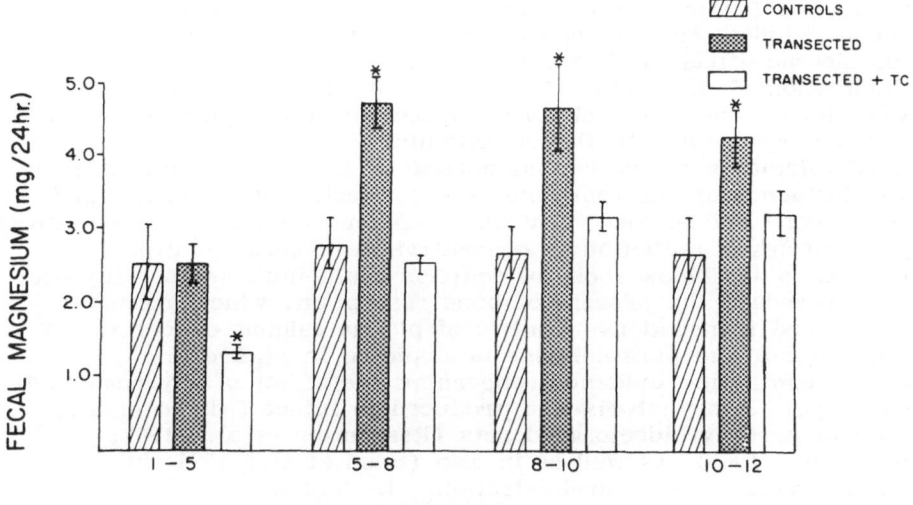

Fig. 4. Fecal excretion of magnesium in controls, transected, and thyrocalcitonin-treated transected rats: the animals were made paraplegic by transecting the spinal cord at the T5 level. Each bar represents mean ± SEM μg of fecal magnesium per 24 hours in 10 rats. TC = 4 MRC units per rat daily. Administration of thyrocalcitonin decreased fecal losses of magnesium in paraplegic rats. (* = p<0.01)

Serum Ionized and Total Calcium

There was a significant hypercalcemia as reflected in elevated levels of both ionized and total calcium in paraplegic rats twelve days after the spinal lesion.   Administration of thyrocalcitonin resulted in a marked lowering of both variables below control levels (Table II).

TABLE II

Effect of Thyrocalcitonin on Changes in Serum Calcium Following Spinal Cord Transection

Group	Serum Calcium (mg/100 ml)	
	Total	Ionized
CONTROLS	9.82 ± 0.18	3.88 ± 0.06
TRANSECTED	11.33 ± 0.19*	4.20 ± 0.04*
TRANSECTED + TC	8.96 ± 0.13*	2.87 ± 0.08*

TC + 4 MRC units of salmon thyrocalcitonin daily
*$p < 0.05$

DISCUSSION

In previous reports, administration of thyrocalcitonin resulted in a decrease in serum calcium levels in patients with Paget's disease Bijvoet et al., 1968; Bell et al., 1970; Gershberg et al., 1973) thyrotoxicosis (Bijvoet et al., 1968), and in women suffering from senile osteoporosis (Caniggia et al., 1970; Jowsey et al., 1971).   Similarly, thyrocalcitonin produced hypocalcemia in the monkey (Bell et al., 1966), in the intact rat (Milhaud and Moukhtar 1966; Alfred et al., 1970; Hirsch et al., 1964), and in nephreceomized rats (Wase et al., 1966). The hypocalcemic effect of thyrocalcitonin was maximal three hours after its administration (Bell, 1966).   Our data show that total serum calcium, which was elevated after spinal cord transection, was significantly reduced after treatment with thyrocalcitonin.

Ionized calcium in serum is that portion of total serum calcium that under the influence of parathormone and thyrocalcitonin is exchanged between the bone and extracellular fluid.   After 12 days of thyrocalcitonin therapy, the marked reduction in concentration of serum ionized calcium to levels far below those of controls could indicate that thyrocalcitonin has reversed the process of bone resorption, which started after spinal cord transection.   Control of plasma calcium concentration by thyrocalcitonin and parathormone is depicted in Figure 7.

There is conflicting evidence concerning the effect of thyrocalcitonin on the kidneys.   Phosphaturia was produced in intact (Alfred et al., 1970), and in parathyroidectomized rats (Rasmussen et al., 1967; Robinson et al., 1966), as well as in man (Hass et al., 1971, in response to thyrocalcitonin administration.   In contrast, an infusion of thyrocalcitonin resulted in a decreased urinary excretion of phosphate rats (Pechet et al., 1967) and an unchanged renal clearance of phosphate in dogs (Clark and Kenny, 1969).   Moreover, injections of thyrocalcitonin inhibited the phosphaturic response to parathyroid hormone in rats (Pechet et al., 1967).   Prolonged treatment with thyrocalcitonin, in this study, did not affect the urinary excretion of phosphorus in the paraplegic rats.   Ziegler et al. (1967) noted that the phosphaturic effect was more pronounced when crude, rather than more purified,

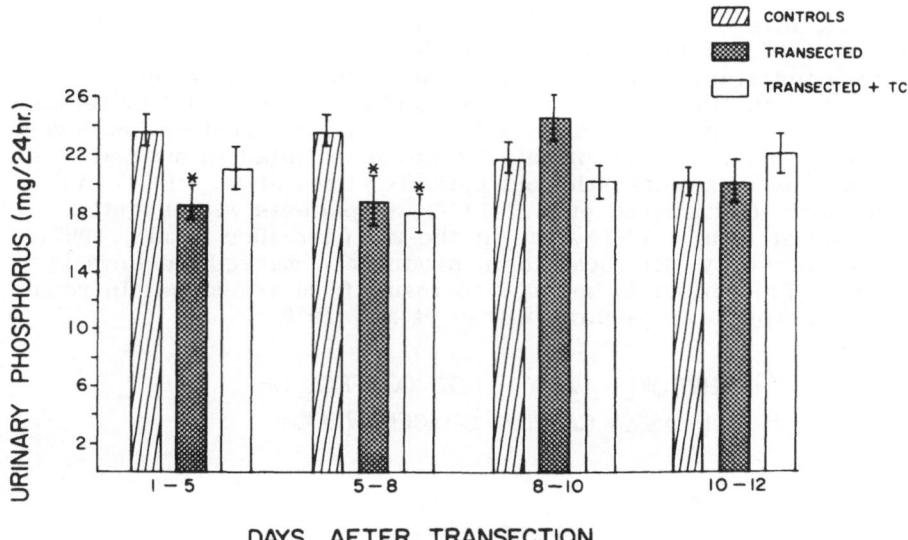

Fig. 5. Urinary excretion of phosphorus in controls, transected, and thyrocalcitonin-treated transected rats: the animals were made paraplegic by transecting the spinal cord at the T_5 level. Each bar represents mean ± SEM μg of urinary phosphorus per 24 hours in 10 rats. TC = salmon thyrocalcitonin, 4 MRC units per rat daily. (* = p<0.01)*

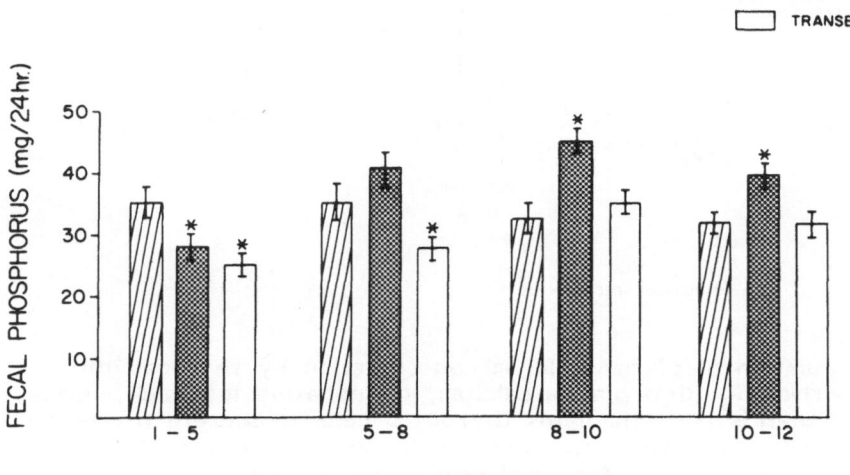

Fig. 6. Fecal excretion of phosphorus in controls, transected, and thyrocalcitonin-treated transected rats: the animals were made paraplegic by transecting the spinal cord at the T_5 level. Each bar represents mean ± SEM μg of fecal phosphorus per 24 hours in 10 rats. TC = salmon thyrocalcitonin, 4 MRC units per rat daily. Note that thyrocalcitonin significantly reduced fecal losses of phosphorus in paraplegic rats. (* = p<0.01)*

Reprinted by permission of Archives of Physical Medicine and Rehabilitation 51:578. 1980

preparations of thyrocalcitonin were administered to rats.   The lack of
phosphaturic effect in our experimental animals is probably due to
administration of purified salmon thyrocalcitonin.

In previous studies, thyrocalcitonin was found to have no
calciuric effect in the rat (Milhaud and Moukhtar, 1966) and in senile
human patients (Caniggia et al., 1970).   Other investigators, however,
reported that administration of thyrocalcitonin resulted in marked
calcium diuresis in hypoparathyroid patients (Hass et al., 1971), in
normal subjects (Rasmussen et al., 1967), in patients with Paget's
disease (Bijvoet et al., 1968), and in the rat (Ardaillou et al., 1967).
In the present study, thyrocalcitonin produced a marked calciuria in
spinal rats.   This effect is believed to result from a decrease in renal
tubular reabsorption of calcium (Alfred et al., 1970).

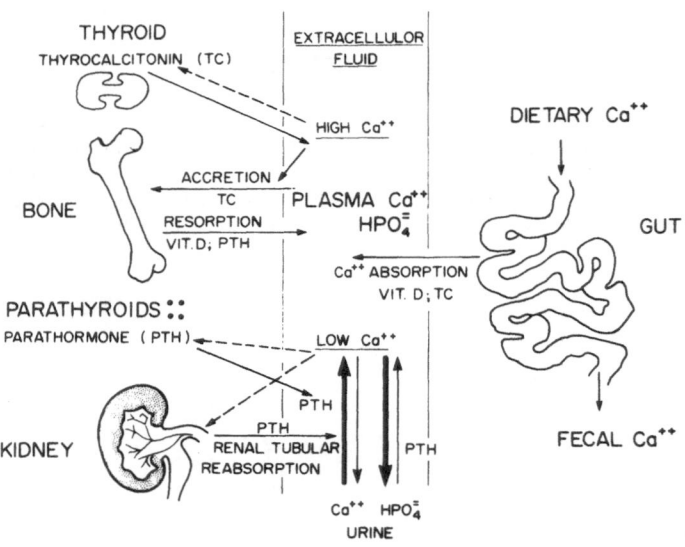

THYROID — PARATHYROID CONTROL OF
PLASMA CALCIUM CONCENTRATION

Fig. 7. Regulation of plasma calcium concentration by thyrocalcitonin
and parathormone. High plasma calcium, by negative feedback, inhibits
parathyroid glands and stimulates thyroid C cells to secrete thyrocalcitonin. The latter hormone suppresses osteolysis and causes bone
accretion, thus controlling hypercalcemia. By contrast, low plasma
calcium stimulates parathyroid glands to secrete parathormone which
increases osteolysis in order to control hypocalcemia and maintain
normal plasma calcium concentrations.
Reprinted by Permission of Archives of Physical Medicine and Rehabilitation 51:578. 1980

Urinary excretion of magnesium was increased after thyrocalcitonin
administration in hypoparathyroid patients (Hass et al., 1971), but
it was decreased in rats three and five hours after a single dose of
thyrocalcitonin (Ardaillou et al., 1967).   Results of the present study

indicate that daily injections of this hormone did not affect the kidney clearance of magnesium during the first nine days of its administration. On days 10 to 12, however, urinary excretion of magnesium was markedly elevated in thyrocalcitonin-treated animals.

Previous reports have shown that thyrocalcitonin had no effect on intestinal absorption of calcium when placed in the stomach of the rat (Wase et al., 1966), during acute perfusion in the rat (Krawitt, 1967), and in thyroparathyroidectomized rats (Milhaud and Moukhtar, 1966). It had a marked influence, however, in reducing endogenous calcium excretion in this animal (Milhaud and Moukhtar, 1966; Wase et al., 1966). It was also shown to improve calcium balance in the rat (Milhaud and Moukhtar, 1966; Wase et al., 1966; Naftchi et al., 1973), in senile women (Caniggia et al., 1970), and calcium and phosphorus balances in patients with Paget's disease (Bell et al., 1970). In our study of paraplegic rats, administration of thyrocalcitonin resulted in a marked improvement of calcium, phosphorus and magnesium balances, which were depressed after spinal cord transection. This improvement was mainly due to a reduction in fecal losses.

In preliminary studies (Viau et al., 1978) we reported that bone demineralization in spinal cord injured man, as evidenced by excessive excretion of urinary calcium and hydroxyproline, started soon after the spinal cord lesion. In the present study, thyrocalcitonin markedly improved mineral balances in paraplegic rats. It may, therefore, be advantageous to treat spinal cord injured subjects with this hormone early after onset of injury in order to prevent bone resorption, which eventually leads to osteoporosis.

Parathormone, thyrocalcitonin, and calcium and phosphate ions affect the rate of conversion of 25-hydroxycholecalciferol (25-HCC) to 1,25-dihydroxycholecalciferol (1,25-HCC). Thyrocalcitonin produces hypophosphatemia and hypocalcemia (Table II). Furthermore, the low levels of calcium and phosphate stimulate, and their high levels suppress renal hydroxylation of 25-HCC to 1,25-HCC. Since the effect of low calcium and not that of phosphorus is dependent on normal function of parathyroid glands, the production of hypophosphatemia by thyrocalcitonin may be an important factor in the final hydroxylation step of vitamin D_3. The action of the latter on increasing the rate of calcium ion absorption is well established.

Our findings demonstrated that long-term adequate administration of thyrocalcitonin caused increased absorption of calcium through the gut. The mechanism of this action may be explained as follows: (1) thyrocalcitonin has a direct effect on absorption of calcium through the gastrointestinal tract; (2) by lowering the plasma calcium level, thyrocalcitonin stimulates parathormone secretion in amounts that enhance calcium absorption through the gastrointestinal tract; the normalization of mineral balance is mainly through the reduction of fecal losses; (3) its enhancement of renal conversion of 25-HCC to 1,25-HCC may be the direct cause of increased calcium absorption; (4) it may act synergistically with 1,25-HCC; (5) thyrocalcitonin affects the solubility product of calcium and phosphate ions in the gastrointestinal tract. As a result calcium phosphate complexes that are not absorbed through the gastrointestinal tract are not formed, thus leaving more of the divalent cation in the free form; and, finally, (6) a combination of several of the above effects.

The actions of thyrocalcitonin and parathormone in calcium homeostasis are illustrated in Figure 7.

REFERENCES

Aldred, J.P., Kleszynski, R.R., Bastian, J.W. Effects of acute
administration of procine and salmon calcitonin on urine electrolyte
excretion in rats. *Proc. Soc. Exp. Biol. Med. 134:*1175-1180 (1970).

Allison, J.B., Wannemacher, R.W., Jr., Banks, W.L., Jr., and Wunner,
W.H. The magnitude and significance of the protein reserves in
rats fed at various levels of nitrogen. *J. Nutrit. 84:*383-388 (1964).

Ardaillou, R., Vaugnat, P., Milhaud, G., and Richet, G. Effets de
la thyrocalcitonine sur l'excretion renale du phosphore, du calcium
et des ions H+ chez l'homme normal. *J. Physiol. (Paris) 59:* Suppl.
1, 204 (1967).

Bell, N.H., Avery, S., and Johnston, C.C., Jr. Effects of calcitonin
in Paget's disease and polyostatic fibrous dysplasia. *J. Clin.
Endocrinol. Metab. 31:*283-290 (1970).

Bell, N.H., Varrett, R.J., and Patterson, R. Effects of procine
thyrocalcitonin on serum calcium, phosphorus and magnesium in the
monkey and man. *Proc. Soc. Exp. Biol. Med. 123:*114-118 (1966).

Bijvoet, O.L.M., Van Der Sluys Veer, J., and Jansen, A.P. Effects
of calcitonin on patients with Paget's disease, thyrotoxicosis or
hypercalcemia. *The Lancet 1:*876-881 (1968).

Braddom, R.I., Erickson, R., and Johnson, E.W. Ineffectiveness of
calcitonin on osteoporesis in paraplegic rats. *Arch. Phys. Med.
Rehab. 54:*170-174 (1973).

Caniggia, A., Gennari, C., Bencini, M., Cesari, L., and Borrello, G.
Calcium metabolism and ^{45}calcium kinetics before and after long-term
thyrocalcitonin treatment in senile osteoporosis. *Clin. Sci. 38:*397-
407 (1970).

Clark, J.D., and Kenny, A.D. Hog thyrocalcitonin in the dog: urinary
calcium phosphorus, magnesium and sodium responses. *Endocrinology
84:*1199-1205 (1969).

Fiske, C.Hl, and Subbarow, Y. The colorimetric determination of
phosphorus. *J. Biol. Chem. 66:*375-400 (1925).

Gershberg, H., Girgis, M., Goldberg, L., Duga, J., and St. Paul, H.
The acute response to calcitonin in Paget's disease: its relationship
to the serum alkaline phosphatase level and the effect of phosphate
treatment. *J. Clin. Endocrinol. Metab. 36:*691-696 (1973).

Hass, H.G., Dambacher, M.A., Guneaga, J., and Lauffenburger, T.
Renal effects of calcitonin and parathyroid extract in man. Studies
in hypothyroidism. *J. Clin. Invest. 50:*2689-2702 (1971).

Hirsch, P.F., Voelkel, E.F., and Munson, P.L. Thyrocalcitonin:
hypocalcemic hypophosphatemic principle of the thyroid gland.
*Science 146:*412-413 (1964).

Jowsey, J., Riggs, P.L., Goldsmith, R.S., Kelly, PlJ., and Arnaud,
C.D. Effects of prolonged administration of procine calcitonin in
postmenopausal osteoporosis. *J. Clin. Endocrinol. Metab. 33:*752-
758 (1971).

Krawitt, E.L. Effect of thyrocalcitonin on duodenal calcium transport.
*Proc. Soc. Exp. Biol. Med. 125:*1084-1086 (1967).

Milhaud, G., and Moukhtar, M.S. Thyrocalcitonin: effects of calcium
kinetics in the rat. *Proc. Soc. Exp. Biol. Med. 123:*207-209 (1966).

Milhaud, G., Moukhtar, M.S., Cherian, G., and Perault, A.M. Effet
de l'administration de thyrocalcitonine sur les principaux parametres
due metabolisme du calcium du rat normal et du rat thyropara-
thyroidectomise. *C.R. Acad. Sci. Paris. Series D 262:*511-514
(1966).

Naftchi, N.E., Viau, A.T., Demeny, M., Sell, G.H., and Lowman, E.W.

Calcium and magnesium metabolism in spinal man and rat. *Physiologist* *15:*224 (1972).

Naftchi, N.E., Viau, A.T., Sell, G.H., and Lowman, E.W. Effect of thyrocalcitonin on calcium and magnesium metabolism in the spinal rat. *Physiologist 16:*405 (1973).

Pechet, M.M., Boradilla, E., Carrol, E.L., and Hesse, R.H. Regulation of bone resorption and formation. Influences of thyrocalcitonin, parathyroid hormone, neutral phosphate and vitamin D3. *Amer. J. Med. 43:*696-710 (1967).

Rasmussen, H., Anast, C., and Arnaud, C. Thyrocalcitonin, EGTA and urinary electrolyte excretion. *J. Clin. Invest. 46:*746-752 (1967).

Robinson, C.J., Martin, T.J., and MacIntyre, I. Phosphoturic effect of thyrocalcitonin. *The Lancet 2:*83-84 (1966).

Viau, A.T., Naftchi, N.E., St. Paul, H.M., Sell, H., and Lowman, E.W. Mineral metabolism in spinal cord injury. *Fed. Proc. 37:*926 (1978).

Wase, A.W., Peterson, A., Rickes, E., and Solewski, J. Some effects of thyrocalcitonin on the calcium metabolism of the rat. *Endocrinology 79:*687-691 (1966).

Ziegler, R., Lemmer, B., and Pfeiffer, E.F. Uber die Einwirkung von Thyrocalcitonin auf die Phosphaturie. *Klin. Wochschr. 45:*34-38 (1967).

15

Mineral Metabolism and the Effect of Thyrocalcitonin on Periarticular Bone in Spinal Cord Injured Man

N.E. NAFTCHI, A.T. VIAU, G.H. SELL, and E.W. LOWMAN

ABSTRACT

In 10 paraplegic and 10 quadriplegic subjects, bone resorption was investigated by determining urinary excretion of hydroxyproline, calcium, and phosphorus. Measurements were performed weekly from the onset to four months after the injury. Compared with control values (100 ± 20 mg/24 hours), urinary excretion of calcium was elevated in spinal cord injured subjects (310 ± 68 gm/24 hours; $p<0.01$) for the entire four-month period. Urinary hydroxyproline was elevated in paraplegic subjects (102 ± 16 mg/24 hours) for the entire 16 weeks following the injury, compared with controls (50 ± 5 mg/24 hours; $p<0.01$). Both paraplegic and quadriplegic subjects excreted more phosphorus (1.6 ± 0.3 gm/24 hours) than controls (0.85 ± 0.1 gm/24 hours; $p<0.01$) only during two weeks following spinal cord injury. Urinary excretion of calcium and magnesium was significantly higher ($p<0.01$) in subjects with complete spinal cord lesions than those with incomplete spinal cord lesions. Sodium fluoride ^{18}F scintimetry was performed on three spinal cord injured subjects with periarticular ossification of the hip and knees before and after one month of treatment with salmon thyrocalcitonin. Thyrocalcitonin therapy caused a marked diminution of ^{18}F uptake in one subject with longstanding periarticular bone of both hips. Clinically, the range of motion in this subject increased by 25 degrees, and there was a marked decrease in pain locally. The results were, however, not duplicated in two subjects with periarticular bone formation of short duration.

INTRODUCTION

One of the sequelae of spinal cord trauma, which starts very soon after the onset of injury, is the loss of calcium from bones (Abramson, 1948). Bone mineral and matrix resorption causes negative calcium balance and, eventually, osteoporosis. Development of hypercalciuria (Naftchi et al., 1972; Claus-Walker, et al., 1972), periarticular bone (Venier and Ditunno, 1971), and renal calculi are common side effects in spinal cord injured subjects.

Periarticular bone formation was reported in 16% to 53% of spinal cord injured subject (Venier and Ditunno, 1971), but its etiology still remains unknown. Most frequently, the hip joints and knees were affected, and, less often, the shoulders, elbows, and spine were affected (Stover et al., 1975). Heterotopic ossification starts as an inflammatory reaction, causing edema, chondrogenesis, and osteogenesis (Rossier et al., 1973).

Early detection of periarticular bone, not visible roengenographically, is readily possible by isotope scanning. Moreover, bone scans facilitate the determination of the maturity of the heterotopic ossification. Bone pain and fractures, as well as restricted joint motion due to periarticular bone formation, limit the rehabilitation, independence, and employability of paraplegic and quadriplegic subjects.

The purpose of the present study was the investigation of bone resorption through determination of urinary excretion of calcium, magnesium, phosphorus, and hydroxyproline, as well as the investigation of the effect of thyrocalcitonin administration on periarticular calcification in spinal cord injured subjects. This hormone is known to inhibit bone resorption (Milhaud and Moukhtar, 1966; Friedman and Raisz, 1965) and to enhance the deposition of calcium into bone (Wase et al., 1966; Foster et al., 1966).

MATERIALS AND METHODS

Ten paraplegic and 10 quadriplegic men with a mean age of 25 years (19-40 years) who suffered complete neurological transverse lesions of the spinal cord were selected for this study. Ten age-matched healthy volunteers who underwent complete physical examination served as controls. During the first two to three weeks following the injury all the subjects were receiving 30-40 mg methyl prednisolone (Medrol) and methyl prednisolone sodium succinate (Solumedrol) daily. They were receiving a diet containing 600 mg calcium and 120 gm protein daily. Twenty-four hour urine specimens for the determination of calcium, magnesium, phosphorus and hydroxyproline were collected from each subject, approximately one week after the onset of the injury and then weekly, thereafter, for a period of four months. Five twenty-four hour urine specimens were collected from each volunteer. In addition, urinary excretion of calcium and magnesium was determined in four paraplegic and 10 quadriplegic, randomly selected subjects with complete spinal cord lesions and one paraplegic and seven quadriplegic subjects with incomplete spinal cord lesions during the acute (0-3 months), subacute (3-6 months), and chronic (over 6 months) stages of the injury.

Urinary calcium and magnesium concentrations were determined by atomic absorption spectrophotometry, and phosphorus concentrations by the method of Fiske and Subbarow (1925). Urinary hydroxyproline was analyzed by the method of Prockop and Udenfriend (1960).

Results are expressed as mean±standard error of the mean. Significance was determined by using the Student "t" test.

In addition, three male subjects with complete spinal cord lesions who exhibited X-ray evidence of periarticular bone formation were investigated in order to determine the effect of thyrocalcitonin on extra-skeletal bone:

T.M.: 45 years old with paraplegia secondary to fracture dislocation at T_{12}-L_1 level, as a result of a car accident on June 19, 1969. One month later he developed periarticular ossification of both hips, which became progressively worse, especially on the left side. In July, 1971, he was admitted to the Institute. At that time the subject was confined to bed and unable to ambulate.

J.B.: 27 years old with quadriplegia secondary to a fracture dislocation at C_6-7 level, as a result of a car accident on June 26, 1971.

In September 1971, he was admitted to the Institute.   In December 1971, he developed periarticular ossification of the right knee.

W.S.:   36 years old with quadriplegia secondary to a fracture dis- location at C_7-T_1 level, as a result of a swimming accident on August 19, 1972.   In October 1972, he was admitted to the Institute.   In October 1973, he developed periarticular ossification of the left hip.

All three subjects were treated for one month with salmon thyrocal- citonin (Armour Pharmaceutical Company, Chicago, Illinois).   During the first two weeks, they received intramuscularly 100 MRC (Medical Research Council) units daily and, during the last two weeks, 100 MRC units every second day.   Treatment with thyrocalcitonin started in the subjects T.M., J.B., and W.S. two years and four months, five months, and three months, respectively, after they had developed periarticular bone.

Three blood samples for determination of ionized calcium were obtained from each subject before the administration of thyrocalcitonin, and seven were obtained during the treatment period.   Ionized calcium was measured potentiometrically by using a calcium specific Orion flow- through electrode.

^{18}F Scintimetry was performed on a Raytheon dual scanner by using a 5" x 5" sodium iodide crystal, according to the method designed by Blau et al. (1972) and Muheim and Crutchlow (1971).   One millicurie of ^{18}F labelled sodium fluoride was administered intravenously and the affected areas were scanned one and four hours later.   The counting time per position was five seconds.   The pelvis and knees were scanned before and after one month of treatment with thyrocalcitonin.

RESULTS

Urinary Calcium

Urinary excretion of calcium was significantly higher in paraplegic and quadriplegic subjects than in controls for the entire 16-week period following spinal cord injury.   There was, however, no significant difference between calcium excretion in paraplegic and quadriplegic subjects.   Hypercalciuria reached the highest levels during the first seven weeks following the injury(Figure 1).

Calcium excretion was significantly lower in subjects with incomplete compared to those with complete spinal cord lesions.   Urinary calcium that was elevated during the acute phase diminished during the subacute phase and then returned to *normal* during the chronic phase of the injury (Figure 2).

Urinary Magnesium

Urinary excretion of magnesium was elevated during three and four weeks following spinal cord injury in paraplegic and quadriplegic subjects, respectively.   Following that period, urinary excretion of magnesium decreased gradually to low control levels in both groups of subjects, and, in quadriplegic subjects during the last three weeks of the study, it became lower than that in controls (Figure 3).

Urinary magnesium was significantly lower in subjects with incom- plete spinal cord lesion, compared with those with complete spinal cord lesions (Figure 2).

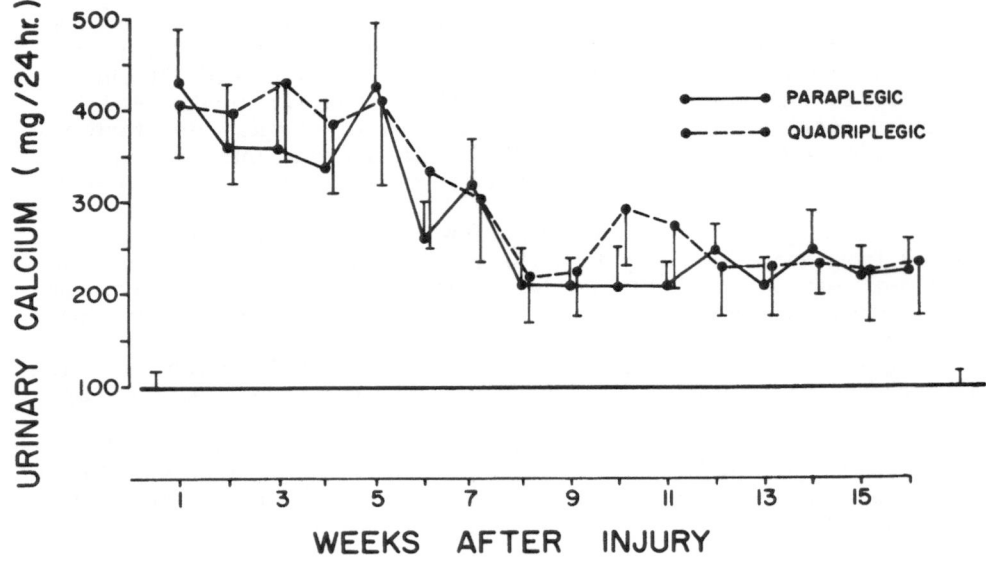

Fig. 1. Urinary excretion of calcium (Mean±SEM) in 10 paraplegic
and 10 quadriplegic subjects from one to 16 weeks following spinal
cord injury. The horizontal line represents urinary calcium in 10
control subjects. All the values obtained in paraplegic and quadriplegic
subjects are significantly (p<0.01) higher than those in controls.
Reprinted by permission of Archives of Physical Medicine and Rehabilitation 61:140, 1980

Urinary Phosphorus

Urinary excretion of phosphorus was significantly higher in paraplegic and quadriplegic than in control subjects for two weeks following
spinal cord injury. After that time it returned to control levels
(Figure 4).

Urinary Hydroxyproline

Urinary excretion of hydroxyproline increased gradually reaching
the highest level at three and four weeks in paraplegic and quadriplegic
subjects, respectively, following the onset of injury. It remained at
the highest level until the seventh week in quadriplegic subjects and
the eighth week in paraplegic subjects. Starting at the ninth week
following the injury, urinary excretion of hydroxyproline in paraplegic
subjects returned to control levels. In quadriplegic subjects, however,
it remained elevated for the entire 16-week testing period (Figure 5).
Four weeks after spinal cord injury, urinary concentration of hydroxyproline in quadriplegic subjects became significantly greater than that
of paraplegic subjects.

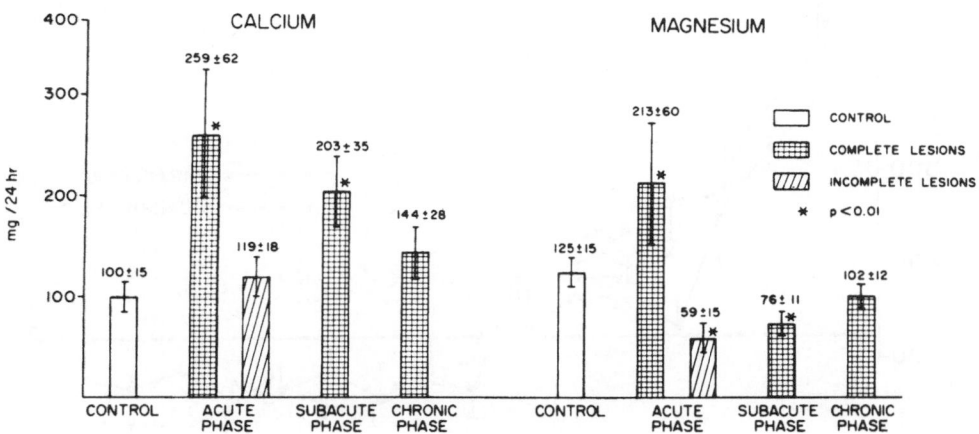

Fig. 2. Urinary excretion of calcium and magnesium (Mean ±SEM) in
14 subjects with complete spinal cord lesions during the acute
(0–3 months), subacute (3–6 months), and chronic (over 6 months)
phases of the injury and in eight spinal cord injured subjects with
incomplete spinal cord lesions during the acute (0–3 months) stage
of the injury.
Reprinted by permission of Archives of Physical Medicine and Rehabilitation 61: 140. 1980

Sodium Fluoride ^{18}F scintimetry

    Scans performed before the administration of thyrocalcitonin
demonstrated marked abnormal uptake of ^{18}F in the affected areas in
all the subjects. Figure 6 shows the results of the scanning of the
hip areas in the subject with long duration periarticular ossification of
both hips (T.M.). High ^{18}F uptake is visible on both hips, especially
on the left hip area with massive periarticular bone. The results of
^{18}F scintimetry performed on the same subject after one month of thyrocalcitonin treatment revealed a marked reduction of ^{18}F uptake in the
affected areas (Figure 7). Clinically, the range of motion in the above
subject increased by 25 degrees (from -35° to -10°), and there was
a marked decrease in pain locally. These results were, however, not
duplicated in the other two subjects with short duration periarticular
ossification who received similar treatment of thyrocalcitonin. In
these two subjects there was no change in ^{18}F uptake before and after
thyrocalcitonin administration, and there was no reduction in local
swelling or pain.

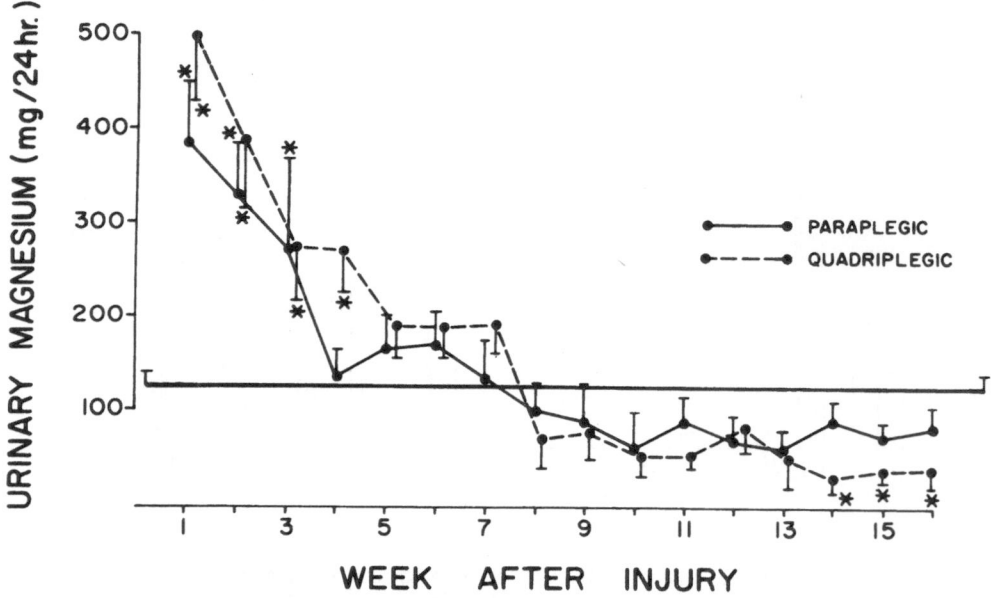

Fig. 3. Urinary excretion of magnesium (Mean ±SEM) in 10 paraplegic and 10 quadriplegic subjects from one to 16 weeks following spinal cord injury. The horizontal line represents urinary magnesium in 10 control subjects. (* = p<0.01)

Serum Ionized Calcium

In the subject T.M. with periarticular bone of long duration, serum ionized calcium was elevated (5.3-5.8 mg/100 ml) before the treatment with thyrocalcitonin. Serum ionized calcium was, however, within normal limits (4.1-5.2 mg/100 ml) in the two subjects with periarticular bone of short duration.

In the subject with long duration periarticular ossification, high serum ionized calcium level was significantly reduced after the treatment with thyrocalcitonin. In the two subjects with normal serum ionized calcium, however, administration of thyrocalcitonin had no significant effect on the serum ionized calcium level (Table I).

DISCUSSION

Hydroxyproline is the major amino acid found in collagen, which is the main component of the bone matrix (Klein, 1967). Total urinary hydroxyproline, therefore, appears to be a sensitive index of bone collagen metabolism (Klein and Curtiss, 1964), and quantitation of urinary

TABLE I

Changes in Serum Ionized Calcium with Thyrocalcitonin Treatment

Subject	Before Treatment	During Treatment
T.M.	5.54±0.20*	4.11±0.±0
J.B.	4.64±0.10	4.19±0.06
W.S.	4.60±0.11	4.00±0.08

Normal Range = 4.10-5.20
Results are expressed as mean±SEM (mg/100 ml)
* p<0.05

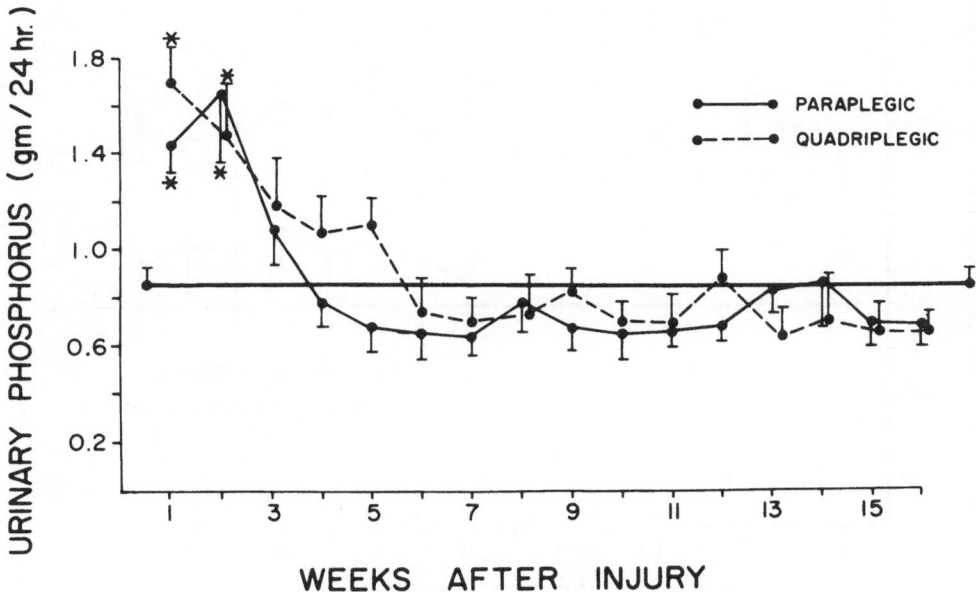

Fig. 4. Urinary excretion of phosphorus (Mean±SEM) in 10 paraplegic and 10 quadriplegic subjects from one to 16 weeks following spinal cord injury. The horizontal line represents urinary phosphorus in 10 control subjects. (* = p<0.01)

hydroxyproline permits a study of collagen breakdown and bone resorption.

An increase in hydroxyprolinuria following spinal cord injury, which was similar to that observed in the present sequential study, was previously reported (Klein, 1967; Claus-Walker et al., 1975; Chantraine, 1970-71; Klein et al., 1966). However, in the present investigation which was contrary to the findings of Chantraine (1970-71) but in agreement with those of Klein (1967), excretion of hydroxyproline was greater and of longer duration in quadriplegic than in paraplegic subjects. The lower collagen breakdown in paraplegic than in quadriplegic subjects, as evidenced by lesser excretion of urinary hydroxyproline in the former group, was probably due to the more suprasegmental sparing and to the active and vigorous exercise regimen in paraplegic subjects; urinary excretion of hydroxyproline was found to be higher in bedridden spinal cord injured subjects, compared with active subjects (Claus-Walker et al., 1975).

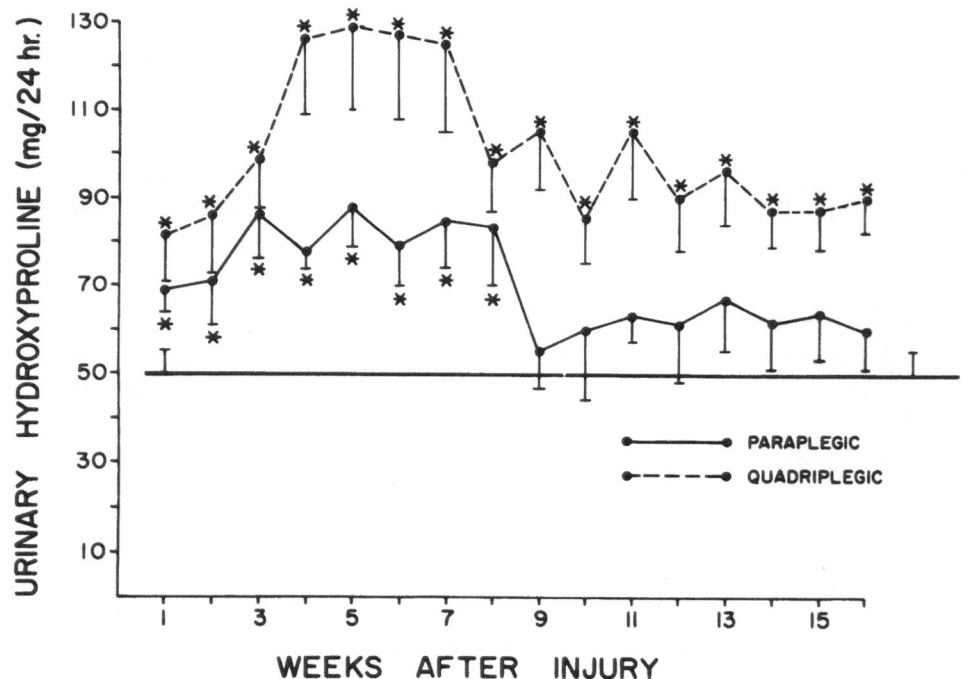

Fig. 5. Urinary excretion of hydroxyproline (Mean±SEM) in 10 paraplegic and 10 quadriplegic subjects from one to 16 weeks following spinal cord injury. The horizontal line represents urinary hydroxyproline in 10 control subjects. (* = p<0.01)

An increased urinary excretion of magnesium, which was similar
to that found in the present study, was previously observed following
soft tissue surgery (Walker et al., 1968) and spinal cord injury
(Broughton and Burr, 1972). It was suggested that increased urinary
magnesium, which follows the onset of paraplegia, is probably derived
not only from bone but also from muscle wasting, as a result of
paralysis (Broughton and Burr, 1972).

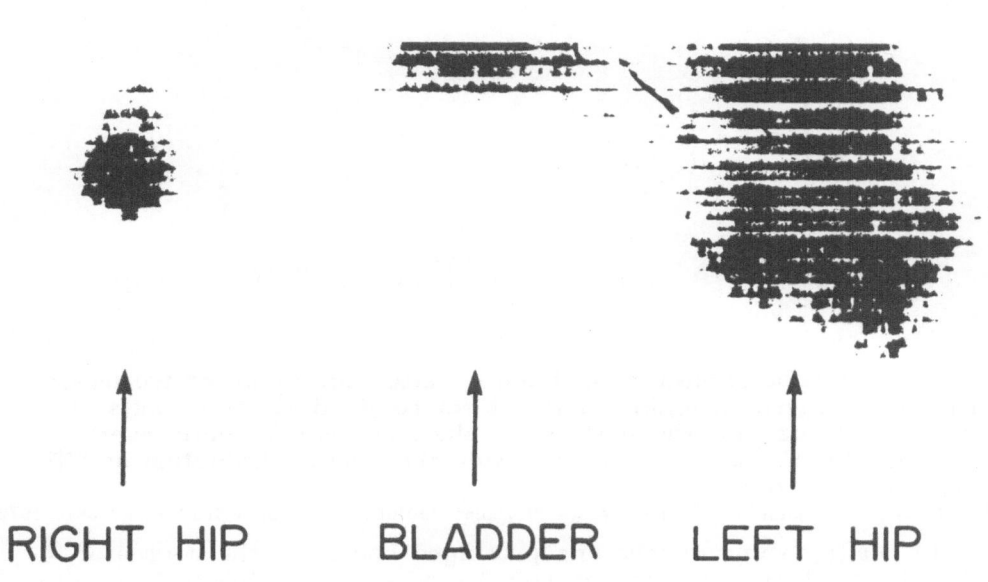

RIGHT HIP   BLADDER   LEFT HIP

Fig. 6. Results of ^{18}F scintimetry performed on a paraplegic subject
with long-standing periarticular ossification of both hips before treatment
with thyrocalcitonin. Bladder is used as a reference point. Note
the enormous ^{18}F uptake especially in the left hip area.
Reprinted by permission of Archives of Physical Medicine and Rehabilitation 60:281. 1979

Elevated excretion of urinary phosphorus observed in this study
was also similar to that reported previously (Broughton and Burr, 1972).
Starting from the first week after the onset of the injury and
continuing through the entire four-month study period, hypercalciuria
was of the sam magnitude in paraplegic and in quadriplegic subjects.
A similar increase in urinary calcium was reported by Klein (1967).
We did not observe a gradual increase in urinary calcium excretion that
was of the same magnitude in paraplegic and in quadriplegic subjects
Broughton and Burr, 1972). On the contrary, the highest concentrations
of urinary calcium were observed during the first seven weeks following
the injury.

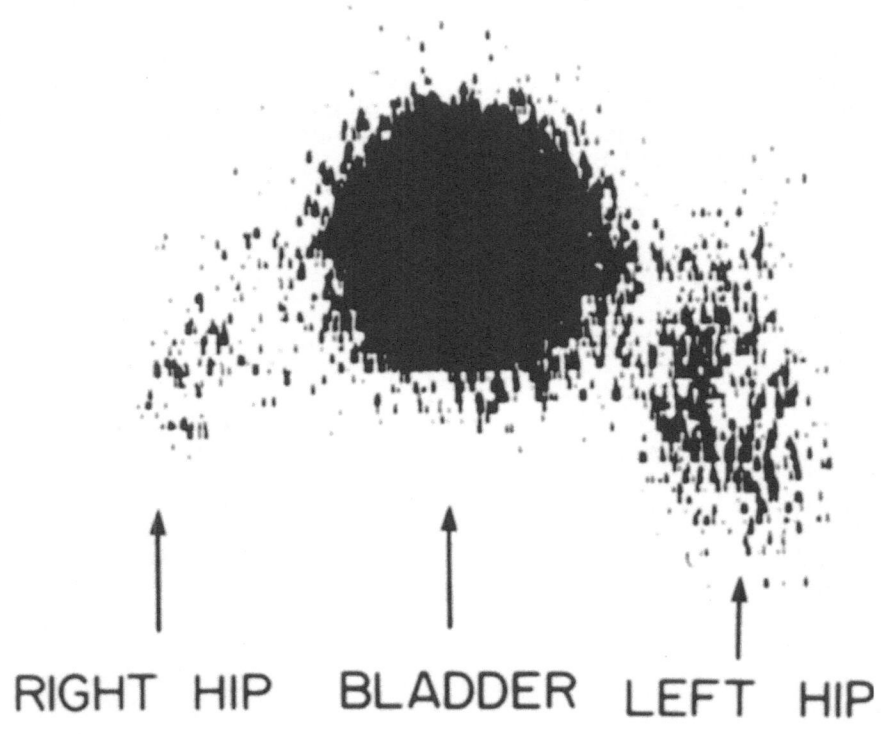

RIGHT HIP   BLADDER   LEFT HIP

Fig. 7. The same subject as in Figure 1 after one month of treatment with salmon thyrocalcitonin. The subject received 100 MRC units of the drug per day for the first two weeks and 100 MRC units every other day for the last two weeks. Note the marked diminution of ^{18}**F uptake in both hips.**
Reprinted by permission of Archives of Physical Medicine and Rehabilitation 60: 281. 1979

In healthy subjects following prolonged bed rest, the degree of calciuria was lower than that in spinal cord injured subjects (Donaldson et al., 1970). Although early rehabilitation exercises shortened the initial period of hypercalciuria in acute spinal cord injured subjects (Claus-Walker et al., 1975), rehabilitation exercises that lead to weight bearing on long bones did not appear to diminish hypercalciuria. The lack of change was thought to be due to interrupted transmission from baroreceptors resulting from severed spinal cord (Claus-Walker et al., 1972). Similarly, in astronauts returning from space missions, the sequelae were comparable to those of acute quadriplegic subjects, probably owing to the lack of baroreceptor stimulation (Leach and Fisher, 1970).

Our findings of a good correlation between hydroxyproline and calcium excretion in spinal cord injured subjects agree with those of Klein and Curtis (1964), suggesting bone resorption. Moreover, the increase in urinary calcium and hydroxyproline excretion without concomitant marked increases in serum alkalaine phosphatase (Klein, 1967; Klein et al., 1966) also indicated that elevated excretion of calcium and hydroxyproline reflected loss of bone mineral and matrix.

Since bone resorption as evidenced by elevated urinary calcium and hydroxyproline excretion started very soon after the injury, any therapy directed against osteoporosis or other complication of disturbed mineral metabolism should be commenced immediately after the onset of paralysis.

In spite of profound changes in calcium metabolism, the occurrence of hypercalcemia is very rare in spinal cord injured adult subjects (Claus-Walker et al., 1975; Steinberg, 1978). The elevation of the serum ionized calcium in the subject T.M. could have resulted from prolonged confinement to bed owing to massive periarticular ossification of both hips. Despite normal total serum calcium, elevated ionized calcium was also reported in nine of the 10 patients who were immobilized for treatment of fractures (Heath et al., 1972). Serum ionized calcium, therefore, seems to be a more sensitive index of bone metabolism than total calcium.

Administration of thyrocalcitonin decreased high serum ionized calcium in subject T.M. to control levels. Similarly, administration of thyrocalcitonin resulted in a drop in serum calcium levels in patients with Paget's disease (Bijvoet et al., 1968; Bell et al., 1970), thyrotoxicosis, and hypercalcemia (Bijvoet et al., 1968).

There was no relationship between the occurrence of periarticular ossification and the level of the spinal cord lesion or the degree of spasticity or flaccidity. Further, the development of extraskeletal bone was not related to inadequate mobilization or lack of physiotherapy (Hardy and Dickson, 1963). Heterotopic bone has never been found above the level of paralysis (Damanski, 1961). Since periarticular bone formation aggravates the disability, its surgical excision increases mobility and independence of the spinal cord injured subjects. The surgery, however, is successful only when the bone is mature, well circumscribed, and trabeculated (Freehafer et al., 1966). Early surgery frequently results in regrowth of the extraskeletal bone. Determination of the maturity of heterotopic ossification, therefore, is of great importance. Bone scans, utilizing isotopically labelled bone-seeking elements such as sodium fluoride (^{18}F) or technetium (^{99}mTc) will facilitate this determination. Their short half-life (110 minutes for ^{18}F and 6 hours for ^{99}mTc) offers the advantage of a lower radiation dose per test and makes frequent repeat measurements feasible.

Since thyrocalcitonin enhances the deposition of calcium into bone, we reasoned that it could possibly accelerate the maturation process. Administration of thyrocalcitonin to one subject with periarticular ossification of long duration did not increase but rather diminished the ^{18}F uptake in two subjects with periarticular bone of short duration.

The results of thyrocalcitonin effect can be interpreted as follows: in the subject with long standing periarticular ossification, the bone was close to maturity and thyrocalcitonin administration speeded the ossification process. When the second bone scan was taken, therefore, the ^{18}F uptake of mature bone was significantly diminished. In the other two subjects with periarticular bone of short duration, the stimulation effect of thyrocalcitonin might have been masked by the maximum growth and turnover activity of the maturing bone. Another explanation for the absence of thyrocalcitonin effect may be the possibility that periarticular ossification lacks the receptors normally present in skeletal bones. The latter hypothesis, however, does not explain the ameliorating effect of thyrocalcitonin on the subject with periarticular bone of long duration. Since in the rat a large dose of thyrocalcitonin (4 mg/kg) administered immediately after spinal cord injury restored the calcium balance (Naftchi et al, 1973; Viau et al., 1974), a larger dose of thyrocalcitonin in the subjects who were not responsive to the presently administered doses might have proved more effective.

REFERENCES

Abramson, A.S. Bone disturbances in injuries to the spinal cord and
    cauda equina (paraplegia). *J. Bone Joint. Surg. 30:*982-987 (1948).
Bell, N.H., Avery, S., and Johnston, C.C., Jr. Effects of calcitonin
    in Paget's disease and polyostatic fibrous dysplasia. *J. Clin.
    Endocrinol. Metab. 31:*283-290 (1970).
Bijvoet, O.L.M., Van Der Sluys Veer, J., and Jansen, A.P. Effects
    of calcitonin on patients with Paget's disease, thyrotoxicosis or
    hypercalcemia. *The Lancet 1:*876-881 (1968).
Blau, M., Nagler, W., and Bender, M.A. Flouride-18: a new isotope
    for bone scanning. *J. Nucl. Med. 3:*332-334 (1962).
Broughton, A., and Burr, R.G. Magnesium metabolism following spinal
    cord injury. *Paraplegia 10:*134-141 (1972).
Chantraine, A. Clinical investigation of bone metabolism in spinal
    cord lesions. *Paraplegia 8:*253-259 (1970-71).
Claus-Walker, J., Spencer, W.A., Carter, R.E., Halstead, L.S. Meier,
    R.H., and Campos, R.J. Bone metabolism in quadriplegia:
    dissociation between calciuria and hydroxyprolinuria. *Arch. Phys.
    Med. Rehabil. 56:*327-332 (1975).
Claus-Walker, J., Carter, R.E., Campos, R.J., and Spencer, W.A.
    Hypercalcemia in early traumatic quadriplegia. *J. Chron. Dis. 28:*
    81-90 (1975).
Claus-Walker, J., Campos, R.J., Carter, R.E., Vallbona, C., and
    Lipscomb, H.S. Calcium excretion in quadriplegia. *Arch. Phys.
    Med. Rehabil. 53:*14-20 (1972).
Damanski, M. Heterotopic ossification in paraplegia. A clinical study.
    *J. Bone. Joint. Surg. 43-B:*286-299 (1961).
Donaldson, C.L., Hulley, S.B., Vogel, J.M., Battner, R.S., Bayers,
    J.H., and McMillan, D.E. Effect of prolonged bed rest on bone
    mineral. *Metabolism 19:*1071-1084 (1970).
Fiske, C.H., and Subbarow, Y. The colorimetric determination of
    phosphorus. *J. Biol. Chem. 66:*375-400 (1925).
Foster, G.V., Joplin, G.F., MacIntyre, I., Melvin, K.E.W., and Slack,
    E. Effect of thyrocalcitonin in man. *The Lancet 1:*107-109 (1966).
Freehafer, A.A., Yurick, R., and Mast, W.A. Para-articular ossification
    in spinal cord injury. *Med. Serv. J. Can. 22:*471-477 (1966).
Friedman, J., and Raisz, L.G. Thyrocalcitonin: inhibitor of bone
    resorption in tissue culture. *Science 150:*1465-1467 (1965).
Hardy, A.G., and Dickson, J.W. Pathological ossification in traumatic
    paraplegia. *J. Bone. Joint. Surg. 45-B:*76-87 (1963).
Heath, H., III, Earll, J.M., Schaaf, M., Piechocki, J.T., and Ting-Kai,
    L. Serum ionized calcium during bedrest in fracture patients and
    normal men. *Metabolism 21:*633-640 (1972).
Klein, L. Metabolic response of collagen to trauma: the relationship of
    urinary nitrogen and hydroxyproline. *J. Trauma 7:*343-356 (1967).
Klein, L., and Curtiss, P.H. Urinary hydroxyproline as an index of
    bone metabolism. In *Dynamic Studies of Metabolic Bone Disease,*
    Pearson, O.H., and Joplin, G.F. (eds.), Oxford, Blackwell, 1964,
    pp. 201-224.
Klein, L., van den Noort, S., and DeJak, J.J. Sequential studies of
    urinary hydroxyproline and serum alkaline phosphatase in acute
    paraplegia. *Med. Serv. J. Can. 22:*524-533 (1966).
Leach, C.S., and Fisher, C. Endocrinologic aspects of manned space
    flight. Paper presented at the 52nd Annual Meeting of the Endocrine
    Society, St. Louis, Mo., 1970.
Milhaud, G., and Moukhtar, M.S. Thyrocalcitonin: effects on calcium

kinetics in the rat. *Proc. Soc. Exp. Biol. Med. 123:*207-209 (1966).

Muheim, G., and Crutchlow, W.P. [18]F and [85]SR scintimetry in the study of primary arthropathies. *Brit. J. Rad. 44:*290-294 (1971).

Naftchi, N.E., Viau, A.T., Sell, G.H., and Lowman, E.W. Effect of thyrocalcitonin on calcium and magnesium metabolism in the spinal rat. *Physiologist 16:*405 (1973).

Prockop, D.J., and Udenfriend, S. A specific method for the analysis of hydroxyproline in tissue and urine. *Analyt. Biochem. 1:*228-239 (1960).

Rossier, A.B., Bussat, P., Infante, F., Zender, R., Courvoisier, B., Muheim, G., Donath, A., Vasey, H., Taillard, W., Lagier, R., Gabbiani, G., Baud, C.A., Pouezat, J.A., Very, J.M., and Hachen, H.J. Current facts on para-osteoarthropathy. *Paraplegia 11:*36-78 (1973).

Steinberg, F.U., Birge, S.J., and Cooke, N.E. Hypercalcemia in adolescent tetraplegic patients: case report and review. *Paraplegia 16:*60-67 (1978).

Stover, S.L., Hataway, C.J., and Ziegler, H.E. Heterotopic ossification in spinal cord injured patients. *Arch. Phys. Med. Rehabil. 56:*199-204 (1975).

Venier, L.H., and Ditunno, J.F., Jr. Heterotopic ossification in the paraplegic patient. *Arch. Phys. Med. Rehabil. 52:*475-479 (1971).

Viau, A.T., Naftchi, N.E., and Lowman, E.W. Effect of thyrocalcitonin on calcium, magnesium and phosphorus balance in the rat. *Fed. Proc. 33:*404 (1974).

Walker, W.F., Fleming, L.W., and Steward, W.K. Urinary magnesium excretion in surgical patients. *Brit. J. Surg. 55:*466-469 (1968).

Wase, A.W., Peterson, A., Rickes, E., and Solewski, J. Some effects of thyrocalcitonin on the calcium metabolism of the rat. *Endocrinology 79:*687-691 (1966).

Naftchi, N.E., Viau, A.T., Demeny, M., Sell, G.H., and Lowman, E.W. Calcium and magnesium metabolism in spinal man and rat. *Physiologist 15:*224 (1972).

16

Urinary Excretion of Collagen Metabolites by Quadriplegic Patients

J. CLAUS-WALKER, J. SINGH, and N. DiFERRANTE

ABSTRACT

Urinary total hydroxyproline, nondialyzable peptide-bound hydroxy-proline, hydroxylysine glycosides, and calcium have been measured in three recently injured quadriplegic patients.

These patients had hypercalciuria and excreted increased amounts of collagen metabolites. The increased metabolism of bone collagen may explain the hypercalciuria and the progressive bone loss. The data indicate that cutaneous collagen is degraded at the same rate as the bone collagen.

INTRODUCTION

The possibility that the hypercalciuria and bone loss occurring in paralyzed patients is secondary to the loss of bone collagen has been supported by the finding of high urinary excretion of hydroxyproline in patients who were recently affected by extensive paralysis (Claus-Walker et al., 1975; Klein et al., 1966; Prockop and Sjoerdsma, 1961).

After two to three years of paralysis, the loss of bone minerals reaches a plateau, although bedrest still leads to a loss of collagen metabolites (Claus-Walker et al., 1975)

A more complete study of collagen metabolism was carried out on three quadriplegic patients who were recently paralyzed by functional transection of the spinal cord at the cervical level. The patients were immobilized in bed at the onset of the study and later were subjected to passive mobilization, verticalization, and wheelchair training.

In this study, we have measured the urinary excretion of total hydroxyproline, which reflects collagen turnover in subjects on a gelatin free diet and a peptide-bound hydroxyproline, which reflects collagen synthesis (Krane et al., 1970). We have also measured two hydroxylysine glycosides, which are excreted in small amounts in urine of normal subjects and are a good index of collagen breakdown because their excretion is not influenced by the diet (Cunningham et al., 1967; Segrest and Cunningham, 1970). Hydroxylysine glycosides are increased in diseases affecting collagen (Askenasi, 1973) and may be modified by appropriate therapeutic management (Askanasi, 1974). The relative proportions of the two glycosides, glucosyl-galactosyl-hydroxylysine, and galactosyl-hydroxylysine may indicate whether bone or skin collagen is preferentially being degraded (Askanasi, 1974).

219

METHODS

   The three male quadriplegic patients (T.J., W.A., and A.H.), were
16, 17, and 19 years old, respectively. They had sustained spinal cord
injury at a level between the 4th and 6th cervical vertebra but had no
previous significant medical problems. During the period of observation,
they received a gelatin-free standard diet, providing an average of
2430 ± 40 calories per day (105 ± 4 g proteins; 276 ± g carbohydrates;
160 ± 15 g fats, 115 ± 4 mEq sodium; 85 ± 3 mEq potassium; and 45 ±
3 mEq calcium).
   Urine was collected daily from cathetherized patients and stored
without preservative at 5°C as soon as possible after the injury: from
the 3rd to the 15th week for T.J.; from the 8th to the 19th week for
W.A., and from the 5th to the 19th and 20th week for A.H. The urine
samples that were obtained from each patient in a given week were
pooled, and the various metabolites were measured on the pooled samples.
   Urinary calcium was assayed by atomic absorption spectrometry
(Claus-Walker et al., 1975) and the values obtained were expressed
as mEq/24 hours. Total urinary hydroxyproline was measured according
to Kivirikko et al. (1967) and expressed in mg/24 hours. Nondialyzable
peptide-bound hydroxyproline was measured according to Krane (1970).
The results were expressed as mg of hydroxyproline in 24 hours. For
the evaluation of hydroxylysine glycosides, 1 ml aliquots of each urine
sample were filtered through a Millipore PSAC membrane, having a
nominal molecular exclusion limit of 1,000; 0.5 to 0.6 ml aliquots of the
filtrate were used for the assay. Galactosyl-hydroxylysine and glycosyl-
galactosyl-hydroxylysine were measured according to Askenasi (1973),
using a 55.5 x 0.9 cm column packed with Beckman PA-28 cation
exchange resin. The column was eluted at 64° C with a pH 5.28, 0.35
M sodium citrate buffer, at a flow rate of 50 ml/hour. The molar
ninhydrin color equivalent of hydroxylysine, as obtained in the 2 column
system employed, was used to calculate the amounts of the hydroxylysine
glycosides (Prockop and Sjoerdsma, 1961). The results were expressed
as micromoles/24 hours.

RESULTS

   The mean urinary excretion of calcium in normal controls is 9.4 ±
0.65 mEq/24 hours (Claus-Walker et al., 1975). The quadriplegic
patients had a constantly elevated excretion throughout the period of
study, with ample fluctuations from week to week (Claus-Walker et al.,
1975) (Figure 1). The urinary excretion of total hydroxyproline in the
three patients was enormously increased, also with ample fluctuations
from week to week (Figure 1). In agreement with these findings, the
urinary excretion of nondialyzable peptide-bound hydroxyproline was
also increased five to 10 times above the normal level (Krane et al.,
1970) (Figure 1). The urinary excretion of both types of glycosides
was more than doubled, compared with normal (Askenasi, 1974) (Figure
2). The ratio of these glycosides, however, was only slightly higher
than normal (Figure 2).

DISCUSSION

   In the three quadriplegic patients, the calciuria exceeded the levels
that were observed during simple bedrest (Claus-Walker et al., 1975)
and was not influenced by the physical therapy that the patients
received.

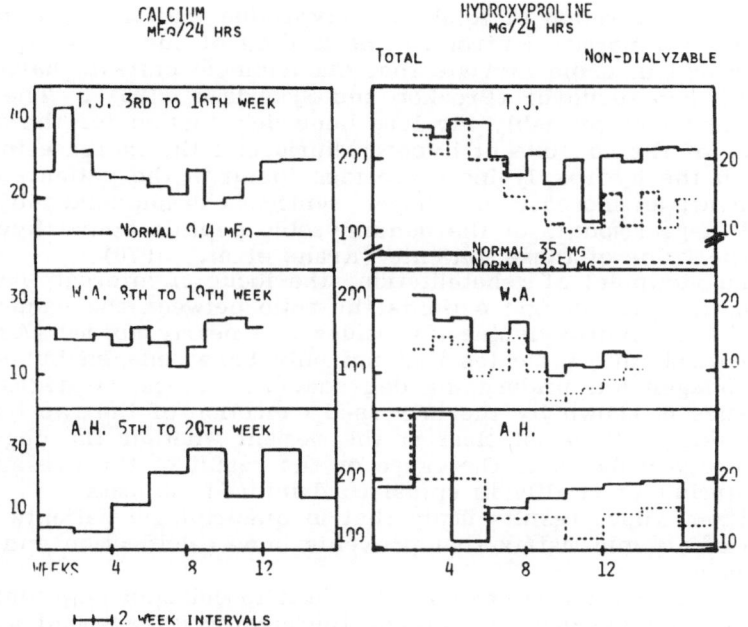

Fig. 1. Urinary excretions of calcium, total hydroxyproline, and peptide-bound hydroxyproline in quadriplegic patients. The respective normal levels of excretion are indicated by the horizontal lines.

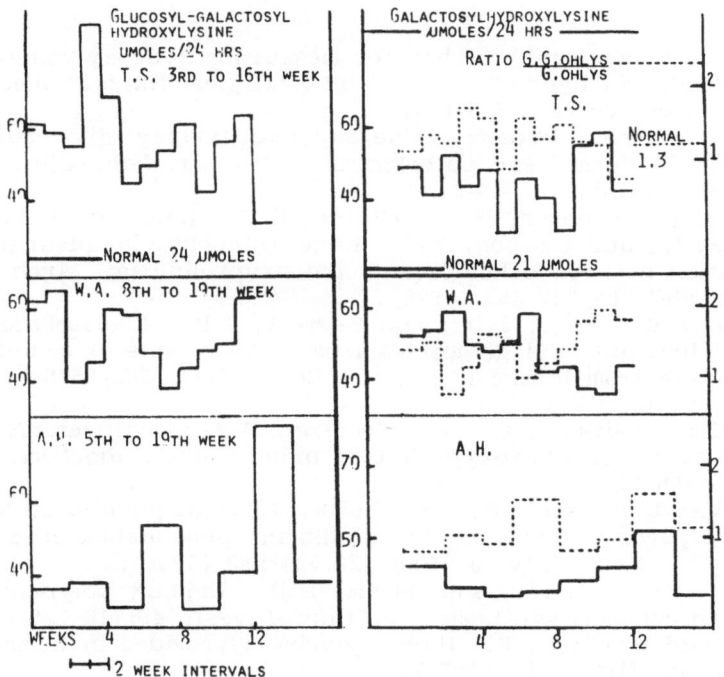

Fig. 2. The urinary excretion of individual hydroxylysine glycosides and their ratio in quadriplegic patients. The normal levels of excretion and the normal ratio are indicated by the horizontal lines.

The urinary excretion of total hydroxyproline was also strikingly different from the normal controls. The finding of such large quantities of this aminoacid in urine indicate that quadriplegic patients have an increased collagen turnover (Prockop and Sjoerdsma, 1961). The increase in turnover probably involves bone degradation for the most part because of the concurrent hypercalciuria and the increase in the urine of both the hydroxylysine glycosides found in the patients. On the other hand, an increase in collagen synthesis is supported by the presence of large amounts of the nondialyzable peptide-bound hydroxyproline in the urine of these patients (Krane et al., 1970).

From the viewpoint of rehabilitation, the focus of interest was to find that in the quadriplegic patients the ratio between the values of excretion of both hydroxylysine glycosides was nearly normal (Askenasi, 1974). A normal ratio indicates that not only bone collagen but also cutaneous collagen was undergoing degradation. Excessive degradation in both tissues is shown by the increased excretion of the two hydroxylysine glycosides. It is not clear at the moment whether the degradation of the cutaneous collagen is the cause or the result of the pressure ulcers, occurring so readily in spinal cord injured subjects.

In addition, these results imply that in quadriplegic patients it may be the loss of organic matrix that prevents bone calcification and leads to osteoporosis.

Until the biochemical mechanism that lead to collagen degradation are thoroughly understood, no rational therapeutic management may be implemented, except to make up for the losses of active wieght bearing and muscular activity by all available means currently used by physical and occupational therapists and perhaps by electrical muscular stimulation.

REFERENCES

Askenasi, R. A new rapid method for measuring hydroxylysine and its glycosides in hydrolysates and physiological fluids. *Biochim. Biophys. Acta 304:*375-383 (1973).

Askenasi, R. Urinary hydroxylysine and hydroxylysyl glycosides excretions in normal and pathological states. *J. Lab. Clin. Med. 83:*673-679 (1974).

Claus-Walker, J., Spencer, W.A., Carter, R.E., Halstead, L.S., Meier, R.H., and Campos, R.J. Bone metabolism in quadriplegia: Dissociation between calciuria and hydroxyprolinuria. *Arch. Phys. Med. Rehabil. 56:*327-332 (1975).

Cunningham, L.W., Ford, J.D., and Segrest, J.P. The isolation of identical hydroxylysyl glycosides from hydrolysates of soluble collagen and from human urine. *J. Biol. Chem. 242:*2570-2571 (1967).

Kivirikko, K.I., Laitinen, O., and Prockop, D.J. Modifications of specific assay for hydroxyproline in urine. *Anal. Biochem. 19:* 249-255 (1967).

Klein, L., Van Den Noort, S., and Dejak, J.J. Sequential studies of urinary hydroxyproline and serum alkaline phsophatase in acute paraplegia. *Med. Serv. J. Can. 22:*524-533 (1966).

Krane, S.M., Munoz, A.J., and Harris, E.D. Urinary polypeptides related to collagen synthesis. *J. Clin. Invest. 49:*716-729 (1970).

Lou, M.F., and Hamilton, P. Hydroxylysine glycosides in human urine. *Clin. Chem. 17:*782-788 (1971).

Prockop, D.J., and Sjoerdsma, A. Significance of urinary hydroxyproline in man. *J. Clin. Invest. 40:*843-849 (1961).

Segrest, J.P., and Cunningham, L.S. Variations in human urinary
    o-hydroxylysyl glycoside levels and their relationship to collagen
    metabolism. *J. Clin. Invest.* *49:* 1497-1509 (1970).

SECTION FIVE

Renal and Urinary Bladder Physiology

17

Electromyography of the Human Urinary Bladder

P.E. KAPLAN

Over 120 years ago, production of electric potentials by the tissue
of a functioning animal heart was demonstrated. Soon afterwards it was
observed that electric potentials developed in abnormal animal tissues
differed from those developed by healthy tissues (DuBois-Raymond,
1860). In 1952, Boyce (1952) studied the electric potentials developed
by bladder, using silver chloride electrodes. Over 100 patients were
studied, and up to five EMG evaluations were recorded per patient.
In the original procedure, the patient was asked to void, and then
a plastic electrocatheter was introduced into the bladder. The electrodes
were engaged on each lateral bladder wall while the bladder was at
capacity. Then the bladder was emptied and remained so for the rest
of the procedure. A series of electric potentials were recorded and
occurred regularly. The frequency was 2.4 spikes per minute; the
electric potentials were diphasic. The average duration was 4.73
seconds, and the amplitude was approximately 400 microvolts. Boyce
in his original work labelled the first deflection on the oscillograph
the A phase and the second deflection the B phase. The entire duration
of both the A and B components averaged 4.73 seconds, as noted
above, the A phase was 1.35 seconds and the B phase was 3.38
seconds. The average peak electromotor force of the B phase was
0.366 millivolts and of the A phase was 0.283 millivolts. Muscular
hypertrophy, "muscular degeneration", and hypoactive and hyperactive
neurogenic bladders were studied. In patients with muscular hypertrophy, the amplitude was increased. In patients with "muscular
degeneration", the amplitude was decreased and the rhythm was
irregular. In patients with hypoactive neurogenic bladders, the amplitude
was decreased and the rhythm was decreased or absent. Patients
with hyperactive neurogenic bladders had variable amplitudes, durations,
and alternate rhythmic activity. It was also determined that maximal
spontaneous bioelectric activity was present near the central portion
of the bladder and much reduced in sections of the dome and the neck
(Corey et al.,1950). Boyce indicated that the electric potentials might
have been artifacted, which resulted from movement of the bladder.
Brunsting also suggested that the waves were mechanical artifacts and
not true electrical potentials, that were produced by the smooth muscles
(Brunsting, 1958). However, several studies between 1950 and 1954
used the same electroencephalographic apparatus and all reported slow
waves that were similar to those found by Boyce (Slater, 1953; Corey
and Vest, 1954; Vest and Corey, 1954).

In 1953 Franksson and Petersen (1953) investigated a series of
patients with normal bladders.   Electrodes were fine sewing needles
that were insulated, except for the tip, and were attached to a thin
stainless steel wire that was passed through a urethral catheter.   In
this way, bipolar recordings were made, using an amplifier and oscillo-:
scope.   Two types of electric potentials were recorded.   One type had
very large amplitudes, up to 400 microvolts, was very slow and appeared
in bursts lasting 0.5 to 3 seconds.   In the interval between the bursts,
there were electric potentials of smaller amplitude of 20 to 40 microvolts
and a frequency of 5 to 25 per second.   The duration of the high
voltage and of the low voltage electric potentials ranged from 25 to
100 milliseconds.   Studies were done to see whether or not segments of
the bladder were firing simultaneously, and it was found that alternating
activity was present.   It was noted that this type of electrical activity
from smooth muscle cells was similar to that in the intestine of animals.

In a recent review of the neurophysiology of the urinary bladder
of the cat, the neural pathway of micturition has been outlined (De
Groat, 1975).   This consists of afferent and efferent sections of the
pelvic nerve connecting the sacral spinal cord and bladder, with
supraspinal pathways (Figure 1).   The electric stimulation of the detrusor

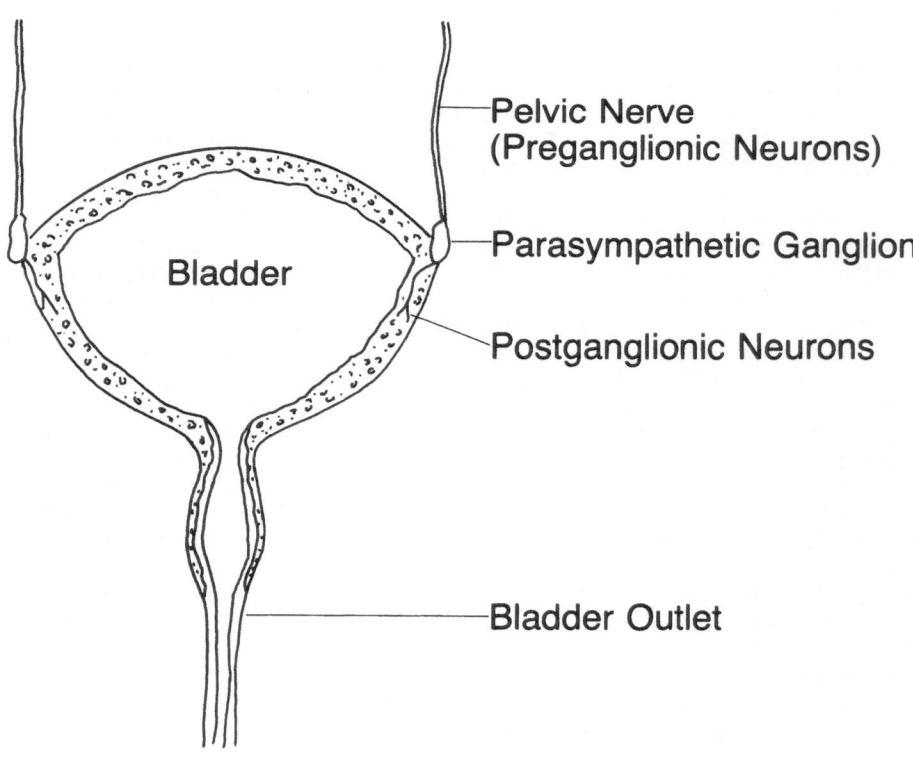

Fig. 1.   Anatomy of the Bladder.

muscle is transmitted by the pelvic nerves. In the cat there is evidence to support the existence of a complex inhibitory mechanism, involving the parasympathetic and sympathetic nervous systems. Under the stimulus of high bladder pressure the pelvic afferent nerves increase the parasympathetic outflow, which excites the bladder. Simultaneous sympathetic outflow is decreased and bladder activity is inhibited. In contrast, lumbosacral root activity can lead to increase in sympathetic outflow, inhibition of the bladder, and a decrease in parasympathetic excitatory activity. This adrenergic inhibition of the bladder can be influenced in the cat by the use of Alpha and Beta adrenergic blocking agents but so far has not been demonstrated in man.

Stanton et al. (1973) studied the electromyographic activity of the bladder, which confirmed the spikes recorded by Franksson and Petersen in 1973. Dysfunction of the detrusor muscle could be distinguished and particularly that involving uninhibited, hypertonic, and hypotonic bladder activity. In addition, increased electric activity was noted in patients just prior to micturition, which included increases in the amplitude and frequency of the electric potentials.

In 1968, several investigators using sensitive electromyographic recording equipment in humans and animals observed that electrical potentials had an amplitude of approximately 20 microvolts and a duration of between 2 and 4 milliseconds. These studies emphasized the need for highly sensitive recording equipment to pick up the electric potentials, and subsequent studies of the normal and the neurogenic urinary bladder confirmed the existence of these electric potentials (Cosgrove et al., 1974; La Joie et al., 1974; Jones et al., 1974). A relationship was found between the potentials' amplitude, duration, and frequency during filling and voiding of the bladder. Resting activity was recorded in normal subjects; it increased in the hypertonic neurogenic bladder and decreased in the hypotonic neurogenic bladder. At rest, the amplitude of the electrical potentials in the normals was between 6 and 12 microvolts, the duration was between 5 and 10 milliseconds, and the frequency was between 0 and 70 spikes per second. This electrical activity was not simultaneous with either peroneal activity or abdominal wall activity but was related to both (La Joie et al., 1974; Kaplan et al., 1975).

Later investigations of a group of patients with spinal cord injury correlated electromyography of the external urethral sphincter and the smooth muscle of the detrusor (Kaplan et al., 1976; Kaplan et al., 1976). The pressures and volumes in the bladder correlated with the amplitude, frequency and duration of the electrical potentials. A statistically significant correlation was found between the increase in volume and an increase in amplitude and frequency and a decrease in the duration of the electric potentials. Also, as the pressure of the bladder increased, the amplitude and frequency increased and duration decreased in patients with hypertonic bladders, bulbocavernosis reflex and positive hypotonic bladders and bulbocabernosis reflex and negative hypotonic bladders. There was a correlation between the results from the control group and from those with neurogenic hypotonic bladders (Figures 2 and 3).

In the patients with hypotonic bladders, the correlations tended to break down, particularly in the group with bulbocavernosis reflex and negative hypotonic bladders. Indeed, in this last group there was no direct relationship between increasing volume and increasing pressure. A summary of these results is presented in Tables I and II.

In conclusion, two types of electrical activity are present in the bladder. One is called Prolonged Electrical Activity (PEA) because the

230 KAPLAN

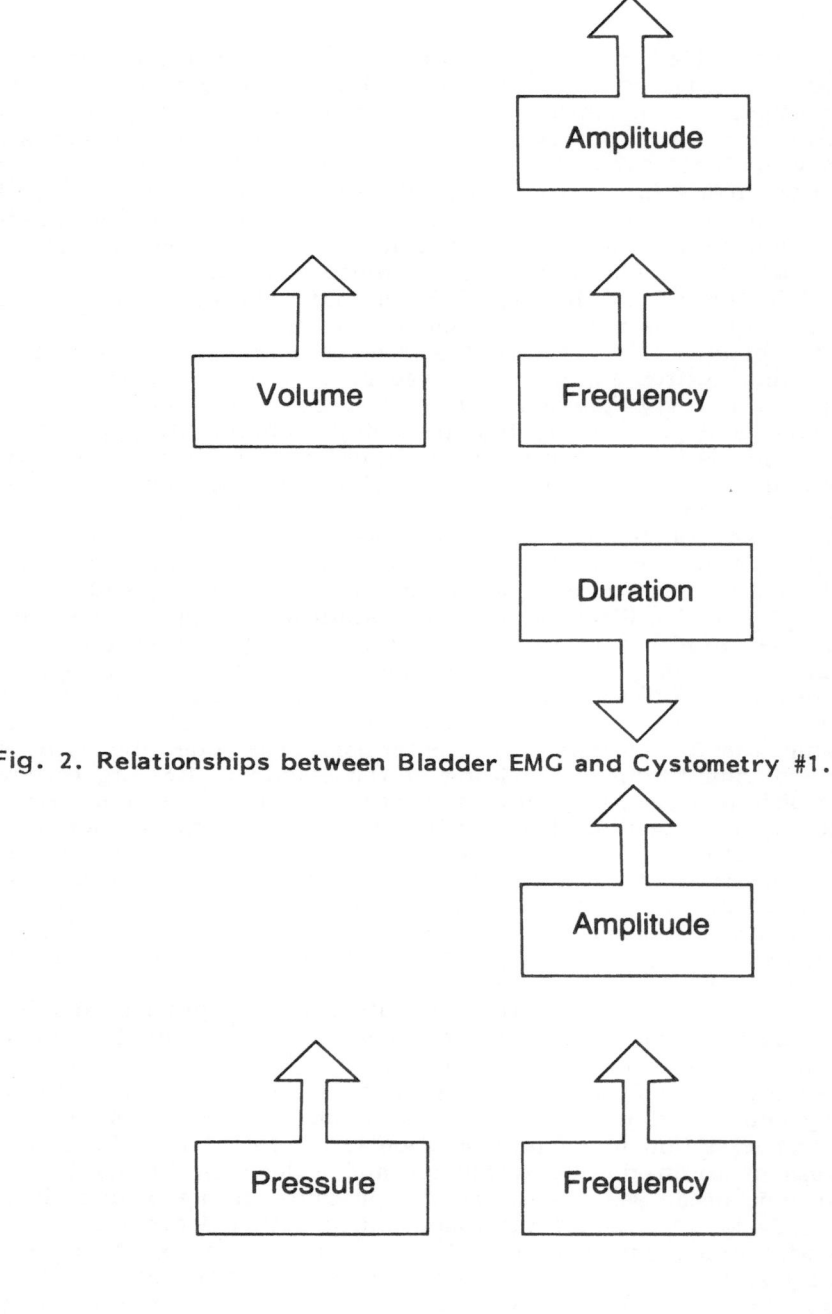

Fig. 2. Relationships between Bladder EMG and Cystometry #1.

Fig. 3. Relationships between Bladder EMG and Cystometry #2.

TABLE I

BLADDER EVALUATION RESULTS #1

Abnormal Bladder	Volume & Pressure Relationship	Frequency Relationship	Amplitude Relationship	Duration Relationship
Lower Motor Neuron, BC/AC	Vol. Very Large, Hypotonic	Nearly Absent	Decreased to 8-10 μV	Decreased to 2 msec
Control	Mean $\frac{25mm\ Hg}{129\ cc}$	Mean 71 cps	Mean 15 μV	Mean 4.6 msec

TABLE II

BLADDER EVALUATION RESULTS #2

Abnormal Bladder	Volume & Pressure Relationship	Frequency Relationship	Amplitude Relationship	Duration Relationship
Upper Motor Neuron,Sp. Cd., Complete	Vol. Small & Hypertonic	Increased to 200 ro 250 cps Freq.	Increased to 40 μV	Decreased to 2 msec
Lower Motor Neuron, BC/AC	Vol. Large & Hypotonic	Decreased to 0-10 cps	Decreased to 8-10 μV	Decreased to 2 msec

duration of the electrical potentials ranges from 0.5 seconds to 4 seconds. This activity is made up of large, relatively slow waves (up to 400 microvolts) and small, faster waves (up to 40 microvolts). The second type is designated Short Electrical Activity (SEA). The duration of SEA ranges between 1 and 12 milliseconds and the amplitude ranges between 8 and 50 microvolts. Whereas the PEA has been recorded on various types of electroencephalographic equipment, SEA can only be observed on extremely sensitive electromyographic equipment. One type of activity is not necessarily exclusive of the other type, and both may be used to more fully understand the electrophysiology of the smooth muscle of the human urinary bladder.

REFERENCES

Boyce, W.H.   Bladder Electromyography: A New Approach to the Diagnosis of Urinary Bladder Dysfunction. *J. of Urol.* 67:650 (1952).

Brunsting, C,D.   An interpretation of the urinary bladder electrocystogram as artefact. *J. Urol.* 79:165 (1958).

Corey, E.L., Boyce, W.H., Vest, S.A. and Franch, C.R. Electro-potential changes in human urinary bladder: A Method of Measurement. *J. Appl. Physiol.* 3:631 (1950).

Corey, E.L., and Vest, S.A. Electropotential changes in the isolated urinary bladder. *Surg. Gyn. and Obst.* 98:91 (1954).

Cosgrove, M.D., Jones, W.G., La Joie, W.J., Kaplan, P.E., and Morrow, J.W. Electromyography of the human urinary bladder. *Urol.* 3:239 (1974).

De Groat, W.C. Nervous control of the urinary bladder of the cat. *Brain Research* 87:201 (1975).

Du Bois-Reymond, R. Untersuchungen Uber Tierische Elektrizitat. Berlin, 1860.

Franksson, C., and Petersen, P.I. Electromyographic recording from the normal human urinary bladder, internal urethral sphincter and ureter. *Ach. Physiol. Scand.* 29:150 (1953).

Jones, W.G., La Joie, W.J., and Cosgrove, M.D. Electromyography in pathologic bladder. *Urol.* 4:186 (1974).

Kaplan, P.E., Nanninga, J., and Lal, S. Bladder evaluation of the abnormal human urinary bladder in spinal cord injured patients. Proc. of Fifth International Congress of EMG, 1975.

Kaplan, P.E., Nanninga, J.B., and Lal, S. Electromyography and Cystometry of the neurogenic bladder - A preliminary report. *EMG & Clin. Neuro. Phys.*, in press, 1976.

Kaplan, P.E., Nanninga, J.B., and Lal, S. The cystometry in electrophysiology of the smooth muscle of the human urinary bladder in healthy patients and in patients with spinal cord injury. *Arch. Phys. Med. and Rehab.*, in press, 1976.

Kolesnikov, G.F., Perogov, V.A., and Fotieva, L.V. Electromyography of the urinary bladder and uretheral sphincters. *Urol. Nefrol.* 33:34 (1968).

La Joie, W.J., Cosgrove, M.D., Jones W.G., and Kaplan, P.E. Electromyography of the human bladder. *EMG & Cl. Neuro. Phys.* 15:191 (1975).

LaJoie, W.J., Cosgrove, M.D., and Jones, W.G. Electromyographic evaluation of human detrusor muscle activity in relation to abdominal activity. *Arch. Phys. Med. & Rehab.* 55:577 (1974).

Slater, E.S. Electromyogram: A Study of bladder contraction measured by differences of electropotential. *J. Urol.* 69:626 (1953).

Stanton, S.L., Hill, D.W., and Williams, J.P. Electromyography of the detrusor muscle. *Brit. J. of Urol.* 45:289 (1973).

Vest, S.A., and Corey, E.L. Electromyography of the urinary bladder. *J. Urol.* 72:361 (1954).

18

Effects of Head-Up Tilt on Glomerular Filtration Rate and Renal Plasma Flow in Spinal Man

K.T. RAGNARSSON, M. KREBS, N.E. NAFTCHI, M. DEMENY,
G.H. SELL, E.W. LOWMAN, and J. TUCKMAN

ABSTRACT

Changes in glomerular filtration rate (GFR), renal plasma flow (RPF) and mean arterial pressure (MAP) were measured in subjects with various levels of spinal cord lesion and thus with different degrees of supraspinal sympathetic vasomotor control. They were tested in supine and head-up tilt positions, and their results were compared with those of normal subjects. The responses of paraplegic subjects to head-up tilt were not significantly different from those of normal controls. On the other hand, in quadriplegics in the supine position, GFR and RPF were significantly lower. When tilted, MAP and RPF decreased significantly, but the fall in GFR was not significant. In all three groups, the GFR during head-up tilt was similar, indicating that in spite of the great loss of supraspinal sympathetic control, quadriplegic subjects apparently equally constrict their afferent and efferent renal arterioles during orthostatic stress and thus prevent excessive fall of GFR.
One of the serious consequences of spinal cord injury is possible progressive deterioration of renal function as a result of an ascending infection from the paralyzed bladder. In order to detect deteriorating renal changes and to determine when to initiate appropriate treatment, a regular urological workup (consisting of an intravenous pyelogram, cystometrics, cystoscopy, urinalysis, urine culture, determination of serum BUN and creatinine, as well as an estimation of the concentrating capability of the kidneys) is of utmost importance. However, it is well known that these methods are relatively insensitive and only detect serious abnormalities. More sensitive methods for studying renal function are measurements of glomerular filtration rate (GFR) and renal plasma flow (RPF) by the standard inulin and paraaminohippurate (PAH) clearance techniques. Price and associates (Price et al., 1966; Price, 1968; Price et al., 1975) reported that these parameters remain within normal limits if complications can be avoided. The level of the spinal cord lesion has not been shown to affect these results (Price et al., 1966; Morales et al., 1956; Doggart et al., 1966).

The head-up tilt position, which spinal cord injured patients are frequently subjected to for shorter or longer periods during their rehabilitation phase, is considered an effective method to reduce orthostatic hypotension by improving circulatory adjustment, improve body balance, limit osteoporosis, prevent urinary calculi and urinary tract infection, and aid morale. The effects of passive head-up tilt upon

GFR and RPF in normal subjects has been extensively investigated by several authors (Thurau, 1964; Smith, 1956). This has not been done in spinal cord injured patients, some of whom have high lesions with loss of supraspinal sympathetic regulation of vasoconstriction, including that of the kidneys. There is evidence that renal circulation is for the most part autoregulated in animals, (Shipley and Study, 1951; Pitts, 1974), as arterial pressure rises from 80 to 180 mm Hg, the renal blood flow (RBF) and the GFR remain essentially constant, regardless of whether the kidney is normally innervated, denervated or isolated. This indicates that an increase in perfusion pressure is accompanied by an equivalent increase in vascular resistance produced by several possible mechanisms (Thurau, 1964; Smith, 1956). It is likely that there is equal contractions of smooth muscles in the walls of the afferent and efferent renal arterioles since GFR remains constant. GFR and RBF vary directly with the mean arterial pressure between approximately 60 and 80 mm Hg, but below 55 to 60 mm Hg filtration ceases.

The kidney is richly innervated by sympathetic post-ganglionic vasoconstrictor fibers derived from the sympathetic trunk, which in turn is considered to receive pre-ginaglionic fibers from spinal segments T5 through L2. In spite of inadequate data, investigators (Thurau, 1964; Smith, 1956) agree that there is little or no neurogenic sympathetic vasoconstrictor tone in the kidney of normal recumbant man. The extent of sympathetic vasoconstriction is normally regulated by vasomotor centers in the brainstem that receive afferent inhibitory stimuli from the baroreceptors of the carotid sinus, aortic arch, low pressure vascular compartments, and higher supraspinal centers. Upon assuming head-up tilt position, peripheral venous pooling of blood with a reduction in cardiac output decreases the rate of afferent impulses from the baro-receptors and thereby their inhibitory effects on the vasomotor centers, resulting in increased sympathetic activity and peripheral vasoconstriction with a slight rise in the mean arterial pressure (MAP) at heart level (Tuckman and Shillingford, 1966). Complete spinal cord lesion at or above the T5 neurotome virtually isolates the major portion of the sympathetic nervous system from supraspinal control, including regulation of most peripheral vasomotor activity.

It has been well documented that during passive head-up tilt in normla human subjects, GFR and RPF decrease significantly (Smith, 1940; King and Baldwin, 1954), apparently due to generalized increased sympathetic activity with peripheral vasoconstriction, including vaso-constriction of renal arterioles, which prevents reduction in blood pressure. Indeed, there is usually a slight increase of MAP at heart level. Therefore, normally during head-up tilt, any possible renal autoregulation is clearly overriden by the sympathetic vasoconstrictor response.

The object of this investigation was to study spinal cord injured subjects with lesions at various levels and, therefore, with different degrees of supraspinal sympathetic control of vasoconstriction, and to compare their renal circulation while supine and during head-up tilt position with that of normal controls.

METHODS

Seventeen spinal cord injured patients, nine quadriplegics, eight paraplegics, and eight healthy control subjects took part in this study. All the spinal cord injured subjects were in good general health and had undergone urological workup, previously described. They all had a normal serum BUN and creatinine and a well functioning upper urinary tract, free of gross infection, urinary stones ureteral reflux, and other potential urological compications that are frequently associated with neurogenic bladder. All the spinal cord lesions were traumatic and physiologically complete. The quadriplegic subjects, eight males and one female were 19 to 30 years old with a mean age of 23.8 years. Their level of lesion varied from C4 to C6-7. Six participated in the study four to eight months after injury, but three were from 2½ to 12 years post-injury. The paraplegic subjects, six males and two females, were 21 to 46 years old, with a mean age of 28.9 years. Their level of lesion varied from T9 to L3-4. Seven participated in the study with within a year of, and one twelve years after, the onset of injury. The controls were healthy volunteers, medical students, physicians, and paramedical professionals, all males 20 to 52 years of age, with a mean age of 32.6 years. One control subject did not tolerate the head-up tilt position owing to physical discomfort.

On each subject, estimation of GFR and RPF were made in both supine and in 45° head-up tilt positions, on a tilt table with a foot board, using inulin and PAH, respectively. The chemical assays were done *colorimetrically* by the methods of Bacon and Schreiner, and the clearance rate was determined by the formula, $C = \dfrac{U}{P} \times V$ [where C = clearance, U = urine concentration of sample (mg%), P = plasma concentration of the sample (mg%), V = volume flow of urine (ml/min.)]. Both inulin and PAH clearances were corrected for the usual 1.73 m^2 body surface area. Filtration fraction (FF), i.e., the ratio of GFR to RPF, was also calculated. All subjects underwent the test in the morning hours after a light breakfast, excluding caffeinated drinks and concentrated carbohydrates, but were well-hydrated after drinking an additional liter of water one hour before the test. With the subject in a supine position, 10 ml of blood for control were drained, centrifuged promptly, and refrigerated. No control urine samples were obtained. Following a loading dose of inulin 50 mg/kg and PAH 8 mg/kg body weight, an infusion was started to maintain an adequate blood level of 20 to 40 mg% of inulin and 1.0-1.5 mg% of PAH. After equilibriation periods of 30 minutes, a liberally lubricated catheter was inserted, the bladder drained, and the urine discarded. To insure complete emptying, the bladder was washed with 2 x 20 ml. increments of sterile normal saline (37°C), followed by 2 x 20 ml increments of air. Thereafter, urine collection was started. At the end of each of three 20 minute intervals in the supine position, the bladder was emptied in the same way, but the entire samples were saved. Beginning 10 minutes after tilt, three additional 20 minute samples were collected in a similar manner. Urine samples were immediately refrigerated, and the exact time of the last air wash in each collection was recorded. Blood samples were collected at the midpoint of the initial discard and collection of the first urine specimen, and at the mid-point of each urine collection thereafter. Blood pressure was determined at frequent intervals by the same investigator throughout each procedure by auscultation of the brachial artery. MAP was calculated as the diastolic pressure plus one-third of pulse pressure.

RESULTS

The values of GFR, RPF, FF, and MAP in supine and tilt positions for the three groups are presented in Table I.

The results of the paraplegics, compared with those of the control subjects, were similar, both in supine and the tilt positions, whereas those of the quadriplegic subjects were different. In changing from supine to head-up tilt positions, the controls and the paraplegics showed the expected and significant reduction in GFR and RPF ($p < 0.01$) documented by various investigators previously (Smith, 1940; King and Baldwin, 1954). There was a small, but statistically insignificant, increase in MAP with the change to tilt position. The change in FF was minimal and not statistically significant.

The quadriplegic subjects showed marked fall in RPF when tilted ($p < 0.001$), but the fall in GFR was much smaller and not statistically significant. However, since there were great fluctuations in the results for this small group of nine subjects, it is possible that in a larger study group the fall in GFR might have been significant. The greater fall in RPF than in GFR produced an insignificant rise in FF. Contrary to the elevation in MAP, which occurred in normal and paraplegic subjects, the MAP fell significantly in quadriplegics.

The comparative analysis of the results between the three groups is presented in Table I. It is clear that the supine values and those in response to head-up tilt were similar in control and the paraplegic subjects, but were quite different from the quadriplegics. In the supine position, the GFR for the quadriplegics was markedly lower, both in comparison with control ($p < 0.001$) and paraplegic subjects ($p < 0.01$), but not in the tilt position. Their RPF was also significantly lower than that of the others, not only in supine but also in tilt positions ($p < 0.05$). No significant difference was found in the MAP between the three groups while supine, but in the tilt position the quadriplegic subjects showed significantly lower values ($p < 0.01$). The FF in the controls and the paraplegics did not show significant variation with the change in position, but rose slightly in the quadriplegic subjects.

DISCUSSION

The supine values for GFR and RPF reported here for the normal, control volunteers are approximately 30% and 7% to 14% greater, respectively, from the usual measurements given in earlier studies (Wasson, 1969; Slack and Wilson, 1976). Those data in "normals" were usually obtained from indigent, hospitalized, convalescent medical patients who did not have renal disease or other similar, pre- or post-surgical operation, asymptomatic patients (Wasson, 1969; Slack and Wilson, 1976). In addition, those earlier clearance studies were almost all done without catherization of the bladder and, therefore, may have been inadequate because residual urine was left in the bladder after voiding at the end of the collection periods. Other possible sources of differences in GFR and PRF values are that previous investigators (Slack and Wilson, 1976) almost always had their subjects fast overnight, and some even administered ADH the night before the studies. Regardless, the methods that were used here to determine the GFR and RPF in the controls and the patients were identical. Also, since the patients had relatively good renal function and proper ranges of inulin and PAH blood concentrations, the relative conclusions presented in this discussion should not be affected by any of the above considered factors.

It is not surprising that in all the parameters measured, there were no statistically significant differences between the controls and paraplegic subjects; since in the paraplegic with low cord lesion, a major part of the outflow to sympathetic nervous system is under supraspinal control. However, it is interesting to note that if there were increased pooling of blood in the paralyzed lower extremities of paraplegics during tilt, the compensatory sympathetically mediated vasoconstriction is adequate to prevent a fall in MAP and a greater than normal reduction of renal

TABLE I

Comparative Analysis of Glomular Filtration Rate, Renal Plasma Flow, Filtration Fraction, and Mean Arterial Pressure in Control, Paraplegic and Quadriplegic Subjects in Supine and Head-Up Tilt Positions

Subjects	Supine				Head-Up Tilt				p Values Supine versus Head-Up Tilt			
	GFR	RPF	FF	MAP	GFR	RPF	FF	MAP	GFR	RPF	FF	MAP
Control N=8	175±37	749±79	0.23±0.03	100±7.8	116±38	514±82	0.22±0.06	104±7.7	<0.01	<0.01	N.S.	N.S.
Para-plegic N=8	187±37 ##	824±247 #	0.24±0.07	93±13.4	145±45	574±138	0.26±0.06	102±9.1	<0.01	<0.01	N.S.	N.S.
Quadri-plegic N=9	130±16 **	620±128 *	0.23±0.05	94±15.3	114±46	387±99	0.26±0.07	78±11.0	N.S.	<0.001	N.S.	<0.01

Data are the mean±SD

Abbreviations:

GRF = glomular filtration rate ml/min/1.73m2
RPF = renal plasma flow ml/min/1.73m2
FF = filtration fraction (GFR/RPF)
MAP = mean arterial pressure
N = number of subjects
* = $p < 0.05$ comparison between control and quadriplegic subjects
** = $p < 0.001$ comparison between control and quadriplegic subjects
# = $p < 0.05$ comparison between paraplegic and quadriplegic subjects
= $p < 0.01$ comparison between paraplegic and quadriplegic subjects

functions.

It is clear from these results that in the tilt position, the MAP decreases in quadriplegic subjects and occasionally produces severe symptoms of orthostatic hypotension. In normal and paraplegic subjects, the MAP tends to rise. In the normal subjects, this is due to peripheral vasoconstriction, medidated through peripheral baroreceptors, the vasomotor centers in the brainstem, and the efferent sympathetic nerves, and in these paraplegics presumably the same mechanisms are responsible. Since blood pressure essentially depends on cardiac output and total peripheral resistance (BP = CO x TPR), it would seem that either one, or both, are decreased in quadriplegic subjects in the tilt position. The changes in cardiac output during tilt in quadriplegics are unknown, but their blood volume has been found to be within normal limits (Naftchi et al., 1978). Although sympathetic tone during tilt has been found to be increased in quadriplegic subjects as shown by elevated plasma norepinephrine concentration and serum dopamine beta-hydroxylase (DβH) activity (Kamelhar et al., 1978), this increased tone apparently is not adequate for producing effective vasoconstriction.

We found that the quadriplegics in the supine position have significantly lower GFR and RPF (Table I) than the control and paraplegic subjects. These lower values for quadriplegic subjects in the absence of known renal disease differ from previous reports, which stated that the level of spinal cord lesion did not affect renal function (Price et al., 1966; Morales et al., 1956; Doggart et al., 1966). Contrary to our results, Comarr (1954) reported an increased incidence of pathological changes of the kidneys with lower levels of spinal cord lesions. It is unlikely that the lower values for quadriplegic subjects could be attributed to unknown renal disease, since the paraplegic subjects who also have neurogenic bladder with all its associated risk and who were managed in an indentical manner have GFR values and RPF values comparable to those of the normal controls. It can be speculated that since the pretilt MAP was essentially the same for all three groups, the renal arterioles in supine quadriplegic subjects are more constricted. Since measurements in our laboratory of serum DβH plasma catecholamine and their metabolites in urine in supine resting quadriplegic subjects have been found to be normal, the vasoconstriction is apparently not due to increased sympathetic activity. A more plausible explanation is that there might be increased vascular reactivity to normal levels of norepinephrine and other vasoconstricting agents (Naftchi et al., 1975), i.e., that the kidney arterioles (similar to digital blood vessel) might be more sensitive to normal levels of norepinephrine, resulting in renal vasoconstriction and decreased GRF and RPF at rest. Denervation hypersensitivity of muscles to acetylcholine in lower motor neuron lesions and increased vascular reactivity of norepinephrine after surgical or chemical sympathectomy have also been documented. Although largely unproven, a similar phenomenon is thought to be operative in suuper motor neuron lesions. Moderate hypersensitivity to intra-arterial injections of acetylcholine has been observed after trnsection of the lower thoracic spinal cord (Cannon and Haimorici, 1939; Solandt and Magladery, 1942). In a previous study (Naftchi et al., 1975) confirmed by others (Debarge et al., 1974), we found increased digital vascular reactivity to intravenously infused norepinephrine in quadriplegic and paraplegic subjects with spinal cord section above T6; there was a twofold augmentation of reactivity, compared with normal and low paraplegic subjects.

In the present study we also found that although the RPF fell significantly for all three groups during tilt, the fall was proportionally

greater and reached lower absolute values in quadriplegic subjects.
The increased renal arterial hydrostatic pressure during head-up tilt
may be partly responsible for renal vasoconstriction and the decrease
in RPF by autoregulatory mechanisms. However, this reduction of
RPF in the control and paraplegic subjects is probably better explained
as being primarily the result of vasoconstriction, owing to increased
reflex sympathetic activity that is evoked by tilt and mediated through
the baroreceptors, supraspinal vasomotor centers, and the peripheral
sympathetic nerves, as indicated by well-maintained or slightly raised
MAP. In the quadriplegic subjects, a different mechanism must be
responsible; the fall in RPF on tilting was accompanied by concomitant
and significant decrease in GFR in the control and paraplegic subjects,
but only by a slight reduction in that of quadriplegic subjects. Therefore, there was no statistical difference in GFR during tilt position
among the three groups. These findings were reflected in a slightly
greater change in FF in the fraction of plasma circulating through the
kidneys and filtrated into the Bowmans space remains essentially the
same regardless of position, neurological injury, and significant
differences in GFR and RPF. This is particularly remarkable in
quadriplegic subjects who have los supraspinal control over sympathetically mediated vasoconstriction but are still able in the tile position to
maintain a GFR comparable to that of normal control and paraplegic
subjects despite a significantly lower RPF. This indicates that the
vasoconstriction of the afferent and efferent arterioles is approximately
equal. Although there is no apparent explanation for the mechanisms
of this vasoconstriction, it should be pointed out that this laboratory
has reported that DβH and plasma renin activity increased in quadriplegic
subjects in tilt position. Thus, it would seem that hypotension stimulates
reflex sympathetic nerve activity despite cervical cord transection
(Kanelhar et al., 1978). However, those measurements did not show
whether all of the sympathetic nerves below the levels of the transection
were stimulated, nor what proportion of the renal arteriolar constriction
was mediated by stimulation of sympathetic nerves compared with
increased vascular reactivity to circulating norepinephrine from other
nerve endings. In any event, despite high cervical cord injury and
loss of supraspinal sympathetic control, the magnitude and type of
renal arteriolar vasoconstriction in quadriplegics adequately prevents
excessive fall of GFR during prolonged orthostatic stress.

REFERENCES

Bacon, J.S.D., and Bell, D.J. Fructose and glucose in the blood of
    the foetal sheep. *Biochem. J. 42:*397-405 (1948).
Bratton, A.C., and Marchall, E.K., Jr. A new coupling component
    for sulfanilamide determination. *J. Biol. Chem. 128:*537-550 (1939).
Cannon, W.B., Haimovici, H. The sensitization of motorneurons by
    partial :denervation." *Am. J. Physiol. 126:*731-740 (1939).
Comarr, E.S. Renal changes in paraplegia as screened by routine
    excretory urography. *J. Urol. 72:*596-605 (1954).
Debarge, O., Christensen, N.J., Corbett, J.L., Eidelman, G.H.,
    Frankel, H.L., and Mathias, C.J. Plasma catecholamines in tetra-
    plegics. *Paraplegia 12:*44-49 (1974).
Doggart, J.R., Guttman, L., and Silver, J.R. Comparative studies on
    endogenous creatinine and urea clearances in paraplegics and
    tetraplegics. *Paraplegia 3:*229-242 (1966).
Kamelhar, D.L., Steele, J.M., Schact, R.G., Lowenstein, J., Sell, G.H.,
    and Naftchi, N.E. Plasma renin and serum dopamine-beta-hydroxylase

during orthostatic hypotension in quadriplegic man. *Arch. Phys. Med. Rehabil. 59:*212-216 (1978).

King, S.E., and Baldwin, D.S. Renal hemodynamics during erect lordosis in normal man and subjects with orthostatic proteinuria. *Proc. Soc. Exp. Biol. Med. 86:*634-636 (1954).

Morales, P.A., Sullivan, J.F., and Hotchkiss, R.S. Renal clearance studies in paraplegics. *J. Urol. 76:*714-722 (1956).

Naftchi, N.E., Demeny, M., Lowman, E.W., and Tuckman, J. Hypertensive crises in quadriplegic patients. *Circulation 57:*336-341 (1978).

Naftchi, N.E., Ragnarsson, K.T., Sell, G.H., and Lowman, E.W. Increased digital vascular reactivity to L-norepinephrine in quadriplegia. *Arch. Phys. Med. Rehabil. 56:*554 (1975).

Pitts, R.F. Physiology of the kidney and body fluids. Year Book Medical Publishers, Chicago, 1974.

Price, M., Tobin, J.A. Reiser, M., Olson, M., Kubicek, W.G., Kottke, F.J., and Boen, J. Renal function in patients with spinal cord injuries. *Arch. Phys. Med. Rehabil. 47:*406-411 (1966).

Price, M. Follow-up studies of renal function in patients with spinal cord injuries of traumatic origin. *Paraplegia 6:*22-28 (1968).

Price, M., Kottke, F.J., and Olson, M.E. Renal function in patients with spinal cord injury: The eighth year of a ten year continuing study. *Arch. Phys. Med. Rehabil. 56:*76-79 (1975).

Schreiner, G.D. Determination of inulin by means of resorcinol. *Proc. Soc. Exp. Biol. and Med. 74:*117-120 (1950).

Shipley, R.E., and Study, R.S. Changes in renal blood flow, extraction of inulin, glomerular filtration rate, tissue pressure and urine flow with acute alterations of renal artery blood pressure. *Am. J. Physiol. 167:*676 (1951).

Slack, T.K., and Wilson, D.M. Normal Renal Function. *Mayo Clinic Proceedings 51:*296-300 (1976).

Smith, H.W. Principles of renal physiology. Oxford University Press, New York, 1956.

Smith, H.W. Physiology and the renal circulation. *Harvey Lectures 35:*166-222 (1940).

Solandt, D.Y., and Magladery, J.W. A comparison of effects of upper and lower motor neuron lesions on skeletal muscle. *J. Neurophysiol. 5:*373-380 (1942).

Thurau, K. Renal hemodynamics. *Am. J. Med. 36:*698-719 (1964).

Tuckman, J., and Shillingford, J. Effect of different degrees of tilt on cardiac output, hart rate, and blood pressure in normal man. *Brit. Heart J. 28:*32039 (1966).

Wasson, L.G. Physiology of the Human Kidney. Grune and Stratton, New York, 84-108, 1969.

SECTION SIX

Hormonal and Behavioral Aspects
of Spinal Cord Research

19

Pituitary-Testicular Axis Dysfunction in Spinal Cord Injury

N.E. NAFTCHI, A.T. VIAU, G.H. SELL, and E.W. LOWMAN

ABSTRACT

Concentrations of testosterone luteinizing hormone (LH), follicle-stimulating hormone (FSH) in serum, and 17-ketosteroids (17-KS) in urine of 10 paraplegic and 10 quadriplegic subjects were measured from the date of onset of the injury and were followed once a week for a period of four months. In paraplegic subjects, serum LH and FSH levels were significantly lower than those of the age-matched, normal controls for a period of two weeks and those of testosterone for six weeks after spinal cord trauma, respectively. Following the above periods of time, serum concentrations of those hormones were not significantly different from those of the controls. By contrast, in quadriplegic subjects serum testosterone concentrations remained significantly lower than those of the controls during the entire four-month testing period. Furthermore, in another group of 10 chronic quadriplegic subjects, serum testosterone and FSH concentrations were comparable to those of the normal controls. Serum LH concentrations were at control levels in chronic paraplegic, but they were significantly depressed in chronic quadriplegic subjects. The concentration of urinary 17-KS exhibited sharp fluctuations over the four-month period and were below control levels in paraplegic but within control limits in quadriplegic subjects. The results indicate that the function of the hypothalamic-pituitary-gonadal axis is disturbed for at least four months in quadriplegic subjects.

INTRODUCTION

Spinal cord injury in the human male results in various degrees of testicular atrophy and sterility in the majority of subjects which may, in some cases, be followed by gynecomastia. The occurrence of mammary hypertrophy, which is occasionally found in men with spinal cord injury (Cooper and Hoen, 1949; Talbot, 1955), may appear as early as three months or as late as five years after onset of the lesion (Cooper and Hoen, 1952). Pathological changes in the testes, reported to occur in over 50% of human males following spinal cord injury, can at times be observed grossly, but usually require confirmation by biopsy (Cooper and Hoen, 1952; Cooper et al., 1950). Ordinarily, microscopic examination reveals marked atrophy of the germinal epithelium of the seminiferous tubules, accompanied by aspermatogenesis (Cooper et al., 1950;

243

Stemmermann et al., 1956; Bors et al., 1950; Horne et al., 1948; Fontaine et al., 1952; Klein et al, 1952) with no alteration (Bors et al., 1950; Horne et al., 1948; Klein et al., 1952) or a marked hyperplasia (Horne et al., 1948; Keye, 1956) of Leydig cells.

Metabolic and hormonal disturbances that cause the impairment of fertility in spinal man are not fully understood. The purpose of this study was to examine the function of the pituitary gonadal axis, as related to testosterone levels in spinal cord injured subjects. Since the changes in the germinal epithelium can occur as early as the fourth day following the injury (Klein et al., 1952) a longitudinal study of serum testosterone, luteinizing hormone (LH), follicle-stimulating hormone (FSH), and urinary 17-ketosteroid (17-KS) concentrations was conducted in subjects with spinal cord trauma, starting approximately one week following the injury.

METHODS

Ten paraplegic and 10 quadriplegic men with a mean age of 25 years (19-40 years) who had suffered complete neurological transverse lesions of the spinal cord were selected for this study. Venous blood samples for the analysis of testosterone, FSH, and LH and 24-hour urine specimens for 17-KS determination were collected approximately one week after the date of onset of the injury and weekly thereafter for a period of four months. Control urine and serum samples were obtained from 10 normal volunteers who were age-matched with the spinal cord injured subjects. In addition, serum FSH and LH concentrations were measured in young, randomly selected chronic (one to six years after the onset of the injury) paraplegic and 10 chronic quadriplegic men. All blood samples were taken between 8-9 A.M.

The separation of unconjugated steroids from the urine for the determination of 17-KS was performed using the Levy and Schwartz (1973) modification of the Bradlow (1968) method. Following acid hydrolysis of the urine samples, the unconjugated steroids were adsorbed onto an Amberlite XAD-2 resin column (Rohm & Hass, Company, purchased from Bio-Rad Laboratories) and then were washed with 1N KOH. The steroids were eluted from the column with 95% ethyl alcohol. The concentration of 17-ketosteroids in the eluate was determined colorimetrically by the Zimmerman reaction. A standardized urine sample (Searle Diagnostic, Inc., Columbus, Ohio) was analyzed each time together with each group of unknown urine specimens. All samples were analyzed in duplicate. The intra- and inter-assay variations in the determination of urinary 17-KS were 7.6% and 8.0%, respectively.

Serum testosterone was determined by a modification of the radio-immunoassay technique of Chen et al. (1971). The sera were extracted with methylene chloride and evaporated to dryness. The samples and standards were then incubated for one hour on ice in phosphate buffered saline, containing bovine serum albumin in the presence of $1,2$-^{3}H testosterone and testosterone antibody. Unbound testosterone fractions were adsorbed on dextran-coated charcoal. An aliquot of the antibody-bound fractions was placed into scintillation vials containing Aquasol (New England Nuclear) and was counted in a liquid scintillation spectrometer (Searle Analytic, Inc., Chicago, Illinois). Testosterone antiserum, $1,2$-^{3}H testosterone, and a standardized serum were purchased from Wien Laboratories, Inc. (Succasunna, New Jersey). Testosterone antibody was highly specific, reacting only moderately with 5α-dihydro-testosterone and delta-1-testosterone. The intra- and inter-assay variations in the determination of serum testosterone were 8.0% and 9.0%, respectively.

Serum LH and FSH concentrations were determined by a modification of the double antibody procedures of Midgley (Midgley, 1966; Midgley, 1967). The samples were incubated for 20-24 hours at room temperature in phosphate buffer pH 7.5, which contained bovine serum albumin in the presence of ^{125}I-labelled human LH (or FSH) and human LH (or FSH) antiserum. The antibody-antigen complex was further bound by the addition of anti-rabbit gamma globulin. The antibody bound radio-activity was separated from the free form by centrigugation and was counted in a gamma counter (Beckman Instruments). The human LH and FSH antisera, ^{125}I-LH, ^{125}I-FSH, anti-rabbit gamma globulin, and standardized serum were purchased from Bio-Ria (Montreal, Canada). A standardized serum was analyzed with each group of samples and all samples and standards were assayed in duplicate. The intra- and inter-assay variations in the determination of serum LH and FSH were 8.0% and 9.0%, respectively. Concentrations of LH and FSH are expressed in milli International Units of the Second International Reference Preparation of Human Menopausal Gonadotropins. One mIU of LH and FSH standard was equivalent to 5ng and 35ng of LER-907, respectively.

The results are expressed as Mean ± SD. Significance was determined by using the Student "t" test.

RESULTS

In paraplegic subjects, average serum testosterone concentration was significantly lower than that found in controls in the six weeks following spinal cord trauma. but it increased thereafter and reached normal levels (Figure 1). Between the fifth and the 12th weeks after the injury, serum testosterone levels in paraplegic subjects were sharply higher than those of quadriplegic subjects. Starting from the onset of spinal cord injury, concentrations of serum testosterone in quadriplegic subjects were significantly lower than those of controls and never reached the control levels during the four-month testing period (Figure 1). None of the subjects studied developed gynecomastia. The average serum testosterone concentration in chronic paraplegic subjects was similar to that in controls. In chronic quadriplegic subjects, however, serum testosterone was lower than in controls, but the difference was not statistically significant.

From the date of onset until two weeks after the injury, average serum FSH and LH levels in paraplegic subjects were significantly lower than those of age-matched, normal controls. Following that time, LH and FSH concentrations reached and remained at control levels (Figure 2 and Figure 3). Average serum FSH (Figure 2) and LH (Figure 3) concentrations in quadriplegic subjects, remained significantly lower than those of the controls during three weeks and 16 weeks, respectively, following the spinal cord trauma. Average serum FSH concentrations in 10 chronic paraplegic and 10 chronic quadriplegic subjects were within control levels; average serum LH levels, however, were similar to those of controls in chronic paraplegic but below control levels in chronic quadriplegic subjects (Table I).

Results in two paraplegic subjects with lesions at the level of T5 and T12 did not follow the usual trend. Testosterone concentrations in one subject (T5) were higher than those of controls, and, in the second subject (T12), testosterone remained at levels lower than those of controls. In this second subject, starting on the tenth week after spinal cord injury, serum LH and FSH concentrations were almost three times higher than those of controls and were not included in the

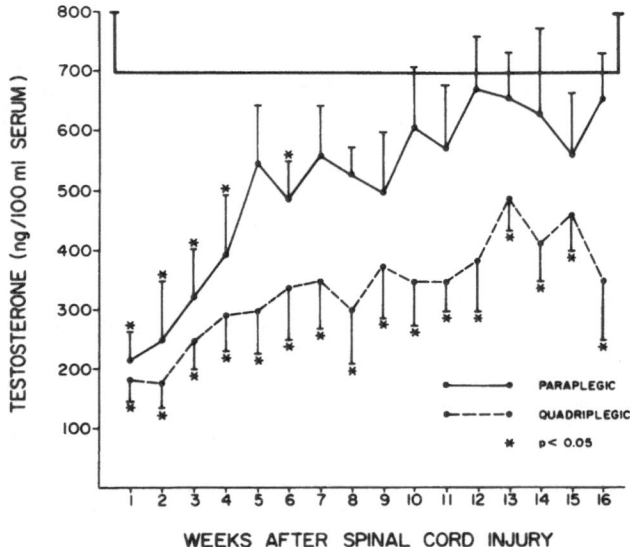

Fig. 1. Serum testosterone concentrations (Mean ± SD) in 10 paraplegic and 10 quadriplegic subjects from one to 16 weeks following the spinal cord injury. The horizontal line indicates average serum testosterone level in 10 control subjects. *

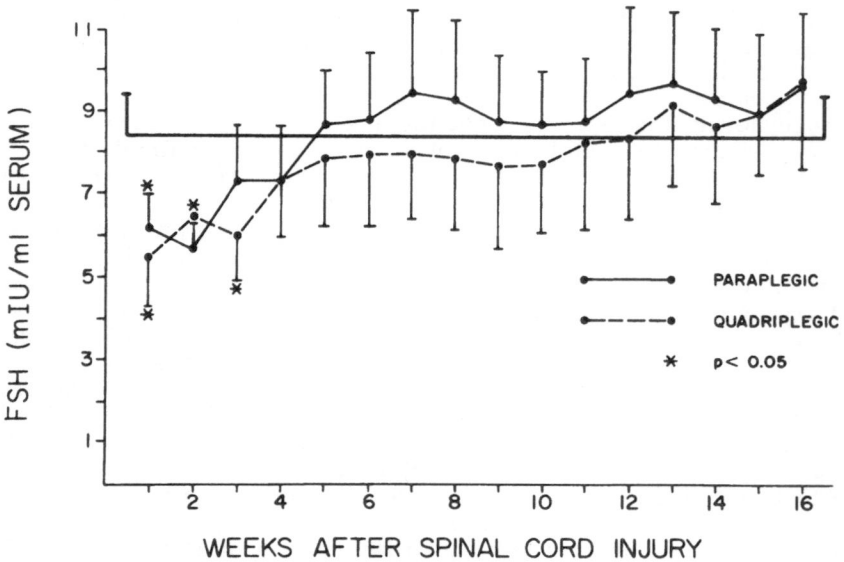

Fig. 2. Serum FSH concentrations (Mean ± SD) in 10 paraplegic and 10 quadriplegic subjects from one to 16 weeks following spinal cord injury. The horizontal line indicates average serum FSH level in 10 control subjects. *

Reprinted by permission of Archives of Physical Medicine and Rehabilitation 61:403. 1980

statistical analysis of the data.

Urinary 17-KS levels exhibited sharp weekly fluctuations from values below normal to normal. The average urinary excretion of 17-KS was within normal limits in quadriplegic and slightly below normal in paraplegic subjects (Figure 4).

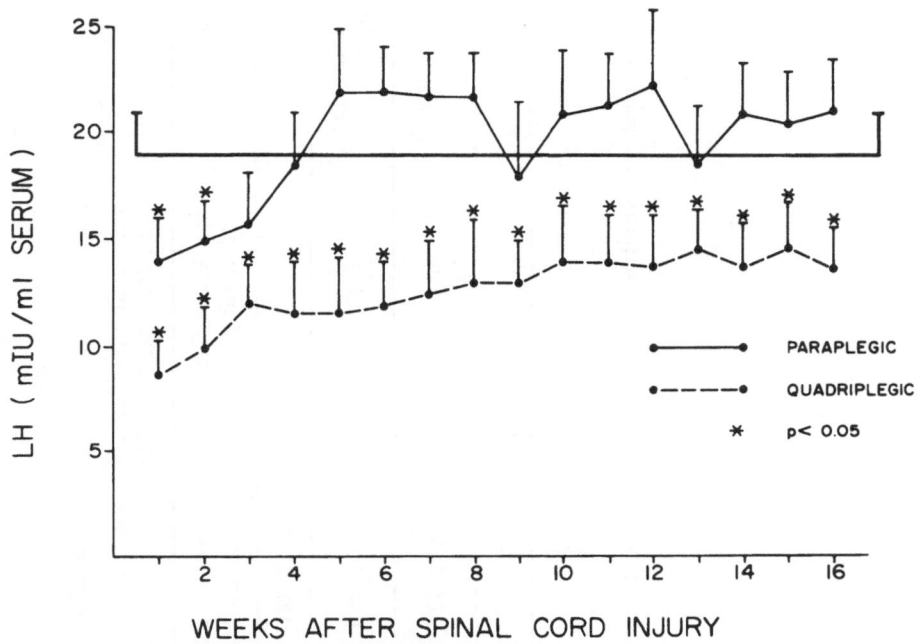

WEEKS AFTER SPINAL CORD INJURY

Fig. 3. Serum LH concentrations (Mean ± SD) in 10 paraplegic and 10 quadriplegic subjects from one to 16 weeks following spinal cord injury. The horizontal line indicates average serum LH level in 10 control subjects.

Reprinted by permission of Archives of Physical Medicine and Rehabilitation 61:403. 1980

DISCUSSION

Previous reports have shown no alteration in plasma testosterone (Mizutani et al., 1972; Kikuchi et al., 1975; Faerman et al., 1970) concentrations following spinal cord injury, owing possibly to a great deal of variation in the age of the subjects studied and in the time following the onset of the injury (a few weeks to over ten years). Furthermore, paraplegic and quadriplegic subjects were treated as one group (Kikuchi et al., 1975). Mizutani et al. (1972) studied subjects from four to 167 months after spinal cord injury and found no correlation between plasma testosterone levels, time following spinal cord trauma, and the level of the lesion. Recently, however, Claus-Walker et al. (1977) reported low testosterone levels in quadriplegic patients.

In all quadriplegic and paraplegic subjects studied in this laboratory, serum testosterone levels were significantly lower than those of control volunteers during the first six weeks following spinal cord trauma. Following this period, average serum testosterone concentrations returned to control in paraplegic but remained below control levels in quadriplegic

TABLE I

Average Serum Testosterone, LH and FSH Concentrations in
Chronic Paraplegic, Chronic Quadriplegic and Control Subjects

Subjects (and Number)	Time After Onset of Injury	Testosterone ng/100 ml (Mean ± SD)	LH mIU/ml (Mean ± SD)	FSH mIU/ml (Mean ± SD)
Control (10)		700 ± 106	19.0 ± 2.0	8.6 ± 2.4
Chronic Paraplegic (10)	1 - 6 years	752 ± 264	18.0 ± 2.3	11.1 ± 2.2
Chronic Quadriplegic (10)	1 - 6 years	609 ± 118	13.0 ± 2.0*	10.9 ± 2.0

*p<0.05

Reprinted by permission of Archives of Physical Medicine and Rehabilitation 61:404. 1980

subjects. These changes cannot be attributed to the stress of the
trauma since the stress, owing to a major surgical procedure, resulted
in a decrease in the levels of plasma testosterone lasting only six days
(Matsumoto et al., 1970) or two to three weeks (Monden et al., 1972).
Moreover, in our study concentrations of serum testosterone correlate
with the time after onset of the injury and with the level of the lesion.

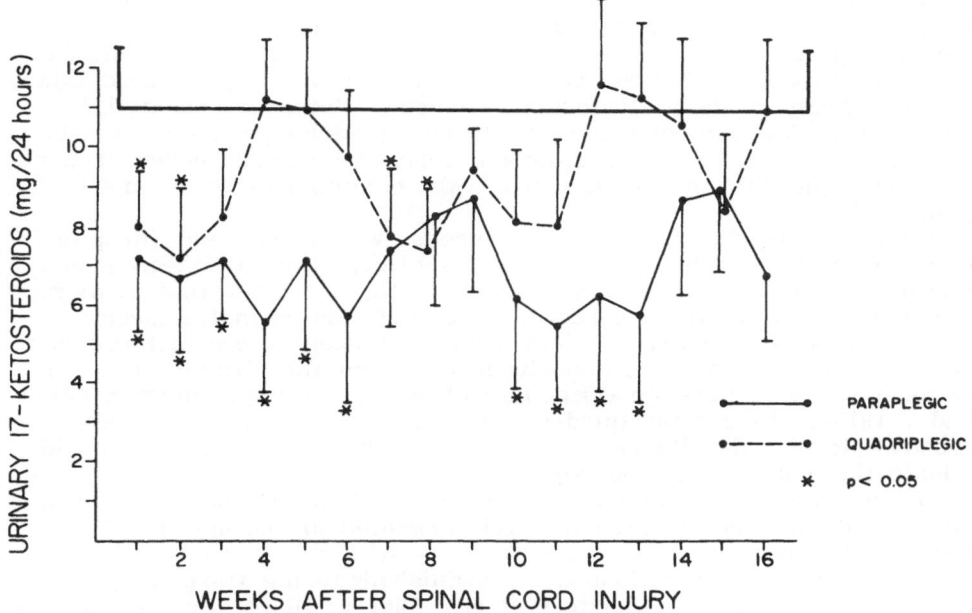

Fig. 4. Average urinary excretion of 17-ketosteroids in 10 paraplegic
and 10 quadriplegic subjects from one to 16 weeks following spinal
cord injury. The horizontal line indicates the average urinary 17-
ketosteroid excretion in 10 control subjects.

Reprinted by permission of Archives of Physical Medicine and Rehabilitation 61:403. 1980

Previous investigators found that following various types of trauma,
urinary excretion of 17-KS fell below normal levels on the fifth day
and remained low for approximately one month (Forbes et al., 1947)
or eight weeks (Monden et al., 1972). Other investigators reported
a temporary elevation of urinary 17-KS from 24 to 48 hours following
spinal cord trauma (O'Connell and Rynearson, 1950) after which time,
the excretion of 17-KS fell to below normal levels (Cooper and Hoen,
1952; Cooper et al., 1950; O'Connell and Rynearson, 1950; Cooper et
al., 1950). Contrary to these reports, urinary excretion of 17-KS
following spinal cord injury was found to be within the normal
(Stemmermann et al., 1950; Cook and Lyons, 1950) and higher than
normal limits (Talbot, 1955; Bors et al., 1950). In the present study,
the average urinary excretion of 17-KS was within low normal range
in quadriplegic, and slightly below normal in paraplegic subjects.
There was no correlation between the time following the onset of the
injury and the amount of urinary 17-KS.

Monden et al. (1972) reported that the decrease in the excretion of 17-KS during the post-operative stage is caused by a decreased excretion of metabolites from adrenal androgens. In paraplegic subjects, therefore, a lower excretion of adrenal androgens could possibly explain the lower excretion of urinary 17-KS than that found in quadriplegic subjects.

Plasma LH levels were reported to be unaltered by spinal cord injury (Kikuchi et al., 1975) and increased significantly for one week, following major surgery (Monden et al., 1972; Aono et al., 1976). In the present study, we did not observe any rise in LH levels one week following spinal cord trauma. On the contrary, serum LH concentrations in paraplegic subjects were below control levels for two weeks and in quadriplegic subjects for the entire four months after spinal cord injury, despite depressed plasma testosterone levels. Moreover, serum LH levels were below control values in chronic quadriplegic subjects. The depressed serum LH levels despite low serum testosteron concentrations in quadriplegic subjects could indicate the condition of secondary hypogonadism.

Depressed levels of serum testosterone, which persisted (despite low levels of serum LH in quadriplegic subjects) two to sixteen weeks following spinal cord injury, may suggest: (a) a certain kind of primary testicular failure in which serum LH does not rise as in the classic form (Kent et al., 1975), (b) that serum testosterone was not reduced drastically enough to exert a feedback effect on the pituitary or, (c) the existence of a possible component of secondary hypogonadism (Kent et al., 1975). In chronic quadriplegic subjects, however, depressed serum LH levels, despite low serum testosterone concentrations, could indicate the condition of secondary hypogonadism.

In one paraplegic subject (T 12) with low serum testosterone levels, gonadotrophins were elevated to levels expected in classical primary testicular failure.

Serum FSH concentrations were diminished during two post-operative days in female patients (Charters et al., 1969). In the present study, serum FSH levels were depressed for two weeks and three weeks following spinal cord injury in paraplegic and quadriplegic subjects, respectively. Serum FSH concentrations were within normal levels in oligospermic subjects (Leonard et al., 1977) and in chronic vitamin A deficient male rats, despite germ cell depletion (Krueger et al., 1974). Moreover, isolated Sertoli cells secreted a factor that selectively suppressed FSH release by cultured rats pituitary cells in vitro (Steinberger and Steinberger, 1976). It seemed, therefore, that the FSH release inhibitor is produced by Sertoli cells and not by germinal cells (Krueger et al., 1974; Steinberger and Steinberger, 1976). In paraplegic and quadriplegic subjects, Sertoli cells are the most prominent constituents of the testicular tubular epithelium despite degenerative changes of the germinal cells (Stemmermann et al., 1950). The lack of a rise in serum FSH levels in later stages of spinal cord injury does not exclude, therefore, the possibility of primary testicular failure in spinal cord injured subjects. Studying the impairment of sweating in the spinal cord injured subjects, Bors and co-authors (Bors et al., 1950) suggested that germinal abnormalities in the testes could be related to poor temperature regulation of the scrotum.

Although the depressed testosterone secretion in quadriplegic subjects may have a primary testicular origin, a component of secondary hypogonadism and an alteration in the hypothalamic-pituitary-gonadal axis is also suggested by the failure of plasma FSH and LH to rise and by the drop in serum LH to below normal levels.

The present study did not include the dynamic testing of the pituitary and testicular responsiveness to stimulating agents. It would be impossible, therefore, to discern whether the depressed serum testosterone in quadriplegic subjects was due to a primary testicular deficiency or to the decreased Leydig cell stimulation, caused by a fall in the secretion of LH. Similarly, the uncertainty remains as to whether low serum LH levels in quadriplegic subjects were due to pituitary deficiency or to a low level of pituitary stimulation by the hypothalamic releasing hormone.

The study now in progress utilizes the hCG stimulation test and stimulation of the pituitary with gonadotropin releasing hormone. It is hoped that analysis of the resulting data will clarify the ambiguities mentioned above.

REFERENCES

Aono, T., Kurachi, K., Miyata, M., Nakasima, A., Koshiyama, K., Uozumi, T., and Matsumoto, K. Influence of surgical stress under general anesthesia on serum gonadotropin levels in male and female patients. *J. Clin. Endocrinol.* 42:144 (1976).

Bors, E., Engle, E.T., Rosenquist, R.C., and Holliger, V.H. Fertility in paraplegic males. A preliminary report of endocrine studies. *J. Clin. Endocrinol.* 10:381 (1950).

Bradlow, H.L. Extraction of steroid conjugates with neutral resin. *Steroids 11:265* (1968).

Charters, A.C., Odell, W.D., and Thompson, J.C. Anterior pituitary function during surgical stress and convalescence. Radioimmunoassay measurement of blood TSH, LH, FSH and growth hormone. *J. Clin. Endocrinol. Metab.* 29:63 (1969).

Chen, J.C., Zorn, E.M., Hallberg, M.C., and Wieland, R.G. Antibodies to testosterone-3-bovine serum albumin, applied to assay of serum 17B-ol androgens. *Clin. Chem.* 17:581 (1971).

Claus-Walker, J., Scurry, M., Carter, R.E., and Campos, R.J. Steady state hormonal secretion in traumatic quadriplegia. *J. Clin. Endocrinol. Metab.* 44:530-535 (1977).

Cook, A.W., and Lyons, H.A. Urinary excretion of 17-ketosteroids in tetraplegic and paraplegic patients. A preliminary metabolic report. *U.S. Armed Forces Med. J.* 1:583 (1950).

Cooper, I.S., and Hoen, T.I. Gynacomastia in paraplegic males. Report of seven cases. *J. Clin. Endocrinol.* 9:457 (1949).

Cooper, I.S., Rynearson, E.H., MacCarty, C.S., and Power, M.H. Metabolic consequences of spinal cord injury. *J. Clin. Endocrinol.* 10:858 (1950).

Cooper, I.S., and Hoen, T.I. Metabolic disorders in paraplegics. *Neurology 2:332* (1952).

Cooper, I.S., MacCarty, C.S., and Rynearson, E.H. Gynecomastia in paraplegic males. *J. Neurosurg.* 7:364 (1950).

Faerman, I., Vilar, O., Rivarola, M.A., Rosner, J.M., Jadzinsky, M.N., Fox, D., Perez Lloret Perez, A., Bernstein-Hahn, L., and Saraceni, D. Impotence and diabetes. Studies of androgenic function. *Diabetes 21:23* (1972).

Fontaine, R., Dany, A., Muller, J.N., and Holderbach, L. Le traitement des paraplegies traumatiques. *Rev. Neurol.* 86:416 (1952).

Forbes, A.P., Donaldson, E.C., Reifenstein, E.C., Jr., and Albright, F.J. The effect of trauma and disease on the urinary 17-ketosteroid excretion in man. *J. Clin. Endocrinol.* 7:264 (1947).

Horne, H.W., Paull, D.P., and Munro, D. Fertility studies in the human male with traumatic injuries of the spinal cord and cauda equina. *New Engl. J. Med. 239:* 959 (1948).

Kent, J.R., Scaramuzzi, R.J., Lauwers, W., Parlow, A., Hill, M., Penardi, R., and Hilliard, J. Plasma testosterone, estradiol and gonadotrophins in hepatic insufficiency. *Gastroenterology 64:* 111 (1975).

Keye, J.D. Hyperplasia of Leydig cells in chronic paraplegia. *Neurology 6:* 68 (1956).

Kikuchi, T., Showsky, R., Eltoraei, I., and Swerdloff, R. The pituitary-gonadal axis in spinal cord injury, *Clin. Res. 23:* 238A (1975).

Klein, M., Fontaine, R., Stoll, G., Dany, A., and Frank, P. Modifications histologiques des testicules chez les paraplegiques. *Rev. Neurol. 86:* 501 (1952).

Krueger, H.M., Hodgen, G.D., and Sherins, R.J. New evidence for the role of Sertoli cell and spermatogonia in feedback control of FSH secretion in male rats. *Endocrinology 95:* 955 (1974).

Leonard, J.M., Leach, R.B., Couture, M., and Paulsen, C.A. Plasma and urinary follicle-stimulating hormone levels in oligaspermia. *J. Clin. Endocrinol. Metab. 34:* 209 (1977).

Levy, S., and Schwartz, T. A simple colorimetric method for the extraction and determination of urinary 17-ketosteroids using styrene divinylbenzene copolymer XAD-2 resin columns. *Clin. Chem. 19:* 679 (1973).

Matusmoto, K., Takeyasu, K., Mizutani, S., Hamanaka, Y., and Uozumi, T. Plasma testosterone levels following surgical stress in male patients, *Acta Endocrinol. 65:* 11 (1970).

Midgley, A.R., Jr. Radioimmunoassay: a method for human chorionic gonadotropin and human luteinizing hormone. *Endocrinology 79:* 10 (1966).

Midgley, A.R., Jr. Radioimmunoassay for human follicle stimulating hormone. *J. Clin. Endocrinol. Metab. 27:* 295 (1967).

Mizutani, S., Sonoda, T., Matsumoto, K., and Iwasa, K. Plasma testosterone concentration in paraplegic men. *J. Endocrinol. 54:* 363 (1972).

Monden, Y., Koshiyama, K., Tanaka, H., Mizutani, S., Aono, T., Hamanaka, Y., Uozumi, T., and Matsumoto, K. Influence of major surgical stress on plasma testosterone, plasma LH, and urinary steroids. *Acta Endocrinol. 69:* 542 (1972).

O'Connell, F.B., Jr., and Gardner, W.J. Metabolism in paraplegia. *JAMA 153:* 706 (1953).

Stemmermann, G.N., Weiss, L., Auerbach, O., and Friedman, M. A study of the germinal epithelium in male paraplegics. *Amer. J. Clin. Path. 20:* 24 (1950).

Steinberger, A., and Steinberger, E. Secretion of an FSH-inhibiting factor by cultured Sertoli cells. *Endocrinology 99:* 918 (1976).

Talbot, H.S. The sexual function in paraplegia. *J. Urol. 73:* 91 (1955).

20

Psychosexual Adjustment to Spinal Cord Injury — An Holistic Approach

J.L. BARDACH and F.J. PADRONE

INTRODUCTION

The incidence of spinal cord injury rises with increasing technological advances in society (Bostrom et al., 1973). The survival rate also increases, for improved technology in medicine is correlated with increased technological advances in general. Unless methods of regeneration of spinal cord tissue are found, we can expect increases not only in the number of paraplegics, but in the number of quadriplegics as well. Estimates of the number of quadriplegics vary, but for a Swiss population, Gehrrig reported (Bostrom, H. et al., 1973) that one-third of the spinal cord injured were quadriplegic, whereas Cheshire (ibid) estimated that 54% of the spinal cord injured in Australia were quadriplegic. Increases in individuals with spinal cord injuries presage a minimally concomitant increase in psychosocial problems.

Experience with reactions to traumatic disability indicates that the severity of disability alone is a poor predictor of subsequent emtional or vocational adjustment, or both. Nevertheless, the psychosocial problems for paraplegic individuals can be somewhat different from those of quadriplegic individuals, with consequent differing patterns of rehabilitation staff-effort and differing patterns of costs. On the practical side, for instance, a quadriplegic individual is apt to need more complex equipment to enable him to function up to optimal indepen-dence; the individual may need a personal aide to help with dressing, feeding, and so forth. A paraplegic individual is not apt to need such elaborate equipment nor need a personal attendent. On the emotional side, both paraplegics and quadriplegics are usually anaesthetic (except for occasional sparing of small areas) in the genital area. But more male quadriplegics are capable of erection than are male paraplegics (Talbot, 1955), thus creating some potential differences in emotional reactions in the two groups.

FACTORS IN EMOTIONAL ADJUSTMENT OF SPINAL CORD INJURED INDIVIDUALS

There are communalities as well as differences in the psychosocial-vocational patterns of adjustment among those whose injuries are in various locations of the spinal cord and among those whose injuries are of varying degrees of severity. The process of coping with problems of adjustment appears to follow a consistent pattern. Knowledge of this

---

The use of the masculine pronoun to encompass the female pronoun as well, was agreed upon only to conform to the other chapters in this book. No sexist philosophy is implied.

pattern is important in understanding the similarities and differences among individuals in the process of adjustment to their traumatic disability in order to know what specific services are needed for particular individuals at particular times, in order to predict length of time necessary for adjustment for particular individuals and in order to predict rehabilitation-outcomes. Such information could minimize unproductive effort, as when a service is offered at a time when the injured individual is psychologically unable to use it (Bardach, 1968); it could help improve deployment of personnel. Knowledge of the process of coming to cope with a traumatic disability could contribute substantially to incrased efficiency, while at the same time obviating disappointments that leave the injured individual discouraged, for in addition to the all-important humanitarian considerations, such discouragement is apt to prolong the individual's process of adjustment.

The description that follows is a kind of natural history of reactions to traumatic disability. The process is considered not only normal but necessary if the individual is ever to come to terms with both his assets and limitations. Such self-knowledge is a *sine qua non* for anyone's successful living, the disabled no less than anyone else.

Most of us do not like to be sick, not only because we may have unpleasant physical symptoms, but also because being ill worries us. At least in the early stages, the psyche does not distinguish between illness and disability. The more serious the condition, the greater the anxiety on the part of both patient and loved ones. When the condition is very serious, as is the case in spinal cord injury, the victim and the loved ones need time to absorb the tragedy. Moreover, traumatic spinal cord injury typically has a sudden onset. A calamity of such major proportions, which appears with little or no warning, gives the individual no time to prepare for it. No wonder, then, that one of the initial reactions is to deny it. The individual may deny that he is disabled; he may deny the permanence of the disability; he may not deny being disabled, but deny the consequences of the disability. Such individuals may say, for instance, that even though they are disabled they can or will be able to do everything just the way they did before the injury.

Though the psychiatric literature (Fenichel, 1945; Freud, A., 1948; Weisman, 1972) generally writes of denial as a psychopathological and infantile mechanism or both, it is one that is used by the normal population to a greater extent than has generally been assumed. For instance, an individual who has just been informed that a loved one has died is apt to say, "Oh, no," or some such equivalent. The denial here is necessary to give the individual time to cope with the unwanted news. Denial is an unconscious mechanism, which protects the individual from a truth that, at the moment, he cannot stand to know. "Denial helps us to do away with a threatening portion of reality, but only because we may then participate more fully in contending with problems" (Weisman, 1972). According to Weisman and Hackett (1967) denial is used not simply to avoid danger but to prevent the loss of a significant relationship. For spinal cord injured persons, it is their way of coping with possible rejection by those who care for them—rejection because they are no longer a whole individual. "Will I be acceptable anyway"? a spinal cord injured individual might wonder. The use of denial may be one factor in the frequently encountered phenomenon of the recently injured that it is easier for some to speak to an aide concerning their condition than to speak to a physician, because to do so will not rupture a relationship that is significant to them. Those who are denying their disability may refuse to go to rehabilitation classes, such as ambulation, for when they are cured there will be no need to taught to walk. Though the use of denial sometimes interferes with rehabilitation procedures, in the early stages after injury it can be essential for the individual's emotional stability. It serves to lessen or even prevent an individual's becoming overwhelmed by anxiety or depression, or both.

The severity of the stress of becoming disabled creates fertile soil for immature behavior. Recently injured individuals are often demanding and self-centered. From the point of view of survival, these individuals are behaving most adaptively, for if a person's life is threatened, or if it is felt that it is, the most sensible thing for these people to do is to focus all their attention and energies on saving it. Thus, for the time being, no considerations are possible for them, other than those perceived as connected with survival.

The intensity of the feelings bring with it a natural anger. "Why should this happen to me"? "It's not fair!" This natural anger may spill over into irritability at staff, at the physicians, at the hospital. But reality dictates that it did happen to the individual and he cannot escape from that unwanted fact. Through rehabilitation training, however, the individual learns that there are many activities that can still be performed despite the disability. Inner strnegth gradually grows. As it does, the individual becomes more realistic and the use of denial begins to decrease. As denial decreases, depression increases, for the individual becomes more and more aware of whatever limitations may remain. There is a reciprocal relationship, then, between denial and depression. The presence of depression, too, is necessary if the person is to make optimal adjustment to the disability. Individuals need to go through a period of mourning for the losses in function they have sustained just as we all must mourn the loss of a loved one. Through mourning, that which has been lost is made psychologically present and therefore not yet lost (Wright, 1960). Mourning continues until the individual has regained enough inner strength to withstand the real loss. Though the person is suffering, the presence of depression, *per se*, is not a sign of emotional difficulties, for it is apt to mean that the person is becoming strong enough to cope with the realities of the condition.

From the point of view of the patient's rehabilitation, there appears to be an optimal time for the depression to appear—when he is still at the rehabilitation center, for instance, where there are trained personnel to help ease the suffering and where the injured person does not have the added load of feelings of guilt if loved ones see him depressed. In addition, the end-point of rehabilitation is returning the individual to as near normal functioning in the community as possible. To have to cope with depression at a time when the person has so many other new adjustments to make can add enormously to the disabled person's problems. Psychodynamically oriented literature frequently views depression as anger turned inward. In that context, depression can be conceptualized as a defense against an anger that is unacceptable to the individual himself. In the case of traumatically injured individuals trying to adjust to what has happened to them, we more often see anger as a defense against depression, for depression comes only when individuals have become able to admit to themselves that they will have at least some permanent residual from their injuries.

But the anger of the disabled person does not diminish his disability. The patient begins to wonder if perhaps being more reasonable might bring about physical improvement. He might, for instance, say that being disabled would be acceptable if he could walk with crutches instead of having to be confined to a wheelchair. The victim would be willing to accept some disability if only it were less than the one he has. He wants to strike a bargain. But because at the present time there is no cure for the condition, there is no bargain that can be made. It is no accident that the appearance of the emotional states of denial, anger, bargaining, depression, and then final adjustment is the same as those reported in relation to dying (Kubler-Ross, 1969), for the spinal cord injured individual is confronted with the death of major functions of his body.

An orderly sequence of emotional events for the traumatically injured individual has been described. The rate at which individuals go through these phases varies with the particular individual. What are the factors that determine that rate? One factor frequently thought of as slowing down the rate of adjustment is the presence of secondary gains. Concerning secondary gains, Fenichel (1945) states, "The symptoms may acquire secondarily the significance of a demonstration of one's own helplessness in order to secure external help such as was available in childhood". We are quick to think of the patient who is not progressing at a rate we would expect in terms of his physical injury as an individual who "just wants a lot of attention." The ease with which this idea comes to the fore suggests that all of us are subject to secondary gains. If we are honest with ourselves, we have to admit that when we are hurting, to be comforted is very satisfying. The difference between the normal use of secondary gains and the maladjusted use of them is that when the normal individual begins to recover, he realizes that much autonomy has to be surrendered in order to continue to receive secondary gains. The spinal cord injured are already struggling with problems of dependence-independence. The possibility of obtaining secondary gains is part of that struggle. Nevertheless, it is much rarer among the spinal cord injured than the uninitiated are wont to believe, perhaps because of the grim reality of some actual physical dependence.

Two other factors are much more salient in determining the rate of adjustment to traumatic spinal cord injury. The first factor is the loss in reality to the individual from the disability. For example, two men, each in their thirties, become paraplegic. One is a lawyer and the other is a house-painter. It would be expected that the house-painter would take longer to adjust than the lawyer, not because the house-painter is less intelligent nor less well educated, but because he is faced with the reality of finding a new livelihood.

The second salient factor affecting the rate of adjustment to traumatic spinal cord injury is what the individual feels is being lost. This factor can be subtle and therefore difficult to come to know. For an individual, for instance, whose self-esteem has been intimately connected with his or her body, a traumatic physical injury can be an especially great narcissistic assault. The professional athlete or the woman who has worked as a model are examples that come to mind. Here, it is not only the reality-toll of the disability itself but the blow in an area so closely tied to the particular individual's self-esteem that is an added burden. The man who pre-morbidly was never sure that he was a manly enough man and who compensated for that anxiety by being especially physically active has a difficult time if he becomes disabled. The individual who tends to handle anxiety by becoming very busy—a common mechanism in our society—is in particular difficulty should he sustain a spinal cord injury. An example is the woman who, when she is anxious, decides to do her spring cleaning, no matter what season of the year it is. There are only two avenues of adjustment open to such an individual, either to find new kinds of business that the injury will still permit or find new ways of handling anxiety. Either of these ways is apt to be prolonged and may require psychotherapeutic help before resolution of the emotional turmoil is obtained.

Admission to a rehabilitation center can be anxiety-provoking, since it may be the first time the patient experiences himself as disabled. Prior to this period the patient may have seen himself as sick and, therefore, convalescing. This idea may be the path by which denial is expressed. In addition, the change in nursing care when one moves from an acute care setting to the more independent style of a rehabilitation center can be frightening and can produce feelings of abandonment. The patient may begin to experience not only additional anxiety but also to feel depressed because self-image begins to be reflected in the disabilities of other patients. The spinal cord injured patient in the next bed may serve as a mirror for the new patient's own disability. Very soon after admission the patient begins to realize that other patients have been in rehabilitation for many months and may still be quite disabled.

Emotional Reactions of Staff

The impact of staff reactions to the newly disabled patient also affects the patient emotionally. The extent of the disability can confuse staff in terms of what the patient has lost. When we compare a young man who is paraparetic with a young man who is quadriplegic, we may feel that the former has only "a minor disability." The greater misfortune here is that the patient may also come to a similar conclusion. As a result, the profound feelings of loss and pain consequent to the disability may neither be fully experienced nor integrated. If, however, one views the disability from the point of view of the victim, it quickly becomes apparent that the extent of the physical disability is neither a measure of the intensity of the actual suffering, nor a measure of the intensity of suffering that the victim *ought* to feel.

To the extent a staff member is involved with a patient, to that extent he may have similar emotional reactions to the patient's progress. Sometimes staff finds it difficult to allow emotional reactions of the patient, especially depression. Often they do not see the usefulness of these reactions. They may also be frightened by them or find it uncomfortable to be around patients who have such feelings. These feelings touch on some of the staff's own difficulties with that emotion or touch on other personal factors. In addition, patients at such times may be tempted to *give up*, which sometimes flies in the face of the staff's personal reasons for going into the field of rehabilitation. The staff wants the satisfaction of seeing the patient improve. Without an understanding of the psychological process involved, to *give up*, then, is experienced by staff as almost a deliberate thwarting of staff's satisfactions on the part of the patient. In reaction to such stress, staff may too quickly push for a patient to work hard toward goals that seem irrelevant to the patient. The goals seem irrelevant in terms of a future the patient cannot envision. Moreover, the goals themselves may be threatening to the patient, for they may imply permanance of the disability. Urging a spinal cord injured person, for example, to practice transfers from bed to wheelchair implies that the individual is going to remain wheelchair-bound. Because, then, of feelings of anxiety, frustration, depression or other personal reactions on the part of staff, staff may resort to *cheering up* the patient in a kind of Pollyanna approach in a misguided attempt to *treat* the depression.

An understanding not only of the psychological processes going on within the patient, but an understanding of those going on within themselves on the part of staff can materially improve patient-staff relations, which will further rehabilitation. Such an understanding can be developed through the use of regular staff group meetings, conducted by a person who is trained in group process and who is knowledgeable in the area of psychodynamics. Such groups work particularly well when they are experiential in nature. Although patient problems can often be discussed, emphasis is placed on the experience of the staff member. The forces at work upon the staff member are explored as well as those at work upon the patient so that a more productive interaction may develop between staff member and patient. For example, the staff member who is entirely focused on the benefits of rehabilitation and the dignity of the work ethic to the exclusion of the recognition of the anguish concerning loss for the patient, may painfully come to the experience his own horror of the pain of loss from a disability. In the process, the staff member also becomes aware of his own form of denial. Out of that experience, the staff member comes to have genuine respect for the patient and for denial as a mechanism of defense. As a result, the staff person is better able to perceive the patient's state accurately and to relate not only more empathically but also more effectively in terms of being perceived by the patient as an ally rather than as an "insensitive slave driver."

Emotional Reactions of Family

The reactions of family members to the disability are very similar to those of the patient. It is axiomatic to say that the closer a person feels to the patient, the more similar the emotional reactions will be. In addition, there are also possible concerns about accepting the responsibility for the physical care of the patient. There are fears of loneliness. There are concerns about financial matters. There may also be concerns about whether or not the relationship can tolerate such a major change in one partner. It is crucial that these concerns be dealth with by trained staff of social workers or psychologists. The counseling should not be confined to family members but should be made available to those individuals who are of major emotional significance to the patient. Such a service is not only important for humanitarian purposes, but, in the final analysis, feelings of those personally close to the patient can hinder or can make possible the optimal reentry of the patient into the life of the community. Implied in the foregoing discussion is the conviction that patients can take optimal advantage of the array of rehabilitation services available only if the emotional reactions of patients, families, and staff are dealt with at the same time that rehabilitation of the physical aspects of the patients are in progress.

Sexual Problems of the Spinal Cord Injured

Despite the fact that the philosophy of rehabilitation has long been to treat the whole person, it is only recently that the sexuality of the disabled has been addressed. Though now sex is emerging as a legitimate concern, in too many quarters it continues to be a neglected area of health care. Most of the work in relation to sex and disability has centered on the spinal cord injured (Cole, Chilgren, and Rosenberg, 1973; Griffith, Tomko, and Timms, 1973; Griffith and Trieschmann, 1975; Held, Cole, Held, Anderson, and Chilgren, 1975; Mooney, Cole,

and Chilgren, 1975), for they tend to be traumatized at an age that is
regarded in our society as the sanctioned peak of sexual activity
(Lowman, 1972). Males outnumber females by far (Smart and Sanders,
1976). Because of that fact, because the mechanics of sexual intercourse on the surface require fewer adjustments for the female and,
perhaps because most of the investigators have been male, the majority
of studies dealing with sexuality in the spinal cord injured have been
concerned with the male. Possibly because of the age-factor and because
of the present freer climate of information about sex, patients began
to express interest in their sexual futures more overtly. Staff also
began to be concerned about the best way of handling the whole topic
of sexuality and disability with the patients.

The exact details of the disability in any one spinal cord injured
person are highly individualized. Nonetheless, some order can be
obtained in the rehabilitation of sexual activity in this group by using
a problem oriented approach. In the spinal cord injured there are a
number of problems that can interfere with sexual activity, and for
each problem there are a number of possible solutions. Though not
every problem will be dealth with (nor will every solution), to look
at the rehabilitation of sexual activity in this way informs patients,
potential sexual partners, and staff of options that do exist. Moreover,
it encourages those concerned to look for options themselves that
might better fit their particular needs.

Bladder Incontinence

Spinal cord injured persons are unable to control their bladder
functioning in the way they could pre-morbidly. Moreover, they do
not sense the need to empty their bladders nor do they feel the
process of emptying. To add to the difficulties, sexual activity may
stimulate bladder-emptying, often a mortifying experience for the disabled
person and an alarming, embarrassing or disgusting one for the partner.
Indeed, a whole host of unpleasant feelings can be elicited from both
individuals.

The primary solution to the problem of bladder incontinence is to
empty it before sexual activity, using the appropriate intact reflexes.
The disabled person or partner can use the Crede maneuver in which
pressure is applied over the bladder area in order to express the
urine into a container. In some cases, tapping or stroking over a
spastic bladder can induce spastic emptying. Intermittent catheterization
is another solution.

Some spinal cord injured persons use devices of various sorts to
handle their problems with bladder incontinence. In connection with
sexual activity, the problem then becomes what to do with the devices.
In some cases they can be removed, but leakage of urine may be a
problem. Catheters can be taped to the side in both males and females.
For the male, they can be folded back on the penis and covered with
a condom after an erection has developed. The presence of a catheter
will not interfere with an erection, nor will the erection interfere with
the functioning of the catheter. Where condom drainage is being used,
the tube can be removed from the collection bag and folded against
the penis, using a second condom to hold the tube in place. This
added bulk sometimes increases sensation for the female partner. For
those individuals who have ostomies of various sorts and who feel the
need to make their device as inconspicuous as possible, it can be
covered, with a sash for women or a cummerbund for men. In addition,
voiding difficulties can be minimized by reducing liquid intake two

hours or so before sexual activity, though before such a procedure, the injured individual should consult with a physician.

Convenience should be a factor to be considered. For instance, a piece of furniture near the bed on which one can place materials can smooth interaction. There may be a need for a place to discard materials and a place from which one can easily obtain materials should the disabled person need to reapply a device either during or after sexual activity.

Even after the most careful preparation, however, *accidents* do occur. The use of such things as disposable "chux" and the placement of a towel under the genital area can be of help. But the most important factor influencing the effect of bladder incontinence on sexual activity is the emotional one for both disabled and able-bodied individuals. One problem has to do with reactions to odor. In some cases the physician may be able to advise medication, such as certain antibiotics, that can change acidification and bacterial action that lead to unpleasant odors. Since most odor comes from contaminated skin or pubic hair, or both, good hygiene is important. Except, perhaps, close to the time of sexual activity, where possible, continual high fluid intake can reduce urine-odor. Odor can also be masked with perfumes and creams.

There may be anxiety concerning whether or not the urine will cause infection. To prevent irritation, it is best not to keep urine on the skin for periods longer than an hour or so. Infection from urine per se, however, is generally not a medical concern.

In addition to emotional reactions to the odor of urine and worry about infection, the incontinent person may have a host of unpleasant feelings, like being an infant or like being a person who is unable to control even so elementary a function as urination. Either or both partners may feel that the incontinent person is dirty. Patients have indicated that for them the most satisfactory way has been to talk about these feelings with their potential sexual partners. Admittedly that has entailed a good deal of self-conquering as well as a good relationship with their partners. It is sometimes easier to begin by acknowledging how difficult the topic is to talk about.

Anal Incontinence

The spinal cord injured person is incontinent of gas. Aside from limiting intake of gaseous foods, there are neither mechanical nor medical solutions at the present time. Both disabled and able-bodied persons are concerned about the smell of gas and the noise of passing gas. The injured person has the further anxiety of not having the physical sensation of passing gas.

Spinal cord injured persons also are unable to control their bowel functioning in the way they could pre-morbidly. And, as with bladder incontinence, they do not sense either the need to empty their bowels nor can they feel the emptying process.

Incontinence of stool is generally managed by the development of a bowel routine, in which the incontinent person has induced bowel movements by the use of rectal suppositories, enemas, etc. at regular times, such as every second or third day at approximately the same hour. In the establishing of a bowel routine, as much consideration should be given to the person's sexual life as is given to the work life or to any other practical consideration. Routines can be upset by changes in diet, by medication, by major variations in physical activity, by illness or by unexpected circumstances that interfere with carrying out the routine. In addition, in some individuals, sexual activity may stimulate bowel evacuation. Many spinal cord injured report such occurrences despite conscientious adherence to bowel routines. The closer one approaches the routine time for bowel evacuation, however, the greater the risk of an accidental bowel-movement. As with bladder incontinence, the use of disposable "chux," towels under the genital area, etc. can aid in clean up should an *accident* occur.

With regard to the whole problem of incontinence, the attitudes toward it and the nature of the interpersonal relationships between the people involved are the major considerations. That many disabled themselves and their partners, whether able-bodied or not, have coped with this problem by working out their emotional reactions to it is a monument to the human spirit.

Spasticity

The involuntary muscle contractions that some spinal cord injured persons have can be interruptive to sexual activity because they are almost always sudden, and they break the rhythm of the on-going activity. Spasm can often be broken by slow, firm pressure. Sometimes, slow, deep breathing of the spinal cord injured person can also relax the spasm. Often medications help prevent spasms. A bewildering number of stimuli such as cold, particular postures, and so forth, can trigger spasticity. The injured individual needs to learn what stimuli trigger spasticity and then take care to avoid them when spasticity is not wanted.

Arousal and Sensation

Sexual excitement usually begins with some kind of stimulation, either external or internal, that is transmitted by the brain through the spinal cord and to the genitals. Such excitement may then proceed through the usual stages of the sexual response cycle. Because of the loss or diminution of sensation with spinal cord dysfunction, most often there is an inability to experience pleasure through the sense of touch below the level of the lesion. The primary erogenous zones have often lost their ability to give direct sensory pleasure through this modality. Such a loss is a major one. The solution to this problem requires some ability to be flexible and to be willing to explore. For the disabled partner there are areas of sensation that remain intact above the level of the lesion. Certainly these areas are as sensitive to touch and as much sites of pleasure as they were preinjury. In addition, these areas can be stimulated with increased attention so that they may become even more pleasurable through practice. For example, the extensive use of light touch or of the tongue to the neck or ears can, for many people, become a more highly erotic experience than it was before the injury. Increased attention directed to the nipples or breasts of both sexes can also become a more highly erotic experience than it was previously. The principle involved here is that when a part of the body is stimulated in a pleasurable way in an erotic context, it is possible for that area of the body to develop erogenous properties.

Below the level of lesion there may be areas in which sensation has been preserved, areas of so-called sparing. It may be helpful for the couple to determine whether or not such areas exist and if they do, to stimulate them during sexual activity. Lastly, it should be noted that the fact of loss of sensation to a part of the body should not exclude that part from stimulation for two reasons: (1) The partner may still derive pleasure, for example, from stroking those parts of the body commonly associated with intimacy and erotic pleasure even though sensation has been lost; (2) The disabled partner may derive considerable pleasure both vicarious and erotic, from witnessing the partner having such an erotic experience with a part of their body. It should also be mentioned that there can be areas of hypersensitivity that the disabled partner experiences as painful or uncomfortable, if they are stimulated at that site. For example, some people report a band of hypersensitivity at the level of the lesion. Once these areas are discovered, the couple can attempt to determine if all forms of stimulation are unpleasant in order to determine whether or not these areas need to be completely avoided.

Motor Losses

The loss or reduction in movement secondary to paralysis or weakness, can lead to problems with holding, touching, thrusting, and positioning, depending on the part of the body affected. Such changes often lead to difficulties in terms of appearing clumsy or incompetent sexually, or both. There may be conflict over sex roles with regard to the stereotype that men are to be the more active partners. Most couples deal with the problem of paralysis or weakness by allowing the partner to assume as much of the responsibility as is possible and as is necessary for their sexual activity. For example, when the disabled person is a male quadriplegic and his partner is a female who has good use of her upper extremities, she may place his arms around her. If able, she may position herself in such a way that any part of her body can be touched by her partner's lips or tongue.

In addition, the use of devices that are sexual in nature, such as dildos and vibrators are also commonly used for sexual pleasure. In terms of sexual intercourse, if physically able, the arms and/or legs of the partner on the bottom may be used to support a disabled partner who could not otherwise tolerate the superior position or one partner may need to straddle the other. In both of these positions, the responsibility for the pelvic thrusts during intercourse will have to be assumed by the partner who has the physical capability rather than by the male, to whom our society has assigned this role.

One of the most significant indicators of arousal in men is the presence of a psychogenic erection, which is an erection that is mediated by the spinal cord as a result of stimulation to the brain. Men who suffer from spinal cord dysfunction (paraplegic or quadriplegic) most often lose the ability for such a psychogenic erection. In its place, however, as a function of spasticity, is a reflex erection, which may be elicited by physical stimulation to the genital region or even by nongenital stimulation. In order to maintain a reflex erection it is necessary that the stimulation be relatively continuous. The stimuli that produce a reflex erection are quite varied, including such input as friction, stroking (light and heavy), the use of heat and cold, scratching, pinching, and oral stimulation. The friction of the vaginal walls during intercourse is usually sufficient to maintain the erection. When it is not, the use of voluntary vaginal contractions is helpful. Another approach to producing an erection is the *stuffing technique* in which the flaccid penis is stuffed into the vagina followed by slow thrusting movements. Even without an erection, the stuffing technique can be used with pleasure by the woman. The same stimuli that produce a reflex erection in men, excluding the stuffing technique, often produce a reflex erection of the clitoris and produce vaginal lubrication in women with spinal cord dysfunction. It is important to realize that erections of either the penis or the clitoris are not felt by the person having them, though the person may receive pleasure indirectly through seeing it, touching the lubrication, directly watching one's partner's increased excitement at the event, and so forth. For those men who cannot attain an erection and for whom it is of paramount importance, the use of penile implants may provide a solution. Some implants lead to a permanent erection while others that are inflatable may be deflated after use. Careful medical and psychological evaluations of both partners beforehand is a must here.

When intercourse cannot take place, the partner can still be satisfied through a host of techniques, such as oral or manual stimulation or with the use of devices. These techniques, of course, are also used by able-bodied individuals even when there is no problem concerning ability to have intercourse.

Positioning

Because of the loss of muscle power concomitant to spinal cord dysfunction, there are often problems with regard to the positions people are able to assume during sexual activity. In order to hold or embrace a partner, a quadriplegic person may need to be sitting up rather than supine. A person with a C_{3-4} lesion can touch the partner and thereby stimulate by using the mouth, head, neck or shoulders. In order to be caressed, if the physical capability is there, the partner can take the spinal cord injured person's hands and use them to touch his body. The disabled person may also be positioned so that he can see the contact. The use of the tongue can be extensive, with partners, if they are able, doing the maneuvering into an accessible position.

For the person with a C_5 lesion, the same solutions as above are applicable, in addition to the ability to stroke with the upper part of the arm and from the elbow to the hand, if the elbow can bend and relax. A person with a C_6 lesion might experiment to see whether or not tenodesis could be used to stimulate a partner. A person with a C_7 lesion can actively bend and straighten the elbow, in addition to being able to move the wrist and to having more finger dexterity. The fewer the physical limitations, of course, the better able is the person to stimulate the partner.

In addition to problems that are created by the limited use of the upper extremities, there are also problems with balance. The solution is to provide for support. Support can be provided either with pillows or bolsters or support can be obtained from the partner. Where there are problems with balance, the positions for intercourse are somewhat less varied than for an able-bodied couple. The partner with balance-problems can assume the supine position. The couple can lie on their sides, face to face or with one partner facing the other partner's back. Where sufficient support can be offered to the person with difficulties maintaining balance, he can assume the superior position. In order to change position, the partner may have to assist or apply leverage so that the disabled person can roll on top of him. In addition, sexual activity can be carried out in a wheelchair. If the man is disabled, intercourse can be carried out in a wheelchair, provided the chair has removable arm rests. The use of devices such as a trapeze or rope tied to the bed can also aid in movement and changing positions.

The epitome of sexual pleasure is often believed to be orgasm. Most often for the person with spinal cord dysfunction the experience of orgasm is considerably changed or it is absent entirely. Reports from the spinal cord injured themselves indicate that at the peak of sexual excitement a type of orgasmic experience occurs that is pleasurable and has as possible manifestations a sudden tingling, a sense of warmth or a sudden decrease in spasticity that is experienced as extremely pleasurable. Such responses are reported to have developed over a period of time and after considerable exploration and practice in sexual activity post-injury.

Ejaculation and Fertility

The process of ejaculation is also often interrupted in men with spinal cord dysfunction. When it does occur, most often the ejaculate is not expelled from the penis but rather passes back down the urethra into the bladder—a retrograde ejaculation. The environment of the bladder is hostile to spermatozoa. Such a factor is one of the reasons for the usual infertility in men with spinal cord injury. In addition, sperm may also be produced in low numbers or not at all and may have low motility. Attempts have been made to preserve sperm by freezing, but so far the technique has not worked well. Some alternatives to the fertility problem in men are artifical insemination or adoption. Counseling for the couple that chooses either of these solutions is certainly necessary.

For a woman with spinal cord dysfunction, there is no problem with fertility. On the contrary, the concern is often with contraception. There is a broad spectrum of opinions by physicians with respect to the types of contraceptives that should be used by the woman with spinal cord dysfunction. In order to choose the appropriate contraceptive, consultation with a physician familiar with the problems of spinal cord dysfunction is necessary. For this same reason, and because of individual differences among women, a physician should be consulted for counseling in regard to pregnancy and delivery. From a functional standpoint, it is important to point out that during the last trimester of pregnancy, the woman may find that her hard-earned independence of functioning post-injury may be considerably reduced. In addition, although labor begins automatically, the woman without sensation will not know when it is occurring. Consequently, she must be closely watched. The pregnant spinal cord woman does have the advantage, however, of being able to deliver a child without physical discomfort.

Attitudes toward sexual practices can often influence the sexual adjustment a couple makes. Such influences can even be more profound when changes in physical functioning, as with spinal cord dysfunction, necessitate changes in sexual practices about which a person may be uncomfortable. For example, an able-bodied woman who has been comfortable being a passive sexual partner may feel that it is improper or she may become quite anxious if she is expected to be more active during sexual acitivty. Sexual practices such as oral genital stimulation or the use of sexual devices may also lead to considerable emotional discomfort. In addition, there may be considerable anxiety over the alteration of the traditional sex roles not only in terms of sexual function per se, but also in terms of a wife or husband acting as a *nurse*. The solutions to such difficulties begin with early sexual counseling for both partners where possible. During such counseling, the partners should not only be given information, but be helped to explore their own attitudes toward the possible changes in their future. In the counseling and in the privacy of their own sexual lives, each couple needs to explore what is best for each individual and for themselves as a couple. If they can have the experience of open communication with each other—their disgusts, their likes, dislikes, their anxieties, and fantasies—they can be free to explore options open to them. Free attitudes and open communication increase the number of options available and therefore increase the possibility of satisfying sexual relationships.

SUMMARY

Adjustment to disability is a process that involves adjustment to loss and change, physically, psychologically, and sexually. There are some relatively common and predictable emotional reactions that are most often necessary for a person to experience in the process of coming to grips with a spinal cord injury. Such experiences are not only difficult for the disabled themselves but are difficult for family and close ones to endure. Often rehabilitation staff also suffer. Psychological exploration is, therefore, indicated not only for patients but for family and staff as well. In addition, the sexual life of the disabled person and his partner is only recently being paid the attention it deserves and needs. A problem-oriented approach to the changes in sexual functioning consequent to a disability seems productive. Such an approach in the context of individual, couple, and group sexual counseling can be an important element in the fostering of adjustment. In general, then, by recognizing, allowing for and caring for the emotional and sexual concerns of the disabled, the ultimate goals of rehabilitation can be furthered.

REFERENCES

Bardach, J.L. Psychological assessment procedures as indicators of patients' abilities to meet tasks in rehabilitation. *Journal Counseling Psychology 15(5):*471-475 (1968).

Bostrom, H., Larsson, T., and Ljungstedt, N., (eds.), *Rehabilitation after central nervous system trauma.* Symposium September 25-27, 1973. Nordiska Baklandelus Forlag, Stockholm, 1974.

Cole, T.M., Chilgren, R., and Rosenberg, P. New program for sex education and counseling for spinal cord injured adults and health care professionals. *International Journal Paraplegia 11:*111-124 (1973).

Fenichel, O. *The Psychoanalytic Theory of Neurosis.* W.W. Norton & Company, New York, 1945.

Freud, A. *The ego and the mechanisms of defence.* (Translated by C. Baines). Hogarth Press, Ltd. and the Institute of Psychoanalysis, London, 1948.

Griffith, E.R., Tomko, M.A., and Timms, R.J. Sexual function in spinal cord-injured patients: A review. *Archives Physical Medicine & Rehabilitation 54:*539-543 (1973).

Griffith, E.R., and Trieschmann, R.B. Sexual functioning in women with spinal cord injury. *Archives Physical Medicine & Rehabilitation 56(1):*18-21 (1975).

Held, J.P., Cole, T.N., Held, C.A., Anderson, C., and Chilgren, R.A. Sexual attitude reassessment workshops: Effect on spinal cord injured adults, their partners and rehabilitation professionals. *Archives Physical Medicine & Rehabilitation 56(1):*14-18 (1975).

Kubler-Ross, E. *On Death and Dying.* MacMillan, New York, 1969.

Lowman, E.W. *Follow-up study of spinal cord injured patients at the Institute of Rehabilitation Medicine 1952-1971 in "Model regional systems of spinal cord injury care."* Grant Application to Social Rehabilitation Service, Washington, D.C., 1972. pp. 20-21. (Available from Institute of Rehabilitation Medicine, 400 East 34th Street, New York, N.Y. 10016).

Mooney, T.O., Cole, T.M., and Chilgren, R.A. *Sexual options for paraplegics and quadriplegics*. Little Brown & Co., Boston, 1975.

Smart, C.N., and Sanders, C.R. The costs of motor vehicle related spinal cord injuries. *Insurance Institute for Highway Safety*, Washington, D.C., 1976, p. 15.

Talbot, H.S. The sexual function in paraplegia. *The Journal of Urology 73(1):*91-100 (1955).

Weisman, A.D., and Hackett, T.P. Denial as a social act. In *Psychodynamic studies in aging: Creativity, reminiscing, and dying*, S. Levin and R. Kahama, eds., International Universities Press, 1967.

Weisman, A.D. *On Dying and Denying*. Behavioral Publications, Inc., New York, 1972.

Wright, B.A. *Physical disability—a Psychological Approach*. Harper Row, New York, 1960.

INDEX

ERRATA SHEET

THROUGH A CLERICAL ERROR THE TABLE OF
CONTENTS WAS PRINTED WITHOUT PAGE NUMBERS.
THEY ARE AS FOLLOWS: